CW01099996

Introduction to Veterinary Epidemiology

Introduction to Veterinary Epidemiology

Edited by

Hans Houe
Annette Kjær Ersbøll
Nils Toft

Division of Epidemiology
Department of Large Animal Sciences
The Royal Veterinary and Agricultural University
Frederiksberg, Denmark

2004

Hans Houe, Annette Kjær Ersbøll and Nils Toft (eds.)
Introduction to Veterinary Epidemiology

1. edition Biofolia 2004

© Biofolia, 2004

Cover: Torben Lundsted and Lene Paz
Typeset: Stallion Press
Print: Narayana Press, Gylling, Denmark

ISBN 87-9131-921-8

Published by:
Biofolia
Rosenoerns Allé 9
DK-1970 Frederiksberg C
Denmark
Tlf: + 45 38 15 38 80
Fax: + 45 35 35 78 22
slforlag@sl.cbs.dk
www.biofolia.dk

All rights reserved.
No parts of this book may be reproduced or transmitted in any form or by any means, electronic or mechanical, including photocopying, recording, or by any information storage or retrieval system, without permission in writing from the publisher.

PREFACE

This book emerged from the desire to have a book that covered the course in Veterinary Epidemiology for veterinary students. However, we also believe that it can serve as a useful textbook for students and researchers who need to refresh the basic concepts of epidemiology.

The textbook will emphasise veterinary epidemiology as an integrated scientific discipline with elements of both veterinary medicine as well as mathematics and statistics. Some chapters have emphasis on describing the biological nature of data followed by a description of the relevant mathematical and statistical procedures. Other chapters dealing with more specialised issues may start the other way round by first introducing the mathematics, which is then followed by biological examples.

After the general introduction to veterinary epidemiology in Chapter 1, we will introduce the establishment of hypotheses including both biological and statistical aspects of hypotheses (Chapter 2). Chapter 3 gives an overview of the relevant biological data. Further, the types of variables and scales of these data will be outlined. Chapters 4 and 5 introduce the two major study types in epidemiology, the observational and the experimental studies. Chapters 6 and 7 describe how the disease occurrence and disease effect can be measured in quantitative terms. Chapter 8 addresses methods for calculating the necessary sample size in epidemiological studies and outlines different sampling methods that can be used in different practical situations. The evaluation of tests used in veterinary medicine for diagnostic, prognostic and screening purposes is described in Chapter 9. Chapter 10 on data management describes the process of the data flow from observing data, through the use of databases and data control, to initial analysis. Dealing with data, special problems such as bias and confounding arise that need to be assessed and adequately handled. Chapter 11 addresses these aspects of data involved in epidemiological studies. A special way of obtaining information and data is through different types of questionnaires, which is covered separately in Chapter 12. Chapter 13 gives a general introduction to data analysis used in veterinary epidemiology including regression and analysis of variance techniques for a continuous and a dichotomous outcome. Methods to assess the possible effects of interaction and confounding as well as methods for assessing agreement between observers or tests are addressed. All the examples used in Chapter 13 are given (with output) as SAS-code in Appendix E and R-code in Appendix F. The programs and data sets can be downloaded from www.itve.dk.

Exercises with solutions to each chapter are given in Appendix A. We hope this will be challenging for further reading of the book.

As with all complex matters it is difficult to decide what should come first. There is not just one logical way to present the subject. We have followed the logical sequence of steps that should be made when performing an epidemiological study. However, being a textbook on basic epidemiology some concepts need to be defined before we can move on to other subjects.

The textbook has been made as a joint effort by the employees at the Division of Veterinary Epidemiology at the Department of Large Animal Sciences at The Royal Veterinary and Agricultural University. We have been through many discussions on concepts and the structure in the textbook. We acknowledge all the feedback we have received from students and other interested readers that has been presented for preliminary editions of this textbook. All chapters have been reviewed by international experts in veterinary epidemiology. We greatly acknowledge the comments and suggestions for improvements we have received from Paul Bartlett, USA; Michel Bigras-Poulin, Canada; Marcus Doherr, Switzerland; Ian Dohoo, Canada; Ian Gardner, USA; Matthias Greiner, Denmark; Ann Lindberg, Sweden; Wayne Martin, Canada; Dirk Pfeiffer, UK; Stuart Reid, Scotland; Peter Sandøe, Denmark, and Henrik Stryhn, Canada.

Hans Houe
Annette Kjær Ersbøll
Nils Toft

Frederiksberg, Denmark
Spring 2004

CONTENTS

1 INTRODUCTION

Hans Houe, Jens Frederik Agger, Annette Kjær Ersbøll and Nils Toft

1.1 Definition

The literal translation of *epidemiology* is the study (logos) of what is upon (epi) the population (demos). Epidemiology has traditionally been defined as *the study of occurrence and distribution of diseases in populations as well as the study of factors that influence disease occurrence*. Also subclinical diseases should be included in the definition (e.g. subclinical infections). In recent years, the definition of epidemiology has been extended to also cover the study of health in populations, where a health characterisation in its broadest sense in addition to absence of disease includes positive health indicators, production variables and behaviour. In this textbook we use this extended definition of epidemiology acknowledging that in most cases, epidemiology is dealing with diseases. Other definitions of epidemiology may be seen in various textbooks on epidemiology, but the essentials are the same as in the definition we use here.

The term disease implies the existence of a sick individual and a disease entity. The *occurrence* of diseases deals with *who has what* and can be described as the frequency of diseases either at a given point in time or as diseases occurring during a defined period. The *distribution* of diseases refers to *when and where* and includes the occurrence in different age groups, among different species and breeds, at different geographical locations at different calendar time, etc. The *factors* or *determinants* that influence disease occurrence include both direct aetiological agents and factors that merely increase the risk of occurrence (risk factors). Thus, these factors refers to *why and how* the diseases occur.

Epidemiology is a population-based discipline. The term *population* can be defined as *the totality of individuals of the same kind that share or have in common certain attributes* (Toma *et al.*, 1999). Examples of populations are: the dogs in Denmark, the cows at a particular dairy farm, or the dairy farms in

Denmark. The size of the population of concern may be finite or assumed infinite, depending on the researcher's specification. In Chapter 2 we will discuss populations in epidemiology further.

It is important to distinguish between study unit and epidemiological unit. The *study unit* describes the entity for which measurements are made, whether it is a measurement of disease status in one animal or a recording of the housing system for a whole herd. Synonymous with the term study unit, unit of concern, sample unit, observational unit (in observational studies), and experimental unit (in experimental studies) are also being used. The *epidemiological unit* defines groups of animals in the population according to certain aggregations such as separate herds, buildings, etc. The term epidemiological unit is especially used in the study of infectious diseases where transmission between animals within an epidemiological unit is higher than transmission between animals from different epidemiological units. Thus, a single cat living in an apartment or 100 dairy cows in the same barn each constitutes one epidemiological unit. The cat will usually also be one study unit, but the 100 dairy cows might constitute between 1 and 100 study units depending on whether the individual cows, groups of cows or the barn is the unit at which measurements are made. Thus, although the study and epidemiological units are extracted from the population the two terms are quite different. Further, the definition of the epidemiological unit and study unit (and to some degree the definition of the population) is context specific. It depends almost entirely on the specific purpose, objective and hypothesis of the study. A herd can be the population, an epidemiological unit or a study unit in a study. Only after stating the hypothesis for the study is it possible to determine the appropriate description of the role of a herd in the study. To avoid unnecessary confusion, we will refrain from using the term epidemiological unit in this book, unless the context is stated specifically.

1.2 Historical background and the need for epidemiology

Epidemiology is an old discipline, which has been practised and developed since ancient times. Hippokrates (approximately 460–377 BC) in his thesis on airs, waters and places described the integrity between human health and the environment (cited in Dohoo *et al.*, 2003) – a view which today is still one of the cornerstones in the understanding of the causal mechanisms for the occurrence of diseases in populations. However, the concept of causality has strongly developed during the recent centuries.

Application of epidemiology in disease control and eradication has been practised for centuries. After the discovery of the importance of micro-organisms, great progress was made and new control methods were developed to deal with diseases like cattle plague, tuberculosis, brucellosis, foot and mouth disease and many others. Quantitative veterinary epidemiology of both infectious and non-infectious diseases has developed significantly since the early 1960s when leading schools of veterinary medicine started to develop the discipline and associated educational programmes.

Veterinary epidemiology is a fast growing discipline. The long lasting trend in animal husbandry towards larger herds and increasing density of production animals, reduction of manpower and increasing use of machinery and other technical support, the continued competition and demand for increased efficiency, productivity and economic outputs, are some of the reasons that the demand for epidemiology is growing. Methods to identify problem herds in public campaigns, to document losses from farm animal diseases, to conduct research in production diseases and to develop herd health programs for veterinary practitioners and farmers in intensive livestock production have become necessary to focus on.

The strong development of information and computer technology has increased the number of data collected and the need for methods to handle data stored in the growing number of databases on, e.g. animal husbandry issues like production, animal breeding and disease occurrence. Further, there are databases on national and international disease control activities and disease outbreaks as well as databases on companion animals with respect to pedigree, location and birth date. Parallel to the increased sampling of data, statistical software packages have been developed with a high impact on the development of quantitative veterinary epidemiology.

The international competition for markets has increased the need for exporters to be able to declare products and the producing country free of certain diseases. The increasing risk of transferring animal and human diseases from one region to another associated with the change in society towards more international trade and travel and the associated risk of inter-species transmission including zoonoses is one more reason for the need of epidemiology. Further, there is a growing concern for the general public's view on animal welfare.

Finally, we need to mention the importance of educating veterinarians in epidemiology to acquire a critical attitude towards research results, and in order to be able to plan and conduct their own studies.

1.3   Epidemiology as a scientific discipline

A scientific discipline can be characterised as having distinct objects (phenomenon and problems), theory and concepts. From the definition of epidemiology the object is clearly the importance of the population in veterinary medicine in the sense that a disease occurrence with its determinants cannot be described and analysed without considering the characteristics of the population. A certain population might result in a specific interaction between the individual animals (the host), the involved disease agents and the environment and, therefore, the disease manifestation will vary from one population to another. Epidemiology uses certain concepts and theories to describe and explain disease occurrence. The disease *incidence*, meaning new cases of disease during a period, is dependent on the *population at risk*, which describes those animals susceptible to the disease in question. The population characteristics have importance for the spread of infection in time and space. An infectious disease propagates differently depending on whether 10% of the population are susceptible, e.g. by having no immunity, or 90% are susceptible. The propagation might also depend on the density of animals in the population. The terms sporadic, endemic, epidemic and pandemic have often been used to describe different kinds of disease occurrence. A sporadic disease occurs irregularly in time and space and generally with a low frequency. An endemic disease is constantly present in a given region and often with a relative constant frequency whereas an epidemic disease (or disease epidemic) occurs in clear excess of what would be expected for a specific region or time (Toma *et al.*, 1999). Pandemic can be used for diseases occurring through several continents affecting a large proportion of the population. The terms point epidemic and propagating epidemic refer to the time duration. A point epidemic includes relatively few individuals getting diseased during a short time period, while a propagating epidemic lasts longer and with many more individuals affected. In epidemiology we use the term *infection dynamics* to describe and explain disease transmission in space and time.

Having developed historically from the need to understand and control infectious diseases a core element of epidemiology is the spread of infectious diseases as being caused by interplay of the host, the agent and the environment. However, the study object certainly also includes the importance of the population for non-infectious diseases.

In the definition of epidemiology is also mentioned 'factors that influence disease occurrence'. Thus, the concept of *causality* is very important in epidemiology, but not unique for the discipline. The concepts of risk factors and causality will be elaborated in Chapter 3.

Other concepts and theories have major importance in epidemiology, but are not unique to the discipline. Assuming that disease can only be fully described and understood by studying a population of animals, and not only individual animals, epidemiology has elements of systems theory. Systems are dynamic entities where changes in one part induce changes in other parts of the system. These changes will again have a feedback effect on the system. Obviously, presence of an infectious disease in a group of animals will influence presence of disease in other groups of animals. This will also be the case for non-infectious diseases. If, for example, a disease causes increased mortality or culling, the age distribution of the population will change and hence the susceptibility to disease may change. It is also characteristic that the same phenomenon may be both cause and effect. In the example where disease causes increased mortality (effect), the increased mortality might subsequently give rise to a younger population that eventually results in a reduced mortality.

In the process of establishing a research question or hypothesis on disease occurrence and the related factors, epidemiology relies on the whole theory in veterinary medicine (immunity, pathology, etc.). A major part of epidemiology is hereafter to design a study, sample relevant data and analyse the data. Mathematical and statistical methodologies have therefore become an integrated part of epidemiology. Probability theory, descriptive statistics (mean, median, standard deviation) and statistical hypothesis testing are all necessary parts of conducting an epidemiological study. Some refer to these methodologies as 'tools' in epidemiology. But one should think of them as an integrated part. Already when formulating a hypothesis, one should think of how the biological information can be transformed into a collection of data that can eventually be formally tested.

In literature, several other subdisciplines of epidemiology have been mentioned. *Clinical epidemiology* applies epidemiological principles and methods to improve medical decision making including aspects of diagnosis, prognosis and decisions on treatments. *Theoretical epidemiology* uses mathematical models to predict the occurrence of diseases and to test the underlying hypothesis. Also, very specific sub-disciplines such as molecular epidemiology and genetic epidemiology are evolving.

As previously mentioned, epidemiology is a fast growing discipline and it seems not clear at the moment whether future development will have emphasis on more advanced mathematical or statistical techniques or there will be more emphasis on interdisciplinary aspects – or maybe epidemiology will still try to keep all these aspects together as necessary prerequisites to study the population. However, no matter what the future brings we believe that the content of this textbook will be central to epidemiology.

1.4 Application of epidemiology

Epidemiological studies provide veterinary professionals (practitioners, laboratories, health services, veterinary authorities, etc.) with knowledge and tools to improve animal health and welfare including better herd health and disease control programmes, increase food safety and improve the economic output from production. As stated in the definition, an epidemiological study investigates the occurrence and distribution of disease and health as well as the factors that influence the occurrence of disease and health. Epidemiology has therefore often been said to consist of two approaches: *descriptive epidemiology* and *analytical epidemiology*. Descriptive epidemiology is concerned with questions such as: Which animals have the disease? Where does the disease occur? When does the disease occur? And what is the frequency of the disease? Descriptive epidemiology is used to summarise the recordings in order to get an overview of the results (e.g. frequencies and mean values). Thus, descriptive epidemiology can be said to be explorative. Analytical epidemiology is primarily concerned with causal questions, i.e. to answer: Why does disease occur? Hence, analytical epidemiology uses statistical inference to test hypotheses and estimate the effect of risk factors on the outcome.

Knowledge based on answers to the above questions is used in disease control, eradication and prevention programmes at various population levels, e.g. herd health management programmes or national disease control programmes. Such activities, however, require more knowledge than epidemiology can provide, and inter-disciplinary collaboration between many disciplines in veterinary and animal science is necessary.

One should be aware that the terms *descriptive analysis* and *statistical hypothesis testing* to some extent can be seen as the statistical counterparts of descriptive and analytical epidemiology. Descriptive analysis is used for statistical summary measures such as mean, median, standard deviation, frequency distribution, etc. of the measures in question. Thus, descriptive analysis refers to descriptive epidemiology. Statistical hypothesis testing is used for making inferences of the associations between variables and thus refers to analytical epidemiology. Especially the use of 'analysis' and 'analytical' for two different things can seem confusing unless one is aware of the meaning.

An epidemiological study gathers data from clinical examinations, pathological examinations, laboratory examinations, production records, etc. and analyses the data in relation to the more applied areas such as disease surveillance, disease control and prevention programmes. Population medicine is the professional domain of application, e.g. herd health, eradication and control programmes, vaccination programmes, preventive veterinary medicine and production medicine. Epidemiology can be seen as a discipline supporting the directed action against diseases or health problems and as a diagnostic discipline for population medicine.

1.5 Outline of the book

The logical sequence in an epidemiological study includes a number of steps starting with first formulation of purpose, objectives and hypothesis until the final conclusions are drawn (Figure 1.1). This book is essentially built up the same way. However, as explanation of some concepts is a necessary prerequisite for others, we cannot follow this principle through all parts of the textbook. We will illustrate the steps in Figure 1.1 by referring to epidemiological studies on bovine virus diarrhoea (BVD) virus (BVDV) before the initiation of the Danish eradication program (Houe, 1996).

In the beginning of the 1990s, the Danish cattle organisation wanted to establish a surveillance programme for herds that contained cattle carrying BVDV. Obviously, the *purpose* was to improve animal health, welfare and production economy. Establishing the surveillance programme can be said to be the *objective* of the project. The hypothesis (Chapter 2) or working hypothesis was that testing a number of animals for *antibodies* could be used to predict whether there would also be *virus* carriers present. Further, it was hypothesised that purchase of animals and having animals on pastures were the main risk factors for herds getting infected. Formulation of the hypothesis is naturally closely linked to an evaluation of the nature of the data (Chapter 3) that we are dealing with. Cattle that get infected with BVDV as adults will often not show any clinical signs. They will develop a strong antibody response and clear themselves for the virus. However, if a cow is in early pregnancy when infected, then the foetus will develop tolerance to the virus for the rest of its life. The calf will be born as so-called persistently infected (PI) and have a high amount of virus in the blood for the rest of its life. It is these calves we

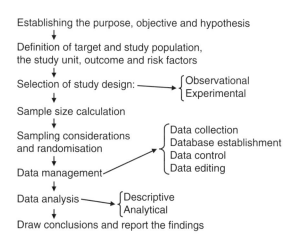

Figure 1.1. *Steps in the conduct of an epidemiological study.*

wanted to trace and remove in a control programme because they are very efficient transmitters of infection. Based on this information the hypothesis was formulated: *PI animals will reveal themselves by infecting all animals in their surroundings*. Usually, there will only be few PI animals present (because few cows have been in early pregnancy at the same time), but there will be many antibody positive around them. Therefore, we can trace PI animals indirectly by testing animals or a sample of animals for antibodies.

The evaluation of the nature of data helped finalising the hypothesis and lead to the conclusion that the important data for the study consisted of the laboratory examinations for virus and antibodies because data on clinics and production are vague and inconsistent.

Once the hypothesis is formulated, it is necessary to define the target population, i.e. the population that we really want to learn about and to which we want to extrapolate our study results, based on the sample of observational units (e.g. animals or herds) that we choose for the study. It is usually neither possible nor necessary to study the whole population in order to obtain the necessary information. In the above example Danish cattle herds were chosen as the target population. The study units consisted of both individual animals that should be blood tested and individual herds on which a disease status was wanted (presence versus non-presence of PI animals). The identified risk factors included the number of purchased animals in recent years and whether animals from the herd came on pasture during the summer.

The next step is to decide on what kind of study is suitable for our hypothesis and how long a study duration is needed. Basically, we can choose between observational studies (Chapter 4) where the investigator observes without intervening and experimental studies with intervention (Chapter 5) where the investigator controls relevant intervening factors. In the present situation an observational study was preferred because it was relevant also to get information about the disease occurrence in a situation without intervention. There are three main types of observational study designs. We could use (1) a 'cohort study' where we select herds according to the presence of risk factors (e.g. select a number of herds using pasture and similar number of herds not having animals on pasture; (2) a 'case-control study' where we select herds according to disease status (i.e. a number of herds with PI animals and a number of herds without such animals); or (3) a 'cross-sectional study' where herds are selected as being representative of the target population and where we at the same point of time (a 'snap shot') examine both exposure level and disease status. To obtain a measure of disease occurrence (or more precise occurrence of infection), it was decided to perform a cross-sectional study.

The decision on the relevant measure of disease occurrence (Chapter 6) as well as measures of association with risk factors (Chapter 7) must then be made. For example, the frequency can be measured in just one examination, which leads to prevalence estimates, or the frequency can be measured as the number of new cases during a period of time – which leads to incidence estimates. As PI animals are virus positive for life, the prevalence estimates were found sufficient for the present study, which again supported the choice of a cross-sectional study.

Before starting the practical part of the study, the sample size must be determined (Chapter 8). In the present situation with two sampling levels it was needed to decide both the number of herds and the number of animals per herd that were needed. As some herds were small and because it was crucial also to know the distribution of antibody carriers in different age groups it was decided to test all animals in each herd. Therefore, the critical sample size was based on the number of herds. Based on prior knowledge or best guesses of what might be a likely frequency of both the risk factors and the infection there are different formulas for calculating sample sizes (Chapter 8). In addition, there are different approaches on how to get a sample of cattle herds that is representative for all Danish cattle herds. In practice, it may not always be possible to follow the scientific optimal procedure, often due to economical constraints. In the present situation it was for example very convenient to select herds on which there were already high quality data in a database on birth dates, purchase of animals, etc. Further, there was not enough manpower and money to select close to 100 herds, which the formulas would recommend. Instead, 19 herds known to represent Danish dairy herds and for which there were high quality data were selected for blood testing. There are no rules for when such compromises are reasonable. In the actual situation there happened to be enough information for most of the hypotheses. But, in many situations we may waste research money if proper sample size considerations are not carried out and followed.

In many studies it is important to obtain more information on how reliable the diagnostic tests are (Chapter 9). Such studies on the sensitivity and specificity of antibody and virus detection were done in parallel with the present study.

Before visiting the herds for blood sampling it must be considered what additional information should be obtained. Here, information on the use of pasturing and also whether there might have been purchased animals that were not recorded in the existing database was wanted. Information on these risk factors was gathered from questionnaires presented to the farmer (Chapter 12).

Once the data have been collected, they should be entered into a database – which today is most frequently on electronic form. It is very important for any investigator to be very precise and also patient in this phase of the project, usually called the data management phase (Chapter 10). There are several software packages available on the market such as, for example, EpiInfo, Statistix, Excel, Access, Oracle, MySQL, Stata, SAS, R and SPlus. Each program has limitations and drawbacks – depending on the purpose and objectives. Some are good for data management, e.g. arranging the data in a logical sequence; others are strong in statistical analyses. Thus, it is quite common to use more than one program for the same study as long as it is possible to export and import data from one program to another. To summarise: the data management steps comprise data collection, database establishment, data control and data editing. All these must be completed before any analyses can be performed. This phase often takes quite some time. However, it needs to be done because you otherwise risk having to redo the analysis if erroneous data are identified in the analytical phase; or you risk making wrong conclusions due to erroneous data. In the BVD example all the blood sample results (virus and antibodies) were initially stored in a separate database. However, in order to utilise the information from the already existing database on birth dates, etc. for the final analyses, the two databases had to be combined.

The analytical phase (Chapter 13) is where you extract the information from the data and test the hypothesis initially stated. The data analysis should always be performed in a systematic way from the very basic descriptive analyses, to the more or less complicated epidemiological and statistical analyses. Thus, it is paramount to develop an analytical strategy. This is also the phase where your imaginations of causal structures are important. Perform the analysis that seems most relevant from a causal point of view to confirm or reject the hypotheses that initiated the study. Multivariable analytical procedures are very common to perform, and confounding factors and interactions (Chapters 11 and 13) should always be searched for. However, much information can be obtained from simple analytical steps. It is also very important to be aware of the balance between the quality of the data, the complexity of the analysis and the conclusions drawn on the basis of the results. In the BVDV example it was shown that presence of PI animals could be predicted by just testing five animals for antibodies. The importance of purchased animals was surprisingly low. In case of 'surprising' results all the steps in Figure 1.1 must be critically re-evaluated. As an example, the importance of purchase is discussed further in Chapter 2 where we discuss the hypothesis.

Finally, the conclusions are made and the study is published.

2 HYPOTHESES, OUTCOMES AND DETERMINANTS

Søren Saxmose Nielsen and Hans Houe

2.1 Introduction

What is the specific question we wish to address in a study? What relations do we wish to draw inferences on? What is the definition of our outcome and our factors of interests? To which extent can we generalise our results? In this chapter we describe some of the basics relating to study hypothesis, outcome, determinants and study population.

2.2 The object and the subject

Scientific studies will generally consist of two components: the object and the subject. The object is what is being studied, e.g. the relations between factor A and factor B, whereas the subject is the researcher or the research community. The subject may be driven by curiosity, belief or needs from the society.

The object is important, because the subject here specifies what particularly is being studied. The specifications relating to the object must be very clear in order to remain objective. If the object is not specific, the researcher may come up with conclusions that have a greater element of subjectivity than objectivity.

In veterinary science and practice, infections, diseases and productivity are the main outcome variables. Causal relations between potential risk factors or determinants and outcomes are determined. These causal relations are often our objects in specific studies. However, a clear definition of the outcome in question is crucial to the design of the study. The production outcomes such as milk yield or number of weaned piglets are often straightforward to define whereas many diseases may be more difficult to define. The definition of a disease could be based on an internationally accepted standard. These

Box 2.1. *Terms and definitions used in the text.*

Definitions and explanations

Aim: An intention of the study, where the object has a central role but is not necessarily specifically a part of it.

Deduction: Subtraction of evidence based on already existing information. Drawing logical inferences from a given set of premises (hypotheses).

Empirical: Experience or experiments are essential.

Experiment: Involves among other things an active intervention in nature.

Hypothesis: A proposition which is supposed. A hypothesis has not been proved but is assumed for the purpose of argument. The proposition of the hypothesis is different from the assumptions which may be used in the study in that the proposition has the status of a proposal which is the focus.

Induction: Inference drawing where single cases are transferred to states of regularity. You add more information than is given in the premises.

Object: Phenomenon which is specifically being studied.

Objective: A specific hypothesis with inclusion of the specific objects in the study.

Observation: The original expression of nature which can be observed or noted. No intervention in the system has been made.

Perceptive subject: The researcher who 'translates' the finding relating to the object.

Purpose: An intention relating to the specific study but not necessarily the specific object of the study.

Subject: The persons involved in the scientific study.

Theory: A formulation of apparent relationship or underlying principles of certain observed phenomena (an explanation of a problem where an acceptable mechanism is incorporated).

standards are often agreed upon in organisations like the Officine International des Épizooties (OIE) of the World Organisation of Animal Health.

However, at times it is more relevant to adapt the disease definition to the specific objective rather than to some standard. The problem of using an internationally accepted definition is not the definition per se, but merely that such definitions are usually created to cover as many situations as possible and they are expressions of specific time-points of the disease. In reality, most diseases follow a dynamic pattern and the study could actually be a part of elucidating this pattern. Therefore, a disease definition that adapts to this situation would apply better. For instance, the dynamics of an infectious disease usually follow a pattern such as: (1) entrance of infectious agent; (2) establishment of the infectious agent; (3) development of an immune response; (4) clinical symptoms; (5) the immune system winning the battle against the infectious agent; and (6) removal of the infection (the sequence and timing of these events are interchangeable depending on the disease and perhaps the abilities of the animal to fight the infection). What would be the true disease definition in these situations? In Toma *et al.* (1999) 'a disease' is defined as 'non-compensated perturbation of one or several functions of an organism'. This is a fairly vague definition, which may be acceptable as a joint designation for various undesirable conditions but not for specific studies of specific conditions.

In this aspect it may be useful to discriminate between two parallel processes: (1) infection, where a pathogen enters and uses a host and (2) pathogenesis, which is the sequential consequence of the entrance of the pathogen. The observed consequences, e.g. clinical signs, lesions (pathology), antibodies (measured by a laboratory test), etc. are diagnostic tests which are not synonymous with 'disease'. Still, the clinician may claim that disease is not present till clinical symptoms have appeared. The pathologist may claim that pathological changes must be present. People involved in preventive veterinary medicine may claim that a population is diseased if an infectious agent is present in one or more animals without all the animals being affected, because of potential passive transmission through carrying the infectious agent (the carrier status). Yet, these diagnostic measures may be more relevant from a utility point of view than from a scientific point of view. The object should be defined, but the subject needs to specify the object prior to conduction of the study.

If we wish to establish the relations between infection with a pathogen and presence of clinical signs, a clear definition of which clinical signs should be present to classify an animal as 'diseased' should then be established. Clearly, 'diarrhoea' could be applicable in some situations but is too broad in other situations. Therefore, it is essential to define the outcome you want to draw inferences on before you undertake the study and make clear whether infection, pathological changes or clinical manifestations are the primary interest. The outcome should be defined before the study is conducted. A practical way of handling this is to create an $n \times 2$ table (Table 2.1), where you have decided

Table 2.1. *An n × 2 table for classification of study outcomes with respect to factors and outcome*

Factor classification		Outcome (disease, infection, etc.)	
		$+$	$-$
Risk factor level	1	a_1	b_1
	2	a_2	b_2
	$\vdots$	$\vdots$	$\vdots$
	n	a_n	b_n

upon a disease definition. If you know how to classify your study animals in such a table before you carry out the study you may be able to actually carry out the study. If you have clear definitions of the outcome and clear definitions of the factors, inference drawing using statistical tests is usually fairly easy to perform. Based on the inferences of the statistical testing, inferences on the biological phenomena can often be made.

Similar to being specific about the outcome, a clear definition of the factors or determinants hypothesised to be related to the outcome is needed. A clear description of a risk factor or determinant is as important as the definition of the outcome. Risk factors are elaborated in detail in Chapter 3.

2.3   The hypothesis

Through experience or experiments we may observe some phenomena which may lead to some kind of knowledge. Knowledge obtained from experience is called empirical knowledge. Pure empirical knowledge disregards theory, reasoning and science. Science should be performed through reasoning; hence, empirical knowledge may seem insufficient due to the disregarding of reasoning. An argument based on single observations which seem to form a state of irregularity is called induction. Induction is the arrival at general principles derived from single observations. Deduction on the other hand is inference drawing based on logical inference on a hypothesis, which states the reasons for single cases. Thus, to make deductions, we need a hypothesis.

The hypothesis is a tool in the construction of arguments behind objects and structures of an observed phenomenon. It is a proposition which has not been proved, but is assumed for the purpose of argument. The difference between a theory and a hypothesis is that the theory is an explanation of a problem, where an acceptable mechanism is incorporated.

The hypothesis is used for making arguments in the exploration of mechanisms or relations underlying what we experience. Through construction of mathematical arguments we can draw inferences that explain single cases. Through a systematic approach we use the deductive structure of mathematics to draw conclusions. It is important to emphasise that final conclusive evidence cannot be obtained through deduction. When a hypothesis is confronted with data, it may at best be falsified. Through deduction you may be able to falsify a hypothesis; you are not able to verify it.

Specifically, we use statistical testing as a part of our mathematical arguments. The consequences (or predictions) derived from a hypothesis are what is being tested. It is not the theory itself. The idea behind testing is to compare the predicted and observed (empirical) data. If a prediction does not agree with an experiment, the theory does not necessarily have to be wrong. The experiment could be, in that it may be subject to criticism as well as the theory could be.

The difference between a theory and a hypothesis is the lack of an acceptable mechanism, in that a theory has the mechanism incorporated. However, various levels of theories exist: some may have only indications of an underlying mechanism whereas others may have an almost fully generalised mechanism that applies in all of the 'known society' as well as in still 'unknown parts of the society'. The domain of a theory is important to define, i.e. it is the theory applicable in general or confined to special situations, where, for instance, certain conditions regarding housing, race, genetic merit, etc. are fulfilled (see Section 2.6).

2.4 Establishing the objective of a study

If our curiosity has driven us to derive evidence on a problem, this problem should be characterised. We should have an intention, an aim, towards where our study should ideally take us. This aim should be specified, along with an objective. The objective of our study relates to our specific object and thus the design of the study. The aim or purpose of a study may be a little bit different, in that they both relate to the intention of the study. However, we may not be able to study the intended aim because our technical methods or study design are limiting factors.

EXAMPLE 2.1. We may have the intention to study if humoral immune responses (the outcome) occur in cows infected with the pathogen X (the determinant). This intention is the aim or the purpose of our study. Current knowledge on the specific infection and the immune responses related with the infection (i.e. the theory) should be obtained from the literature. It has been determined, that there are no descriptions on the relations between humoral immune responses and X-infection. Yet, we assume that infected cows will develop humoral immune responses and formulate a hypothesis: 'Cows infected with X develop humoral immune responses'.

However, specifically we are only able to detect IgG in serum samples as a measure of humoral immune responses and we are only able to determine infection status in the cows by detection of the pathogen in faeces. Thus, our object is the relation between pathogens in faeces and IgG in serum. The objective can be formulated: 'The objective of our study is to compare the proportion of cows with IgG among X-infected cows shedding pathogen X in faeces relative to the proportion of cows with IgG among non-infected cows'. This is also an object which can be submitted to statistical testing and subsequent inference drawing. The subject (the researcher) has decided that humoral immune responses should be substituted by the presence/absence of IgG and infection should be substituted by shedding of X, irrespective of whether these measures are not really what we wish to study. It is merely what we can study given the situation, and our current belief renders us to think it is sufficient.

2.5   Inference drawing on the hypothesis

When an appropriate hypothesis is stated for a conceptual model, and an objective has been formulated, we can carry out the study. First, a study design is chosen (see Chapters 4 and 5). We then submit our hypothesis to a statistical test. Based on the statistical test, we can draw inferences on the hypothesis. The hypothesis can be formulated mathematically, i.e. with a null hypothesis H_0: The proportion of cows with IgG among infected cows is the same as the proportion of cows with IgG among non-infected cows, or:

$$H_0: \quad Pr\{IgG + |X+\} = Pr\{IgG + |X-\}$$

where the vertical bar (|) means 'given that'. Recall that through mathematical arguments we are using the deductive principle and we can therefore only falsify the null hypothesis. We may therefore wish to have an alternative hypothesis (H_A):

$$H_A: \quad Pr\{IgG + |X+\} \neq Pr\{IgG + |X-\}$$

A p-value can be obtained to express the probability that H_0 is true. The magnitude of the p-value will then be submitted to a subjective interpretation of the researcher who will then determine if H_0 can be rejected and H_A should be accepted (a threshold of 0.05 for the p-value is often chosen, but depending on the given situation, we may use a different threshold).

EXAMPLE 2.2.   Paratuberculosis is a chronic disease in cattle and other ruminants. The disease is normally considered incurable and the end manifestations are chronic diarrhoea and death. The incubation period (from infection to clinical manifestations) is typically 2–4 years. A veterinarian was told in vet school that paratuberculosis is more frequent among Jersey cows than among Holstein cows. Why would one breed be more prone to develop paratuberculosis than another breed? The hypothesis is that Holsteins have a genetic composition that renders them more resistant to infection.

She (the subject) decides to investigate if this is true among her patients. She knows that the farmers cull all cows manifesting diarrhoea for more than 2 weeks. Therefore, only few cows with clinical paratuberculosis are available. Instead, she decides to carry out two diagnostic tests, one to detect antibodies (an ELISA) and one to detect bacteria shed in faeces (faecal culture (FC)). She decides that both tests should be positive in order to classify a cow as a 'paratuberculosis case'. Thus, being positive in only one test defines a cow as a non-paratuberculosis cow. The definition of the outcome has been made. Her object is thus specified to be the relation between serial test positivity and breed. Her objective thus becomes to study if cows of the Jersey breed have a higher probability of being positive in both ELISA and FC, than cows of the Holstein breed. This is her object. The associated mathematical specification is:

$$H_0: \quad Pr\{FC + \text{ and ELISA} + |\text{Holstein}\} = Pr\{FC + \text{ and ELISA} + |\text{Jersey}\}$$

against

$$H_A: \quad Pr\{FC + \text{ and ELISA} + | \text{Holstein}\} \neq Pr\{FC + \text{ and ELISA} + | \text{Jersey}\}$$

where Pr is the probability of event (here, FC+ and ELISA+) given being one or the other breed. The statistical hypothesis that will be tested in the end is: The probability of being a paratuberculosis case is the same in Jerseys and in Holsteins. The alternative hypothesis is: The probability of being a paratuberculosis case is different among Jerseys than among Holsteins. The study was conducted and the cows classified as shown in Tables 2.2 and 2.3. Since the study was cross-sectional with comparison of two groups with investigation of the difference in the proportion of 'disease' in the two groups, a relative risk (see Chapter 7) can be calculated along with statistical tests (here, the χ^2-test was used to test the association between outcome and risk factor). The relative risk estimates reveal that the risk of Jerseys being FC positive is 1.6 times the risk of Holsteins being FC positive (Table 2.2, $p = 0.30$) and the risk of being positive in both tests as a Jersey is 2.2 times the risk of being positive in both tests as a Holstein (Table 2.3, $p = 0.10$). Neither is statistically significant at the usual 5% level of significance, but the results are not exactly the same. The most correct result in the present situation is the one in Table 2.3 because the veterinarian defined a paratuberculosis case based on the definition used in that table ahead of performing the study. It should be emphasised, that this is the correct paratuberculosis definition in this study because it was the starting definition. A more suitable biological definition could have better general use. The result of the hypothesis testing is that at a 5% level of significance the veterinarian could not demonstrate any difference in the occurrence of paratuberculosis among Jerseys and Holsteins. The statistical hypothesis cannot be rejected! The biological hypothesis has not been proven correct. However, it has not been rejected either, and we may wish to follow up on the results in a different study. If the breeds in addition to Jersey and Holstein also had consisted of various cross-breeds, a clear definition of breed classification would also have been necessary.

During the study, a different problem has arisen: What difference in proportion of infected cows would be acceptable to be considered 'a difference'? Was our sample size big enough to draw the inferences we wish? This will be covered in Chapter 8.

Table 2.2. *Paratuberculosis is defined by an animal being positive in a faecal culture (FC) test*

Number of cows	Study outcome (FC+)		Total	Risk	RR
	+	−			
Jersey	9	122	131	9/131	
Holstein	11	241	252	11/252	1.6
Total	20	363	383		

Table 2.3. *Paratuberculosis is defined by an animal testing positive in both faecal culture (FC) and ELISA*

Number of cows	Study outcome (FC+ and ELISA+)		Total	Risk	RR
	+	−			
Jersey	9	122	131	9/131	
Holstein	8	244	252	8/252	2.2
Total	17	366	383		

EXAMPLE 2.3.   Bovine virus diarrhoea (BVD) virus (BVDV) can infect cattle and a number of other ruminants. In cattle the disease is characterised by transient diarrhoea and reproductive disorders in cows and severe diarrhoea and death among young stock. The different clinical manifestations in cows and young stock are due to two different types of infection:

- Cattle that are infected as adults will get no or few symptoms followed by antibody production 2–3 weeks later. Hereafter, the virus will disappear and the cow will have antibodies for life. The cows will be immune subsequently. If the cow is pregnant when becoming infected, the foetus becomes infected.
- Foetuses of cattle that are infected in the first 3 months of pregnancy may develop 'tolerance' to the virus. In calfhood, they are not able to produce antibodies and they will carry the virus for the rest of their lives. We therefore refer to these animals as persistently infected (PI). Most die at the age of 6–18 months.

Farmers are interested in avoiding infection with BVDV. Especially, the PI animals are unwanted because they will shed a large amount of virus in the surroundings and they have a high risk of dying. One of the major risk factors of introducing the infection into the herd is believed to be purchase of animals. In a study it was therefore hypothesised that purchase of animals in recent years would be a risk factor for presence of PI animals (Houe, 1996). Houe as the researcher was in this instance the subject. In 19 herds of which 10 herds had PI animals and nine herds did not have PI animals the farmer was asked if he had purchased any animals in the past 3 years. The object studied was thus presence of PI animals and purchase of animals within the past 3 years. The result is shown in Table 2.4.

The null hypothesis (H_0) in Table 2.4 is that there is no association between presence of PI animals (the outcome) and whether the farmer had purchased any animals during the past 3 years.

$$H_0: \quad \Pr\{PI+ \mid \text{purchase}\} = \Pr\{PI+ \mid \text{no purchase}\}$$

against

$$H_A: \quad \Pr\{PI+ \mid \text{purchase}\} \neq \Pr\{PI+ \mid \text{no purchase}\}$$

The p-value is calculated as 0.09. Thus, the null hypothesis could not be rejected. The researcher is disappointed because intuitively it makes sense that purchase of animals would influence the presence of infection. There might be several different reasons for this failure of rejecting the hypothesis, such as: the hypothesis itself, the design, the sample size and the definition of the outcome. Nineteen herds is a small number and therefore it would be difficult to show significance. However, there may also be severe problems with the hypothesis. The question that should be asked is really: Will purchase of animals increase the risk of introducing the infection? However, presence of PI animals may not be a good measure for that. The infection may have been introduced to the herd 4–5 years ago and been present in the herd since. Measuring only purchase in the last 3 years will not tell anything about the risk of introducing the infection 4–5 years ago. A future study should therefore be designed to relate purchase of animals to the exact time of introducing the infection, for example, measured as when the first seroconversions would occur among cows.

In epidemiological literature there will be many examples of sub-optimal biological hypothesis simply due to lack of the data that are really needed. In the BVD example it would be very costly to test cows repeatedly for sero-conversion.

2.6   Target population, study population and study unit

In preparing the epidemiologic study, the target population, the study population and the sample unit must be defined. If we want to make a study of a risk factor for occurrence of BVDV in Denmark, then all cattle herds in Denmark

Table 2.4. *The importance of having purchased any animals the last 3 years on presence of animals persistently infected (PI) with bovine virus diarrhoea virus*

Number of herds	Study outcome		Total
	+PI	−PI	
Purchase			
Yes	10	6	16
No	0	3	3
Total	10	9	19

constitute the target population, i.e. the population we want to draw conclusions on. The study population on the other hand is the population from which a sample is taken, whereas the specific cows, that samples are obtained from, are the study units. In the case where samples are obtained repeatedly from a cow, it is the test-day sample which is the study unit.

It is essential that the study population is representative of the target population. This is the basis for our statistical testing and therefore subsequent inference drawing on the hypothesis. If the sample comprising our study population is obtained through a study design where selection of specific animals has been included, this has to be taken into account in the statistical procedures, which often makes these much more complicated. Therefore, randomisation is the easiest and most reliable method of sample collection, though this is often ignored because the sampling itself is cumbersome. Yet, the results may have no value if the sampling is done incorrectly and not handled appropriately in the subsequent statistical testing.

3 NATURE OF DATA

Hans Houe, Annette Kjær Ersbøll
and Liza Rosenbaum Nielsen

3.1 Introduction

Veterinary epidemiology utilises many types of biological data to study animal health and the associated determinants. Health is a difficult issue to measure as it includes many different variables such as the occurrence of disease, presence or absence of positive health indicators (such as fertility, hoof wall quality, body conditions score, appetite, etc.), production and abnormal behaviour. The definition of health often depends on the context in which it is used and may range from presence or absence of specific diseases or clinical signs to a total measure of the animal's performance or well-being.

Disease determinants are characteristics that affect health in the population. We will refer to determinants or disease determinants in this book, although it should be recognised that these determinants also include measures of health, animal well-being or productivity and not just the narrow definition of disease. Determinants can be described according to their association with the host, the agent or the environment. The host determinants include characteristics such as genetic composition, immunity, age, breed, sex, etc. These are also referred to as intrinsic determinants. The agent can refer to any immediate or primary cause of disease, but often it relates to infectious agents (bacteria, viruses, prions, fungi and parasites). The agent determinants include the ability of the agent to enter the host, to cause disease and to spread to other hosts. Environmental determinants include production system, management, climate, etc. The agent and environmental determinants are also referred to as extrinsic determinants.

Biological data should always be critically evaluated according to how well they are defined and how well they can be measured. In this chapter, we will start with some considerations on when a relation between an exposure or event and occurrence of disease (or other outcome) can actually be seen as a causal relationship, i.e. when is a factor a disease determinant. Hereafter, the intrinsic and extrinsic disease determinants and data on animal performance are briefly characterised with focus on their epidemiological importance. Finally, an overview is given of how to characterise and illustrate the data in mathematical and statistical terms.

3.2 Disease causation

In epidemiology, there are several expressions (aetiology, agent of disease, risk factors and others) for the relation between an exposure and the ensuing outcome.

Often the use of these terms depends on the certainty and the strength of the relation between cause and effect. Furthermore, the exact definitions may vary in literature. The terms are really dealing with the same thing, but which one is used depends on the context. Thus, the *aetiology* or *agent of disease* is often used when the exposure is the immediate cause of disease. Disease agent means a 'biological, mechanical, social, or behavioural entity for which the presence, the excess, or deprivation influences the occurrence of disease' (Toma *et al.*, 1999). For example foot and mouth disease virus is the aetiological agent for foot and mouth disease (FMD) and bovine virus diarrhoea (BVD) virus (BVDV) is the aetiological agent for mucosal disease. Many times the word *agent* means infectious agent, but it also includes toxins, hormonal imbalances, allergens, physical injuries and many others.

A risk factor is a factor that is associated with an increase in the probability of occurrence of an outcome of interest (e.g. disease, reduced performance or productivity). Sometimes a risk factor is used for the opposite situation when the factor reduces the risk of an outcome (also called a protective factor). Sometimes risk factors are used for any factor that is statistically associated with an outcome without knowing whether there is a causal relationship. Other authors consider risk factors to imply a certain degree of causality. This means that the term risk factor is generally not as strongly associated with causality as disease agents. A typical example of a risk factor is high humidity that increases the risk of pneumonia.

It also complicates the picture that an exposure factor that in one disease situation is considered to be aetiological, may be considered as a risk factor in another situation. For example, BVD virus is the aetiological agent for development of mucosal disease in cattle. On the other hand, BVD virus is only a risk factor for development of pneumonia, since here it merely acts as one of several possible causes and is not a specific cause of pneumonia. Therefore, the distinction is not always clear as it relates to the complicated issue of *causality* of diseases or other outcomes. When exposure is considered a causal factor for disease, the frequency of disease among exposed animals should clearly be higher than the frequency in non-exposed animals. However, statistical association is not enough to determine the factor as causal. For example, some diseases may be statistically associated with season. However, it may not be the season per se that is the reason an animal becomes ill. It may be that animals are getting less exercise or different feed stuffs during winter. Therefore, we must be sure that the factor is not only associated with the disease, but actually determines the disease. Finally, a causal factor must of course occur before the disease (Figure 3.1). This leads to the following definition of causal association: Association between a variable X (exposure or event) whose variations precede and determine the status of another variable Y (disease or production outcome): $X \Rightarrow Y$ (Toma *et al.*, 1999).

Although the definition may look simple, it is in practice often very difficult to establish clear evidence of a causal relationship. Apart from the statistical association and time relationship, one should also consider the following conditions that are required or at least increase the likelihood of a causal relationship:

- The relationship should be found between studying different populations and populations under different circumstances (consistency and repeatability).
- Removal of the factor should decrease the probability of the disease (reversibility).
- If possible, a dose–response relationship should be established (e.g. an increase in the amount of a poison will increase the severity of disease).
- As far as possible, a biological explanation should be identified.
- The stronger the statistical association, the lower is the probability that the association is due to chance (but remember that statistical association in itself does not reveal any causal relationship).

As mentioned already, there are different certainties regarding the importance of an exposure factor in relation to disease outcomes. These differences are closely related to the concepts of necessary and sufficient causes of disease. A *necessary cause* is one without which the disease will not occur.

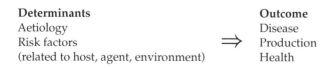

Determinants		Outcome
Aetiology		Disease
Risk factors	$\Rightarrow$	Production
(related to host, agent, environment)		Health

Figure 3.1. *The causal association between determinants and outcome.*

Mycobacterium paratuberculosis is a necessary cause of paratuberculosis. Without the bacteria, the disease will not occur. It is still discussed whether the bacterium, by itself, is also a sufficient cause, as the infection may be subclinical. On the other hand, the necessary cause is always a part of sufficient causes. For many respiratory viruses, we know that they are involved in pneumonia. However, they are not by themselves sufficient to produce disease. Pneumonia in calves, for example, is usually the result of virus infections followed by secondary bacterial infections and the presence of suboptimal environmental factors (crowding, high humidity, etc.). All these elements together make up the sufficient cluster of causes. A *sufficient cause* of a disease always produces an effect. There may be many different clusters of causes for a particular disease, but the agent (the necessary cause) is a member of all sufficient clusters. Unfortunately, we never know all the sufficient clusters for a disease, but at least this approach gives us a conceptual structure for understanding causal structure.

Often the sufficient cause (or sufficient cluster of causes) consists of several components and the disease is then called a *multifactorial disease*. The components of sufficient causes of multifactorial diseases often include aspects of the host, the agent and the environment. Both specific aetiology and risk factors are called disease determinants. Often, the host, agent and environmental determinants act together in a very complex interplay and they are often called the 'triad' of disease causation. This means that occurrence of respiratory viruses in one herd may not have importance whereas in another herd with a different climate they have a very severe effect. Therefore, it is difficult to evaluate one determinant alone as it often depends on the occurrence of the others.

3.3 Host determinants

Host determinants have significant influence on the occurrence of disease in animals. In epidemiological studies, it is important to have good knowledge of important host characteristics in the sampled individuals, the study population and the target population. Some host characteristics are well defined and easily obtained, such as age, sex and breed. When studying other host characteristics such as physiological, hormonal and immunological status, different tests need to be performed. The host characteristics are often related to each other. For example, physiological measures are related to sex, age, body condition, etc.

3.3.1 *Age*

Age is one of the most important host characteristics. Diseases such as diarrhoea and pneumonia are much more likely to occur in young animals, although the diseases are also strongly related to environmental risk factors. Milk fever in cattle is rarely seen among first-lactation cows, whereas annual incidences of more than 10% are seen in cows at second lactation or older in intensive production systems. Some chronic diseases like paratuberculosis (Johne's Disease) or bovine spongiform encephalitis (BSE) have very long incubation periods and are more likely to be found in older animals.

The fairly short lifetime of production animals as compared to companion animals affects the disease pattern. For example, the occurrence of different types of cancer is much more frequent in companion animals than in production animals. Often it is relevant to measure disease occurrence as age-specific prevalence or incidence.

3.3.2 *Sex*

Difference in disease occurrence between males and females are often self-evident when they are directly linked to the sexual organs, e.g. endometritis, mastitis and orchitis. The high milk production in cows predisposes for metabolic diseases, e.g. ketosis. Other differences between the sexes may be related to hormonal, physiological, genetic and behavioural differences. Some male animals get more physical injuries than females, e.g. male dogs and cats. Studying whether sex is a risk factor for a certain condition in production animals may be complicated by the fact that male animals are of little value to the farmer and may often be given less attention and care, and are sold, slaughtered or killed at a young age.

3.3.3 *Species and breed*

Some diseases are only seen in one or a few species. Closely related species like cattle and sheep are more likely to be susceptible to the same infectious agents and the same pathological conditions as remotely related species. For example, infectious microorganisms need to attach to the cell surface and some also enter the host cells. These infection mechanisms are highly dependent on the receptor-types of the host. The difference in susceptibility to infectious disease between species may be caused by differences in receptor-sites for the agent.

The number of host species susceptible to the different micro-organisms varies considerably. For example, most species can be affected by rabies and tetanus, whereas only ruminants and pigs get FMD. Some breeds may be more severely affected by certain infectious diseases than other breeds within the same species, e.g. the Doberman and Rottweiler dog breeds are more susceptible to Parvovirus diarrhoea than most other dog breeds (Ettinger and Feldman, 1995).

Non-infectious diseases may also be more prevalent in some species and breeds, e.g. 'Sweet Itch' is more frequent in Icelandic horses than in other horse breeds. The apparent effect of breed is often influenced by other risk factors such as age or geographic location. For example, Jersey cows have often been said to have a higher incidence of milk fever than other breeds. However, the mean age of lactating Jersey cows is higher than for other breeds. If the effect of breed on milk fever is corrected for the age effect, the breed effect diminishes. The higher prevalence of paratuberculosis in Jersey cattle may also be due to the fact that Jersey cattle are over-represented in high-prevalence areas (e.g. Funen in Denmark).

3.3.4 *Size and conformation*

Chronic sinusitis (inflammation of the sinuses and bony structures of the nasal cavity) caused by herpes virus, calici virus and chlamydia infections is more

Box 3.1. *Definitions of some of the diseases mentioned – see also textbooks in Veterinary Medicine.*

Ketosis: Accumulation of ketone bodies (e.g. acetone, acetoacetic acid) in blood and body tissues due to fatty acid metabolism in the liver. Occurs when cows are in severe negative energy balance. Symptoms include lack of appetite and neurological symptoms.

Mastitis: Inflammation of the mammary gland, usually infectious.

Metritis: Inflammation of the uterus.

Milk fever: Metabolic disease occurring just before or soon after calving. Lack of calcium in the blood and tissues leads to muscular weakness, circulatory failure with cold skin, weak pulse, recumbency and drowsiness.

Orchitis: Inflammation of the testes.

Rabies: A highly fatal viral infection of the nervous system which can affect all warm-blooded animal species, usually infected by bites from other infected animals.

Rhinitis: Inflammation of the mucous membranes of the nose.

Sweet itch: An intensely itchy skin disease in horses caused by hypersensitivity to the bites of insects of the *Culicoides* spp.

Tetanus: A highly fatal disease occurring in all animal species caused by the neurotoxin of the bacteria *Clostridium tetani*. Symptoms are related to the extensive muscle spasms in parts of or the entire body.

severe and problematic in Persian cats than other cat breeds. Although this can be said to be a breed effect, it seems more likely to be directly associated with the conformation of the head of Persian cats which predisposes these cats to infections in the upper airways and eyes.

3.3.5 *Immunity*

The immune system is a complex matter of great importance for disease pathogenesis. It influences susceptibility to disease and ability of the host to survive an infection. It also influences the ability of the animal to clear the infection or to become an asymptomatic carrier of an infectious agent. Some substances of the immune system (e.g. antibodies and cytotoxins, such as interferon and interleukin) can be used in epidemiology as health measures and to describe dynamics of diseases. Therefore, the immune system has elements of importance for measuring determinants for disease and health and for measuring the disease outcome itself (Figure 3.1).

The immune system can be divided into several entities as illustrated in Figure 3.2. The unspecific immunity (also called the innate immunity) is a

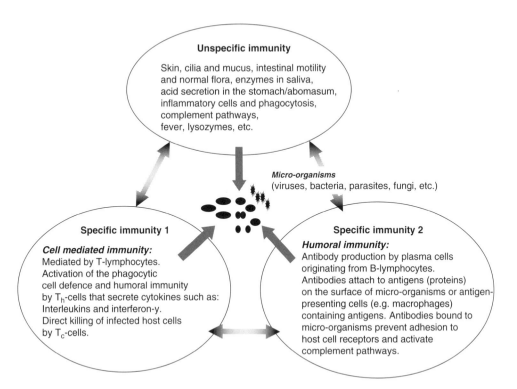

Figure 3.2. *The immune system. Schematic representation of the battle against intruding organisms.*

general defence mechanism against infectious agents, poisons and injuries. It consists of mechanical barriers (e.g. skin, gastrointestinal lining), chemical barriers (e.g. acid secretion in the stomach) and inflammatory reactions that immobilise and eliminate foreign agents in the body tissues. In general, these mechanisms are difficult to quantify and therefore not used much in epidemiological studies. An exception is the somatic cell count in dairy cows, which is used extensively all over the world to evaluate the health status of the mammary gland in cows, and as an indicator of subclinical mastitis. The somatic cell count indicates the concentration of inflammatory cells in milk.

The specific immunity (also called the acquired immunity) consists of two parts, the so-called cell mediated immune response and the humoral immune response. The specific immune system recognises the micro-organisms as foreign to the body and therefore directs its defence mechanism specifically to the intruding pathogen.

Antibodies produced by the humoral immune system are widely used in epidemiology as indicators of disease and health status of animals and herds. They are indicators of whether an animal has been infected or not. The amount of antibodies in the individual animal can be quantified. This is useful for gaining knowledge about stage or dynamics of disease. The amount of antibodies present can be expressed as a titre or an OD-value (OD = optical density). An animal is said to seroconvert if it changes from not having antibodies to having antibodies directed against the pathogen. If the animal already has antibodies but becomes infected again, it may change from having low levels of antibodies to having high levels of antibodies. As a rule of thumb, a four-fold rise in antibody titre is said to be indicative of a recent infection.

The humoral immune system has a delayed response. It usually takes 2–3 weeks for an animal to produce antibodies following an infection with

Box 3.2. *Definitions of common terms used to describe immunity.*

Antibody titre: The highest dilution of a sample where antibodies are still detectable.

Herd immunity: The ability of a group of animals to resist becoming infected or to minimise the effect of an infection in severity and incidence.

Optical density: A photometry measure of the amount of light absorbed by a sample in an ELISA-reader.

Seroconversion: Development of antibodies to an infectious organism in response to natural infection or to the administration of a vaccine.

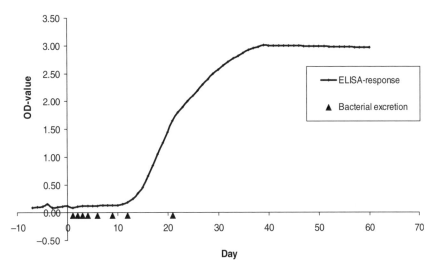

**ELISA-response (OD-values) and faecal excretion
of salmonella bacteria following infection on day 0**

Figure 3.3. *A typical course of the immunoglobulin G (IgG) response measured by an indirect O-antigen-based LPS ELISA-test after infection with Salmonella Dublin in cattle. Note that the faecal bacterial excretion stops after the first 3 weeks post-infection, whereas the humoral antibody response (in this case measured by IgG) is delayed 2–4 weeks (modified from Robertsson (1984)).*

virus or bacteria. However, the response varies a lot between individual animals. Generally, very young animals have slow or little antibody response to infections. The response also depends on the infectious agent. The antibody response to infection by mycobacteria may be delayed several years. Figure 3.3 shows a typical antibody response to salmonella infection in animals. Note that when the animal is excreting bacteria in the faeces, it may not yet have produced measurable antibodies against salmonella. Also note that the antibody level remains high even after the animal stops shedding the bacteria and is no longer infected.

For some infections, the antibodies continue to be detectable for the rest of the animal's life, whereas for others they will slowly disappear. If these individual disease and host characteristics are taken into consideration, antibodies can be useful tools in epidemiological studies of occurrence and dynamics of disease.

3.4 Agent determinants

The term *agent* means any immediate cause of disease including a biological, mechanical, social or behavioural entity that influences the occurrence of disease. However, due to the special role of infectious agents in the host–agent–environment triad, we will only deal with infectious agents in this section.

The most important properties related to the living agents concern infectivity, infectiousness, pathogenicity and virulence. The *infectivity* is the ability of the agent to enter and multiply in the host. One way to quantify the infectivity of an agent is to establish the number of infectious particles necessary to establish infection. The infectivity may vary with the host characteristics. For example it requires more salmonella bacteria inoculated orally in calves aged 8–12 weeks than in calves aged 2–6 weeks in order to produce the characteristic disease patterns in the animals.

The *infectiousness* is the ability of the agent to be transmitted from one host to another. For instance, transmission may require direct contact, or it may spread by air, sexual contact or food. *Pathogenicity* denotes the possible pathological changes the agent may inflict on the host. Pathogenicity is a qualitative measure as it describes the possible outcome and not the severity of the outcomes. *Virulence* indicates the severity of the pathological changes. For example, the case fatality rate can be a measure of severity.

Infectious agents may cause persistent infections despite the immune response of the host. The persistent infections are often subclinical and hard to recognise. There are different categories of persistent infections and the definitions may vary between authors. One way of categorising may be as follows:

1. *Latent infections (the hosts may be called latent carriers)*: The agent is difficult or impossible to detect, except under reactivation. The reactivation may be associated with recurrent disease. A commonly seen example is herpes virus infections, which occur in most species.
2. *Chronic infections (the hosts may be called active carriers)*: The agent is detectable and the host may be shedding the agent continuously or frequently. The host may be healthy or diseased, or disease may develop at a later point in time. An example is calves persistently infected (PI) with BVDV due to immunotolerance. Many of these calves are clinically normal; some are chronically unthrifty. Such PI-animals can develop acute disease with a sudden onset and die within a few weeks.
3. *Slow infections*: The number of pathogens and pathological lesions gradually increases. After a long subclinical phase, the infection leads to a slowly progressive and lethal disease. Feline leukaemia (FeLV), feline infectious peritonitis (FIP), paratuberculosis in cattle, enzootic bovine leukosis and mad cow disease are examples of slow infections.

If the host does not respond to the infection at all and the bacteria simply pass through the body and leave the host then the host is called a *passive carrier*.

Box 3.3. *Definitions of terms used when characterising infectious agents.*

Agent: (Syn: pathogen) Biological, chemical, physical, mechanical, social or behavioural entity for which the presence, excess or deprivation influences the occurrence of disease.

Infectivity: The characteristics of a micro-organism that allow it to infect and subsequently survive and multiply within a susceptible host. The degree of infectivity is the number of micro-organisms necessary to provoke an infection in a particular host.

Infectiousness: A relative quantification of the ease with which a disease organism is transmitted from one host to another.

Pathogenesis: The way the disease develops in an organism, organ or tissue.

Pathogenicity: The host-specific ability of an agent to cause disease or otherwise induce pathological change in a susceptible host.

Virulence: The host-specific ability of an infectious agent to multiply in the host while inducing lesions and disease.

Subclinical infection: Infection that does not produce clinical signs but generates detectable biological reactions.

Immunotolerance: Infection is present but the immune system of the infected animal is not able to produce a normal response because the immune system does not recognise the micro-organism as foreign. For instance, no rise in antibody titre occurs in response to infection.

This may be seen in animals grazing at pasture where, for example, parasites and bacteria may pass through the host and be transported passively from one location to another.

3.5 Environmental determinants of disease

Risk factors in the immediate environment of the animals include the production system, the climate and the handling of the animals. Further, the presence of reservoirs is important. Data on production system and climate are generally easily obtained with high accuracy and precision. On the other hand, several of the elements of husbandry can only be vaguely defined and, further, they are very difficult to quantify. For example: How can thoroughness

Table 3.1. *Important risk factors in the immediate environment of animals*

Production system
Housing type (single stalls, loose housing, tie stalls, etc.)
The sizes and shapes of pens, boxes, beds and stalls
Floor and bedding type (concrete, slatted floors, rubber, straw, etc.)
Density of animals in the barn area of interest (animals per square metre or animals per cubic metre)
Pasture characteristics
Feeding equipment
Light sources
Construction of facilities (e.g. placement of separation bars)

Climate
Temperature
Humidity
Dust
Polluting gasses (ammonia, etc.)
Draught
Ventilation

Handling – husbandry/management
Feeding procedures
Insemination, reproduction control
Procedures at parturitions
Movements of animals (in groups, single-animal movement, isolations procedures, etc.)
Purchase policy
Hygiene (all-in all-out, cleaning procedures, changing clothes, washing hands, dip baths for boots, sharing equipment with other farms, etc.)
Treatment and prophylactic routines
Routines at milking
Isolation of sick animals
Advisory agreements with veterinary and agricultural consultants
Continuing education

Reservoirs
Rodents
Wildlife

---

and patience in calving assistance be measured and its effect on calf mortality be evaluated? A list of important risk factors for development of disease related to the environment is given in Table 3.1. In order to identify risk factors for occurrence of pneumonia in calves, several of the risk factors mentioned in the table are needed. The production system, including number of animals and housing density will affect the risk of transmission of pathogens among the calves. Further, poor climate with high humidity and draught will increase the likelihood that the available pathogens will cause disease. Several management factors may affect the likelihood of disease. Thus, feeding too little colostrum causes a lack of protective colostrum antibodies, moving and mingling of calves will increase the general stress level and also increase the probability of encountering pathogens against which the calf has no protection. For some diseases, the occurrence of reservoirs (see later) is also of importance for the risk of introduction of infectious diseases. It would be necessary to include all these (and even more) environmental components to get a good model for predicting occurrence of pneumonia. Even though several risk factors are obtained, the ability to explain disease occurrence has sometimes been disappointing. When studying occurrence of mastitis, several risk factors including housing type, floor type, bedding, climate, feeding, hygiene and milking routines have often been obtained. Still, it is often only possible to explain a minor part of the mastitis occurrence. This may be due to circumstances that are difficult to measure. For example, handling the animals in a calm way may be as important as the physical conditions. It is outside the scope of this textbook to give a description of all possible environmental risk factors; the reader is referred to textbooks on animal production, housing and management.

For many diseases, it has become evident that both the prevalence of disease and the severity of disease is highly dependent of the interplay between environment, host and agent. Therefore, risk factor studies often need to include several of these factors in a statistical/epidemiological model.

3.6 Transmission of infection

The transmission of infections is related to the host, the agents and the environment. The transmission pathways can be divided into: sources of infection, shedding of agent, mode of transmission, mechanisms of invasion and susceptibility of the host.

3.6.1 *Sources of infection*

The sources of infection may be a host, object or environment. The host origin of infection may be:

1. Diseased animals
2. Carriers
3. Reservoirs (can also include non-animal substances such as water).

When the source consists of diseased animals, the advantage is that it is possible to identify the source solely based on clinical investigations. A carrier animal belongs to the species that may show clinical signs, but the carrier animal is clinically normal. The carrier animal may be transiently or persistently infected. The carrier animals are shedding the pathogen, and they are important epidemiologically because they can go unnoticed in the population. Reservoirs are animal species or inanimate substances serving as a habitat for the pathogen and upon which the pathogen depends for its survival.

3.6.2 Shedding of agent

The methods for excretion or shedding of infectious agents depend on the pathogen. Excretion can occur through the respiratory and gastrointestinal system, through the urinary and genital tract and through lesions in the skin. Many disease symptoms cause increased excretion of pathogens, for example, during coughing, sneezing and diarrhoea.

3.6.3 Mode of transmission

Modes of transmission can be classified as horizontal or vertical. Horizontal transmission implies transmission among animals of the same generation. Vertical transmission implies transmission among animals of different generations. Horizontal transmission is again subdivided into direct, indirect and airborne. Vertical transmission is divided into transovarial, in utero and colostral (Table 3.2). However, these subdivisions may vary.

Direct transmission occurs by direct contact between infected and susceptible hosts, by the animals touching, licking, scratching or biting each other or by sexual intercourse. Droplet spread from coughing is also considered direct contact. This so-called direct projection is usually limited to approximately 1 m. No intermediate biological or mechanical element is involved in direct

Table 3.2. *Mode of transmission (after Smith (1991)).*

Horizontal	Direct	Direct contact
		Droplets
	Indirect	Vehicle borne
		Mechanical $\Big\}$ Vector
		Biological
	Airborne	Droplet nuclei
		Dust
Vertical		Transovarial
		In utero
		Colostral

transmission. Direct transmission implies immediate transmission from the infected to the susceptible animal.

Indirect transmission of a pathogen between two individuals involves an intermediate animal, object or substance. The indirect transmission can be vehicle borne, for example, bedding (straw), instruments, clothes, soil, water, food and biological products (milk, blood, urine, semen, etc.). Vector-borne transmission is another form of indirect transmission and involves invertebrates (flies, ticks, etc.) carrying infectious agents between vertebrate hosts. Vector-borne transmission can be either mechanical, where the agent is simply carried between two animals, or biological, where the agent multiplies in the vector. Indirect transmission depends on the capability of the pathogen to survive in the environment, which may vary considerably between pathogens. For example, the survival of salmonella in the environment increases the importance of indirect transmission of this type of pathogen. Salmonella bacteria survive and multiply best under wet conditions and when organic material is present in the medium of growth, such as faecal material and contaminated water. This means that it can survive well in the barn environment and on pastures. *Salmonella* Dublin, for instance, has been shown to survive more than 6 years in faecal contaminations of barn facilities in cattle herds. Even though vertical transmission from mother to foetus during pregnancy or to the newborn at birth is possible, horizontal transmission of salmonella bacteria from the environment is an important indirect route of transmission between animals (Hardman *et al.*, 1991). Lowering of the environmental contamination level by manual cleaning and disinfecting is essential in control of salmonella infections in both cattle and pig herds and poultry flocks.

Airborne transmission consists of small particles (microbial aerosols) with diameters of approximately 1–100 µm. They can stay in the air for long periods and thus also be transmitted over long distances (e.g. foot and mouth disease). The particles can consist of droplet nuclei, which are created after evaporation from droplets shed from an infected host. Alternatively, they can consist of small dust particles that contain micro-organisms.

Vertical transmission is transmission of agents from one generation to the next. Transmission can thus occur via transovarial or transplacental infection (BVD-infections) or it can occur via colostrum (e.g. paratuberculosis).

3.6.4 *Invasion of the host*

Typical mechanisms for invasion of the host are droplets entering the respiratory organs, oral transmission or invasion through skin via insects or wounds. Also, the genital organs are important routes for micro-organisms.

Whether a new host is actually infected depends on whether the number of live pathogens that reaches the new host exceeds the infectious dose.

3.7 Animal performance

The definition of epidemiology is changing towards dealing with animal health and disease in their broadest sense, thus including diseases, production, behaviour as well as positive health indicators. This textbook emphasises occurrence of disease when evaluating animal performance.

In order to describe disease occurrence, a clear definition of the disease of interest is necessary. Although the medical textbooks may give long descriptions of diseases, identifying a clear definition that is uniformly used is often one of the biggest challenges in epidemiological studies. We have already described the importance of disease definition in Chapter 2. In order to characterise the data, it is convenient to divide disease classification into three levels (Thrusfield, 1995):

1. Presenting problems
2. Lesions or deranged function
3. Specific causes.

The definitions may be overlapping, and definitions may depend on the nature of the disease. Thus, many well-defined infectious diseases are named by their specific clinical appearance, which also gives name to the specific causal agent, e.g. FMD caused by FMD virus, and infectious bovine rhinotracheitis (IBR) caused by IBR virus. Sometimes it is indicated in the name the disease that the animal is actually diseased from the infection. Thus, in paratuberculosis and salmonellosis, the ending 'osis' indicates that the animals are diseased from the infection and not just subclinically infected.

Multifactorial/multicausal diseases are often named according to the *lesions* found. Enteritis, dermatitis or hepatitis indicates inflammation of the gut, the skin or the liver, respectively. These characterisations are broader as there may be several possible causes in each case. The characterisation becomes even broader when describing the condition as a *presenting* symptom such as diarrhoea, nasal discharge or coughing.

The reason for using different levels of disease characterisation is lack of knowledge at the moment of establishing the diagnosis. An initial clinical examination of a cow may show that it has fever and nasal discharge ('presenting problem'). A closer examination then reveals that the cow has rhinitis ('lesion'). A blood sample examined for IBR virus or antibodies may later establish the exact diagnosis that the cow suffers from IBR infection ('specific cause'). Thus, the data obtained are often a sequential process trying to identify the diagnosis in greater detail. The sequential procedure also shows that the data typically come from clinical, pathological or laboratory examinations. Further, they can come from extended examinations such as X-ray, endoscopy, electrocardiogram, etc. Some clinical data such as heart rate, respiratory rate and temperature can be obtained with high precision. However, many other clinical variables are more subjective and dependent on the examiner. It may vary among clinicians when a lung sound is considered 'rough'. Further, symptoms may be stated as present or not present without stating the degree of the abnormality (i.e. diarrhoea versus no diarrhoea). Sometimes a scoring system for clinical conditions is used. For example, from 1 to 5 where 1 is mild and 5 is severe. Pathological examinations are more precise and can often describe the degree of the condition. For example they can be used to record the percentage of the lung that is affected. Laboratory tests and extended examinations are used to give a more precise diagnosis and will, therefore, give additional information to the clinical and pathological examination. The evaluation of tests for making a diagnosis is covered in detail in Chapter 9.

The nature of the data is obviously very different from one health problem to another with respect to how precisely the data describe the underlying condition. Epidemiological studies should therefore always be concerned about the origin and definitions of the data sampled and hence the data quality. This issue will be covered further in Chapter 10 on data management.

Important production measures are pelt production from mink, eggs from poultry, meat from poultry, swine and cattle and milk from cattle. Many production parameters can be described in more detail such as annual yield of energy corrected milk, weight gain or number of piglets per litter. Compared to the problems of disease definitions, most production variables are very well defined and also recorded with reasonably high accuracy and precision. Therefore, they will not be described further here.

Figure 3.4 illustrates the relations and overlaps between intrinsic determinants, extrinsic determinants, disease mechanisms and animal performance. As described in the previous section, measuring the factors shown in the figure may be problematic as there is a large variation in how well single factors can be measured. This is why disease occurrence may be described as specific causes, lesions or deranged function or as presenting problems.

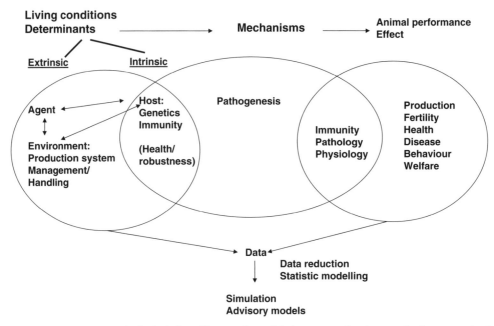

Figure 3.4. *Important biological data illustrated as risk factors, mechanisms and effect on animal performance.*

3.8 Types of variables and scales

Data for an epidemiological study usually consist of a number of measurements for each animal or observational/study unit. These measurements can be grouped into two types of variables: quantitative and qualitative. Each variable is measured on a specific scale. The types of variables and scales are important to identify as part of the design of an epidemiological study. It has an influence on, e.g. calculation of sample size, choice of descriptive measures and choice of analytical method. An overview of the different types of variables and scales is given in Table 3.3.

Quantitative variables consist of numerical values on a well-defined scale, which can be either a continuous scale or a discrete (discontinuous) scale. Measures on a continuous scale have no limitations; they can (in principle) take all possible values, positive or negative. An example is the daily weight gain of piglets. On average, it is approximately 550 g/day; however, a negative daily weight gain (e.g. −50 g/day) is also possible, for instance, if the piglet is diseased. Measures on a discrete scale can only take integer values or can be transformed to do so. Typical measures on a discrete scale are counts such as number of parasites in a faecal sample and number of bacteria on an agar plate.

Qualitative variables can take one of two or more specified values. A qualitative variable is also called a categorical variable, as the animals are grouped

Table 3.3. *Types of variables and scales with examples*

Variables	Scale	Examples
Quantitative	Continuous	Milk yield (kg) Daily weight gain (g/day) Concentration of calcium in a blood sample (mmol/l)
	Pseudo continuous	Summary measures of qualitative variables, for example, percent jersey cows among all cows in a herd (In essence any continuous variable that is defined on a closed interval)
	Discrete	No. *Ascaris suum* in a faecal sample (No./g) Number of times a pig is tail biting during a day Litter size (No. piglets/sow)
Qualitative	Ordinal	Body condition (1–5, with 1: very thin cow, ..., 5: very fat cow) Pain evaluation (1–5, with 1: no pain, ..., 5: severe pain) Gait score (0–5, with 0: walk without problems, ..., 5: unable to walk)
	Nominal	Housing system (tie stall, loose housing, etc.) Breed (Jersey, Holstein, Red Danish, etc.) Region (Northern Jutland, Southern Jutland, Funen, Zealand, etc.)
	Dichotomous (binary)	Infection (yes, no) Gender (male, female) Pregnancy (yes, no)

into one of a number of possible categories. Qualitative variables can be on an ordinal or a nominal scale. Values on an ordinal scale have some order. As an example, the body condition scores of cows are given on a scale from 1 to 5. The scale is defined in more detail in other textbooks, but 1 denotes very thin cows and 5 very fat cows. Another example of an ordinal scale is gait scoring of broiler chickens, with a scale of 0–5: 0 is given to a normal walking chicken, 1 is given when the chicken has a slightly affected gait and 5 is given when the chicken is unable to walk. A nominal scale is used for variables such as breed, housing system, type of diet and season. There is no order implied between values on a nominal scale. A dichotomous scale (also called binary) is a special case of a scale for a qualitative variable with only two possible values, e.g. infection or no infection.

The classification of variables determines which methods to use for analysis of the data. It is always possible to categorise a quantitative variable to a qualitative variable on an ordinal scale by defining a number of intervals. The type of variable and scale of the data influence the ways of performing the descriptive analyses of data, as illustrated later in the present chapter, as well as the statistical hypothesis testing (Chapter 13). Throughout this textbook, we will refer to variables and scales as presented in Table 3.3. However, it should be noted that additional terminologies have been used to describe different data such as interval and ratio scales.

3.9   Variation in observations

Repeated observations of the same trait are rarely identical, even when we perform the measurements under similar conditions. An example is estimating the weight of broiler chickens (Example 3.1).

EXAMPLE 3.1 (Weight of broiler chickens).   Chickens from the same house are usually at the same age, same breed, originate from the same parent flock, are fed and bred in a similar manner. We therefore expect the weight of the chickens to be very similar, but not exactly equal. However, if we take a random sample of 50 chickens, the weights are not always similar. The variation between the weights of the 50 chickens can be explained by different sources of error. There are two obvious sources of error in the broiler chicken example: animal variation and measuring error using a scale.

The variation in recorded observations can be explained by different sources of error. These include: variation among animals, variation in the laboratory (e.g. variation between repeated analyses using the same instrument or procedure on the same sample) and errors introduced by humans (e.g. handling and recording measurements, etc.). Generally, the variation in the observations can be ascribed to *random error* and *systematic error*. The systematic error is also called *bias*. Systematic error is seen when measures are consistently above or below the true value. When the measures are evenly distributed around the true value, the error is random. An example of random and systematic error is given in Example 3.2.

EXAMPLE 3.2 (Random and systematic error of weight of broiler chickens).   A producer of broiler chickens would like an estimate of the mean weight of the chickens in one of his houses, all aged 42 days (ready for slaughter). He has 20,000 chickens in the house. In order to obtain a precise mean weight of the chickens, the producer can measure the weight of all chickens. However, we will often prefer to select a sample and estimate the mean weight of the chickens in the house by the mean weight of the chickens in the sample. The producer randomly selected 50 chickens. He expected the mean weight to be 1550 g. However, the mean weight of the 50 chickens was 1450 g. If the true mean weight of chickens in the house is 1550 g, the deviation between the true mean weight and the estimated weight using the sample could be due to different sources of error. As mentioned in Example 3.1, the two types of error are: the variation among chickens and measuring error using a scale. The

---

animal variation will be a random error, whereas an error due to problems with the scale is systematic (e.g. always measuring 10 g above the true value or measuring 5% more than the true value). Another systematic error could be due to an unbalanced sample in relation to gender. Males are growing faster than females. Therefore, a difference in weight is seen between chickens of different gender at the same age. We expect the distribution of gender in the house to be 50% males and 50% females. However, if the sample of 50 chickens has a gender distribution with 45 females and 5 males, the mean weight will be lower than the expected weight due to a skewed distribution of gender in the sample. This error is a systematic error, as we would conclude that the mean weight of the chickens was 1450 g and not 1550 g.

The quality of recorded observations can be evaluated by accuracy and precision. *Accuracy* refers to how well the observed values agree with the true value and is a measure of the systematic error. *Precision* refers to how well the observed values agree with each other and is a measure of the random error or repeatability. Accuracy and precision are illustrated in Figure 3.5. Figure 3.5(a) represents poor accuracy and poor precision, as the measurements on average are different from the true value (systematic error) and the measurements are very scattered (random error). Figure 3.5(d) represents both good accuracy and good precision as the mean value is close to the true value and the measurements are close together. Note that the systematic error (bias) can be corrected for as long as the error is known (e.g. a scale that always measures 2 kg above true level). The random error can be minimised by increasing the sample size, whereas bias is never corrected by increasing sample size. An example is given in Table 3.4 with the milk yield for the four combinations of high or low accuracy and precision. The true (but unknown) milk yield is 30 kg.

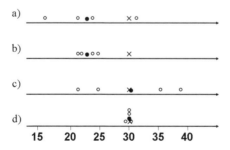

Figure 3.5. *Illustration of the accuracy (systematic error – also called bias) and the precision (random error). Observations are coded as* ○, *the sample mean as* ● *and the true mean as* ×. *The four situations are: (a) low precision, low accuracy; (b) high precision, low accuracy; (c) low precision, high accuracy; and (d) high precision, high accuracy.*

Table 3.4. *Accuracy and precision of the milk yield. Accuracy is a measure of the systematic error (bias) and precision is a measure of random error*

	Accuracy and precision			
	Low, low	*Low, high*	*High, low*	*High, high*
True value	30	30	30	30
Measurements	24, 32, 22, 16	22, 24, 23, 25	22, 39, 36, 25	31, 29, 30, 30
Mean (Std)	23.5 (6.6)	23.5 (1.3)	30.5 (8.3)	30.0 (0.8)

3.10 Descriptive analysis of qualitative and quantitative variables

Usually, a study is performed in order to gain some new information by testing a hypothesis. In the initial phase of the evaluation of the study results, we need to get an overview of the results. If we have more than just a few animals, it is not possible to summarise the information simply by looking at the numbers. The descriptive analysis is used to summarise the results obtained into few and simple descriptive measures such as the mean, standard deviation and frequencies, and to illustrate the tendencies in data by graphical illustrations.

Further, the descriptive measures can be used to indicate the expected outcome of the hypotheses, e.g. a difference between treatment groups. If the mean values for the treatment groups are very similar, we will not expect to see a difference when testing the hypothesis. The descriptive analysis includes calculation of descriptive measures (mean, standard deviation, frequencies, etc.), and use of different graphical illustrations (e.g. box plot, scatter plot and histogram) in order to obtain an overall impression of the data. An overview of the descriptive measures and graphical illustrations is given in Table 3.5.

Table 3.5. *Descriptive analysis of measurements for quantitative and qualitative variables given by descriptive measures and graphical illustrations*

Type of variable	Descriptive measure		Graphical illustration
Quantitative	Location	Mean	
		Median	Box-and-whisker plot
			Histogram
	Spread	Standard deviation	Dot plot
		Standard error	Scatter plot
		Quartiles	
Qualitative	Number		Bar chart
	Percentages		Pie chart

Different descriptive measures are used for categorical and quantitative variables. For quantitative variables, such as milk yield and daily weight gain, we calculate the location (central tendency) and spread of data. The location of data is calculated by the mean value and the median. The spread of data can be measured using the standard deviation, standard error and quartiles. If the measurements of the variable are skewed, then the median and quartiles are preferred, as they are not influenced by a few extreme values like the mean and standard deviation. However, measurements with a normal distribution (bell-like form/not skewed) can be summarised using mean, standard deviation and standard error. Qualitative variables like breed and body condition should only be summarised using frequency distributions (number and percentages of animals in each category). For example, the mean of body condition score should not be calculated because it is a qualitative and not a quantitative variable. However, based on a qualitative variable, e.g. body condition score for individual animals or breed, we can calculate a summary measure for the herd, e.g. percentage of animals with body condition score equal to 3 or percentage of Jersey cows. The derived variables are quantitative variables on a continuous scale although they are limited to the interval 0–100% (defined as pseudo-continuous variables in Table 3.3). If we have a number of herds in the study, we can calculate the usual descriptive measures for the derived variables using mean and standard deviation, etc.

The choice of graphical illustration of the results depends on the types of variables. For quantitative variables, the following plots can be used: scatter plot, dot plot, box-and-whisker plot and histogram. Qualitative variables can be illustrated using a bar or pie chart.

EXAMPLE 3.3. In a study of Danish dairy cows, 1141 cows were selected from the Danish Cattle Database. Information on breed, parity, milk yield (kg) and fat content (%) was extracted from the database. In Figure 3.6 and Table 3.6 an example of descriptive analysis of the milk yield is given (a quantitative variable on a continuous scale). In Figure 3.7 and Table 3.7 an example of descriptive analysis of breed and parity is given (two qualitative variables on a nominal and an ordinal scale). Note that the histogram (Figure 3.6) and bar chart (Figure 3.7) look very much the same, but they are different in that the histogram illustrates a quantitative variable (that is categorised) whereas the bar chart illustrates a qualitative variable.

3.11 Data levels

Data in veterinary epidemiological studies may originate from animals selected from a number of herds randomly selected in the country.

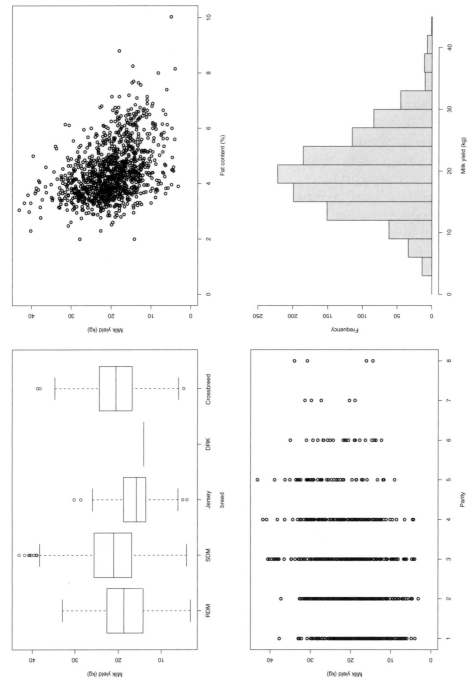

Figure 3.6. *Graphical illustrations of the milk yield of Danish dairy cows: box-and-whisker plot (top left), scatter plot (top right), dot plot (bottom left), histogram (bottom right).*

Table 3.6. *Descriptive analysis of the milk yield of Danish dairy cows*

	All cows	Stratified (grouped) by breed				
		RDM	SDM	Jersey	DRK	Crossbreed
N	1141	161	518	196	1	265
Mean	19.9	18.5	21.4	16.2	14.1	20.7
Std	6.5	6.4	7.0	4.4	–	5.5
SE	0.19	0.51	0.31	0.31	–	0.34
Minimum	3.2	3.2	4.1	4.0	14.1	4.8
Q1	15.4	14.4	16.9	13.6	14.1	16.8
Median	19.6	18.8	21.1	15.8	14.1	20.6
Q3	23.6	22.5	25.6	18.8	14.1	24.4
Maximum	43.1	33.0	43.1	30.0	14.1	38.8

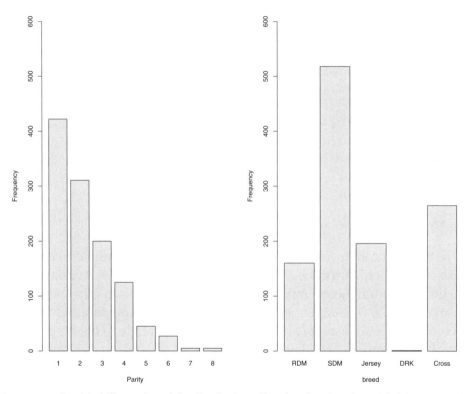

Figure 3.7. *Graphical illustration of the distribution of breed and parity of Danish dairy cows using bar charts.*

Furthermore, we are often not able to investigate all animals, so we randomly select a number of animals within each herd. This selection could be a number of litters and a number of animals within each litter. The structure is hierarchical (also called multilevel or nested).

Table 3.7. *Descriptive analysis of the parity and breed of Danish dairy cows*

	Frequency (%)	*Cumulative frequency (%)*
Parity		
1	422 (37.0)	422 (37.0)
2	311 (27.3)	773 (64.3)
3	200 (17.5)	933 (81.8)
4	125 (11.0)	1058 (92.8)
5	45 (4.0)	1103 (96.8)
6	27 (2.4)	1130 (99.1)
7	5 (0.4)	1135 (99.6)
8	5 (0.4)	1140 (100.0)
Missing	1	
Breed		
RDM	161 (14.1)	161 (14.1)
SDM	518 (45.4)	679 (59.5)
Jersey	196 (17.2)	875 (76.7)
RKD	1 (0.1)	876 (76.8)
Crossbreed	265 (23.2)	1141 (100.0)
Missing	0	

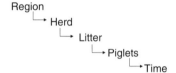

Figure 3.8. *An example of the hierarchical levels in a study of piglets.*

The basic concept in a hierarchical data structure is that animals within the same level (e.g. herd) are more alike compared to other animals. Animals in the same litter are often more similar compared to animals from different litters. Similarly, animals within the same herd are more alike, compared to animals from other herds. An example of the hierarchical structure in data is given in Figure 3.8. Measurements taken at the same level (i.e. same epidemiological unit) are expected to be more alike compared to measurements taken at different levels. This hierarchical structure of data is important in relation to design of the study, calculation of sample size and selection of analytical methods for evaluation of the hypotheses. When designing the study and calculating the necessary sample size, we have to assess the variation in measurements at the different levels in the data structure and allocate more animals at levels with larger uncertainty.

4 OBSERVATIONAL STUDIES

Annette Kjær Ersbøll, Nils Toft and Jeanett Bruun

4.1 Introduction

One of the cornerstones of veterinary epidemiology is the study. By study we refer to a scientific activity aiming at generating information thereby recording the relevant properties regarding the hypothesis of our study. For the epidemiologist, the study is aimed at generating information at the population level. This population may vary from all dairy cattle in a country, to the kittens in a litter. Traditionally, we differentiate between two branches of study: the observational studies, where the investigator observes without intervention, and the experimental study, where the investigator intervenes (e.g. allocates treatments). In an observational study, the researcher has little or no control over events and the association between risk factors and outcomes is studied without intervention. In an experimental study, the researcher can deliberately influence events and hereby investigate the effect of intervention on the outcomes. In this chapter we will introduce the observational study and the next chapter will address the experimental study.

Generally, the epidemiologist conducts a study for one of two reasons: for descriptive purposes or analytical purposes. The descriptive study characterises the population with respect to various traits such as occurrence of disease, milk yield or other variables of interest. The analytical study aims at identifying one or more risk factors, as the possible cause of a disease. While the descriptive study is observational by nature, the analytical study can be either observational or experimental. To appreciate the difference between these, we consider as an example, a study regarding the effect of milking procedure (robot versus traditional semi-automatic) on the occurrence of mastitis. To carry out an experimental study to evaluate this effect we could choose a design where we instal both systems in a dairy herd and then randomly allocate the individual cows to one of the milking procedures. The study should be repeated in a number of herds. The advantage of such a study would be that we could balance the study with respect to all other factors, such as age of dairy cows, management factors since these traits are all believed to have an influence on the occurrence of mastitis. The disadvantage of this approach is the relative high cost of installing the different systems, keeping track of cows, etc. As an alternative to the experimental design we could carry out an observational study, where data recordings are made on farms already using one of the systems. This approach makes it harder to control the other factors, but allows a lot more study units (cows) and possibly also herds at the same cost.

Traditionally, we distinguish between three different basic designs of an observational study: cross-sectional, cohort and case–control. This chapter outlines the differences between these three basic designs. The choice of an appropriate design for an observational study depends almost entirely on the hypothesis motivating the study. However, other elements in planning a study might also influence the choice of study design.

4.2   Design of epidemiological studies

Design of a study (observational and experimental) covers in principle all considerations from establishment of the hypothesis to the start of data collection. A list of the main items is given in Table 4.1. Proper planning of the study is very important as it will increase the quality and reliability of the collected data and the result of the study. Statistical methods cannot compensate for a poorly planned and conducted study.

The hypothesis is the base of the study. Therefore, it is important to establish and describe the hypothesis as precisely as possible. Formulation of hypotheses was described in Chapter 2 and is further discussed in Chapter 13 in relation to data analysis. The hypothesis should be clear and precise. By defining the hypothesis many of the considerations listed in Table 4.1 are already handled. An example of a hypothesis is 'Vaccination of piglets against *Actinobacillus pleuropneumoniae* increases the daily weight gain compared to non-vaccinated piglets'.

When the hypothesis is defined, we proceed to define the target population, the study population, the unit of observation, the outcome and the risk factors (if relevant).

The target population is the population we would like to draw conclusions about (see Chapter 2). However, the sample is usually taken from a limited part of the target population called the study population. Assume that the target population is all cows in Denmark. However, the cows in the study are selected solely from herds in the Kongeå region (a region in the southern part of Jutland in Denmark). The study population is therefore cows in the Kongeå region.

Table 4.1. *The main items in design of epidemiological studies with reference to relevant chapters, a short description and an example based on a cross-sectional study*

Item	Chapter	Description	Example
Establishing the hypothesis	2	The hypothesis is fundamental for the study	'Jersey cows have fewer hoof lesions than Holstein cows'
Target population	2	The population we would like to draw conclusions on	Dairy cows in Denmark
Study population	2	The population we select the animals from	Dairy herds in the Kongeå region
Unit of the study or sample unit	1, 2	The observation level recordings are made on (region, herd, cow, quarter)	Cow or individual hoof level depending on the definition of the outcome
Definition of the outcome	3	The outcome variable is used to measure the effect (disease, infection, . . .)	Hoof lesions (yes/no) measured either on the individual hoofs or aggregated on the cow so that yes means hoof lesion(s) on one or more hoof(s)
Definition of risk factors and additional explanatory variables	3	If associations are evaluated, the risk factors have to be identified	Risk factor: breed (Jersey, Holstein). Other explanatory variables: grazing (yes/no), housing (tie stall/loose), floor type (slatted/straw)
Duration of the study	4	The study can, e.g. be a longitudinal study or a single point in time	'A single point in time', herds visited once in May 2002
Selection of the study design	4, 5	The above listed items are used to guide the selection of study design	Cross-sectional study, as we have a single point in time
Sample size	8	Sample size is calculated with a specific purpose, e.g. detecting a difference or estimating a proportion with a specified uncertainty	Thirty herds and 20 cows within each herd

(continued)

Table 4.1. (continued)

Item	Chapter	Description	Example
Sampling	8	A strategy for selection of animals/herds is important in order to limit bias	Two-stage sampling, e.g. first herds are randomly selected, then cows are randomly selected within these herds
Randomisation	8	The procedure for inclusion of animals/herds in the study should be random. In observational studies animals should generally be randomly selected. In experimental studies animals are generally randomly allocated to treatments	Herd (CHR) and cow (CKR) identification numbers are used to randomly select herds and cows within selected herds
Methods for data collection	3, 8	Description of the collection procedure is important in order to ensure high validity of data	Cows are examined by a visiting veterinarian in a separation box and a blood sample is obtained for virological examination
Methods for data analysis	13	Considerations regarding which statistical methods to use are important in order to evaluate how it is possible to analyse data in the study	χ^2-test or logistic analysis

The unit of the study (observational unit, experimental unit, unit of concern, unit of observation or sample unit) describes the entity for which measurements are made (see Chapters 1 and 2). Recordings can be at animal level, litter level, pen level, herd level, etc. When calculating sample size, the number of observational units is calculated (e.g. number of animals or number of herds).

The outcome and the risk factor(s) should be clearly described and defined by types and scales. The type of the outcome is crucial in relation to sample size calculation, as the formula to use depends on the type of outcome and the hypothesis to test. The outcome and the risk factors are also important in relation to the method(s) for data analysis, when data have been collected. If factors other than the risk factor hypothesised by the study are known to influence the outcome of the study, variables describing these factors should also be defined and collected.

Studies can be prospective and retrospective. In a prospective study data are collected forward in time from study onset. In a retrospective study, data have already been collected (partly or completely). Figure 4.1 illustrates the difference between a prospective and a retrospective study.

The duration of the study has to be considered. There are basically two options: (1) a study with a single point in time or (2) a study across time. In a single point in time study (cross-sectional) all recordings (on outcome and exposure) are made at one single point in time. In a study across time (e.g. a cohort or a case–control study) we investigate changes over time with at least two points in time. These will be discussed further in the following sections. Advantages and disadvantages of the three basic designs are listed in Table 4.2.

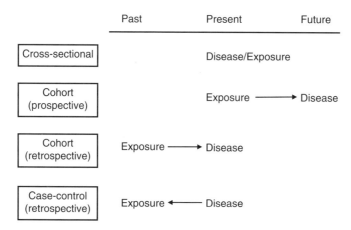

Figure 4.1. *Overview of the commonly used designs in observational studies in relation to the present time of the study.*

Table 4.2. *Advantages and disadvantages of the three basic observational studies*

Design	Description	Advantages	Disadvantages
Cross-sectional	Animals are included at random without considering exposure or disease status. After inclusion, the animals are grouped according to exposure and disease. A snapshot in time	Proportion of exposed and non-exposed animals in the population can be calculated. Proportion of diseased and non-diseased animals in the population can be calculated. Relatively inexpensive and quick to conduct. Useful for descriptive purposes	Incidence rate and risk of disease among exposed and non-exposed animals cannot be calculated. Not useful for analytical purposes because causality might be difficult (or impossible) to establish
Cohort	Animals are included in the study based on their exposure status (inclusion of exposed and non-exposed animals)	Incidence rate and risk of disease among exposed and non-exposed animals can be calculated. Useful for analytical purposes. Gives direct information of causality (sequence of exposure and disease). A number of diseases can be studied simultaneously	Relatively expensive and time-consuming. Large number of animals or long duration are required to study rare diseases. Not suitable for diseases with a long incubation period. Withdrawal a problem due to reduction of sample size. Proportion of exposed and non-exposed animals in the population cannot be estimated. Basically, only one risk factor can be studied (exposure and non-exposure) unless more cohorts are made
Case–control	Animals are included in the study based on their disease status (inclusion of cases and controls)	Proportion of exposed and non-exposed animals in the population can be calculated. Relatively inexpensive and quick to conduct. Useful for analytical purposes. Many risk factors can be studied simultaneously. Well suited to study rare diseases and diseases with long incubation periods. Relatively small sample size compared to an equivalent cohort study	Proportion of diseased (prevalence) and non-diseased animals in the population cannot be calculated. Incidence rate and risk of disease among exposed and non-exposed animals cannot be calculated. Causality might be difficult to establish. Can usually only investigate one disease outcome. Problems with bias due to selection of controls

4.3   Cross-sectional study

The key to understanding a cross-sectional study lies in two things: (1) the sample must be representative of the target population and (2) the sample is taken as a *snap shot* of the population. The first property is what basically names the study, since we require that samples are taken across all sections of the population to reflect the variation (Figure 4.3). The second property reflects that samples ideally are obtained at the same point in time (Figure 4.2). In practice a duration of a short period is often necessary and accepted. If the cross-sectional study is conducted to estimate the proportion of disease in the population (i.e. the prevalence) then we often refer to the study as a prevalence study. Usually, the exposure status (of one or more exposures) of the animals is measured simultaneously with disease status. Thus, disease prevalence may be compared across sub-populations with different exposure status, e.g. geographic location. Since the exposure status is determined at the same time as disease status, we have the same problems with causality as in the case–control study: did the exposure occur prior to disease or vice versa. Whenever there is strong evidence of the exposure being present prior to disease, (e.g. risk factors such as breed or sex), we can make an inference concerning the exposure as a risk factor.

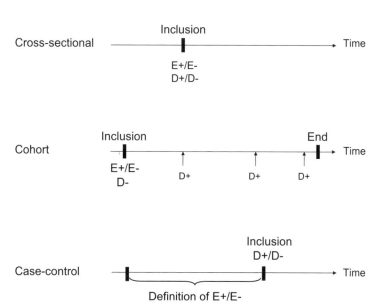

Figure 4.2. *Illustration of the three basic observational studies. (Exposure E+/E−, disease D+/D−.)*

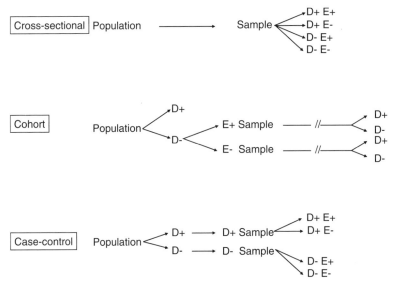

Figure 4.3. *Illustration of the sampling procedure used in the three basic observational studies. (Exposure E+/E−, Disease D+/D−.)*

EXAMPLE 4.1. An example of a prevalence study is given in Nielsen *et al.* (2000) where the herd level prevalence of paratuberculosis in Danish dairy herds was investigated. The objective of the study was to determine the proportion of Danish dairy herds with paratuberculosis infected cows using a bulk tank milk sample. Paratuberculosis is a chronic untreatable infection in cattle, which makes it a suitable disease to detect using a cross-sectional study. The target population is the Danish dairy herds. The study population is assumed to be the same. The unit of the study is the individual dairy farm. A sample of bulk tank milk from 900 herds was obtained through six different milk collecting centres located in different parts of Denmark. The outcome of the study was paratuberculosis status (positive or negative) and the exposure was geographic region (six different regions were defined by the milk collecting centres). The main conclusion of the study was that paratuberculosis was present in 47% of the farms with variation between 0% on Bornholm (a small Danish island) and 91% on Zealand (a large Danish island).

4.4 Cohort study

The word cohort is the Latin word for one of the 10 divisions of a roman legion. Hence, a cohort of animals is a group of animals that have something in common. A classic cohort study defines two or more cohorts that differ according to their exposure status regarding a risk factor, e.g. if the risk factor is sex, then the two cohorts would be a group of males and a group of females. Suppose that herd size was expected to be a risk factor, then cohorts of sizes 0–50, 50–150 and >150 could be defined. In this example part of the study design would be to justify why exactly the split into these three distinct groups is relevant to consider. Regarding the outcome, it is required that all study units are disease free (or in general that the condition we investigate is absent) at the onset of the study (see Figures 4.2 and 4.3).

Since we define the sample by selection based on exposure status we cannot estimate the prevalence (proportion of diseased animals) in the target population. We can, however, estimate the proportion of animals that develop the disease (or outcome) for given levels of exposure status. Furthermore, since we know that animals are initially disease free, we can use the study to make an inference about the causality of the risk factor, i.e., we know that exposure happens prior to disease.

The problem of the cohort study lies in ensuring that individuals in the cohorts actually develop disease during the study period. For rare diseases, this might be a problem. To ensure that enough cases (i.e. diseased animals) will be included, the study period must be long or a large number of animals have to be included in the study. This increases the expenses, and a case–control study might be considered. Another problem is withdrawals, as withdrawn animals reduce the sample size and hereby diminish the possibility for the study to establish a significant association between the exposure and the outcome. Reasons for withdrawal include that the animal is sold, dies or is culled (the latter two for reasons other than the outcome of the study) during the study period. Advantages and disadvantages of the cohort study are summarised in Table 4.2.

The traditional cohort study establishes the cohorts (groups with different exposure status) and then follows them onwards in time for a predefined specified period (e.g. 3 months). This is usually called a prospective cohort study, as opposed to the retrospective cohort study, where the cohorts are included at a point back in time and followed forward from that point in time (Figure 4.1). A study where observations are made at more than one point in time is often called a longitudinal study or a study with follow-up. Hence, reference might be made to a longitudinal prospective cohort study, which simply means that the study was a study in which the cohorts were defined at the start of the study and then followed for a period onwards. Since we are required to follow the animals regularly for some time (e.g. each week), the study is time consuming and often quite costly. Note that we must monitor the cohorts during the study rather than just follow up at the end of the period in order to ensure that all relevant observations are made. Regular observations are needed in order to calculate time at risk for each animal as precisely as possible.

EXAMPLE 4.2. Endometritis in dairy cows is an important disease, that results in a reduced milk yield and an increased calving to conception interval. The incidence risk (proportion of new cases of endometritis among all cows in the study) of endometritis was in 1993–1994 in Denmark estimated as 0.7% (modified after Bruun *et al.* (2002)). It is therefore a relatively rarely diagnosed disease. Different categories of endometritis are seen. Acute endometritis and intermediate endometritis are often diagnosed within the first 10 days and around the first 30 days after calving, respectively. Endometritis is a multifactorial disease. Mastitis prior to endometritis is one of the expected risk factors for endometritis (in other studies, mastitis could be the outcome). However, in the present example, we focus on endometritis as the outcome (the disease) and mastitis prior to endometritis as the risk factor (exposure). In order to evaluate the association between mastitis and endometritis, a number of cows with and without mastitis (exposure) were included in the study. For calculation of a relevant sample size and random selection of animals, see Chapter 8. No cows had endometritis at the time of inclusion. The cows were followed for a 2 month period after calving and development of endometritis (the outcome) was recorded. Based on this study it is possible to estimate and compare the number of new cases of endometritis for cows with and without mastitis. However, based on this study it is not possible to estimate the proportion of cows with mastitis in the population of cows.

4.5 Case–control study

In a case–control study the animals are sampled according to their disease status, i.e. a group of cases (diseased) and a group of controls (disease free). These two groups are then further divided according to their exposure status (see Figures 4.2 and 4.3). This approach has several advantages compared to the cohort study as it is cheap, usually a lot faster to do and will ensure that a certain number of cases are present. These advantages are accompanied by a set of disadvantages (see Table 4.2 for a summary of the advantages and disadvantages). The sample strategy of selecting according to outcome status prevents us from direct inference of the obvious question of the study: *What is the probability of disease given absence/presence of exposure.* Instead we must settle for: *What is the probability of exposure given absence/presence of the disease (the outcome variable).* This means that we seek to answer the hypothesis of the exposure being a risk factor for the outcome of the study by testing if chance of exposure is higher in the diseased than the non-diseased group of study units. As we cannot determine the causal relationship between exposure and disease (see Chapter 3.2), the case–control study requires that there are strong indications that the risk factor was present prior to disease. Permanent traits of animals and many management practices (rarely changed) are good examples of exposure or risk factors that precede the outcome. A bad example could be stress-related observations as exposure variables for diarrhoea in piglets. It is not obvious if stress induces diarrhoea or diarrhoea induces stress.

Often, available cases are selected for the study, especially when the disease under study is rare. The control group is less obvious to select. Woodward (1999) discusses how to select controls and emphasises the following four general principles for selecting controls:

(1) Controls must be selected amongst those that are free from the disease (or in general the condition) being studied. Whether any animal which is presently disease free, but at sometime has had the disease can be used as a control depends on the specific circumstances of the disease and the study in general.
(2) Controls should be drawn from the same general population as gave rise to the cases. Thus, if the cases are from the entire horse population, then a poor choice of controls would be thoroughbred race horses, as it might introduce possible confounders (see Chapter 11).
(3) The source from which controls are selected should not give rise to bias (see Chapter 11). A good choice of source for the controls is one where the chance of exposure is roughly equal to the general chance of exposure among the non-diseased population.
(4) Controls should have some potential for the disease, i.e. bulls are a poor choice of controls for cases of mastitis.

To illustrate the above principles we use a study of diabetes in dogs as an example. The cases (dogs with diabetes) might be all the diabetic dogs diagnosed at the Small Animal Hospital at The Royal Veterinary and Agricultural University. How should the controls be defined and selected? A convenient approach is to select among the non-diabetic dogs at the hospital. These dogs can easily be established as non-diabetic (or included as cases if they are diabetic) and sampled so that they reflect the same general properties as the cases. However, it might be that dogs admitted to the hospital generally have a different chance of exposure to the risk factors for diabetes than the general dog population. The problem is that selecting controls in the general dog population might solve this problem, but at the cost of making the chance of exposure among cases much different from that of the controls. There might be potential risk factors for diabetes, that are closely related to whether or not owners will consult the hospital in the first place. Hence, no general advice on how to select controls for a case–control study can be given. The best choice depends on the specific circumstance for the individual study. Thus, a central part of the design of a case–control study is to establish a well-justified procedure for selecting controls.

EXAMPLE 4.3. In the previous section, a cohort study of risk factors for endometritis in dairy cows was described. Endometritis is a rarely diagnosed disease and using a cohort design will therefore result in an expensive study as the number of cows should be large. Now a case–control design with mastitis prior to endometritis as the proposed risk factor (exposure) will be used. It should be stressed that mastitis should precede endometritis in order to be able to evaluate the casuality of mastitis as a risk factor for endometritis. In the case–control design a number of cows with endometritis (cases) and a number of cows without endometritis (controls) are included in the study. After inclusion, it is evaluated if the cow had mastitis prior to endometritis or not. Based on this study, the association between mastitis and endometritis can be evaluated. Furthermore, it is possible to estimate the proportion of cows with mastitis within the group of cows with endometritis. However, the study does not enable us to estimate the proportion of cows with endometritis in the population of cows. The advantages of using a case–control design for evaluating mastitis as a risk factor for endometritis are shorter study duration and lower number of cows to be included in the study.

4.6   Other observational study designs

In the previous sections the three basic designs used in observational studies have been discussed. However, the design used is often none of the three basic designs but rather a combination of two of them. In general, these types of studies are considered to have a hybrid design. In this section, three types of hybrid designs are described: a cross-sectional study with follow-up, a nested case–control study and a repeated cross-sectional study. Examples of the three hybrid designs are given.

4.6.1   Cross-sectional study with follow-up

A commonly used design in many epidemiological projects is a cross-sectional study with follow-up. This is an example of longitudinal study. A longitudinal study is a study with repeated recording on the same animals. We select animals from a single baseline sample without considering the exposure or disease status. In a typical cohort study we would include a number of exposed and a number of unexposed animals. In the cross-sectional study with follow-up, information on disease status and a number of possible risk factors (exposures) is collected across time by repeated sampling (see Figure 4.4). In order to estimate the proportions of diseased animals and the proportion of exposed animals in the population, the study should be based on a random sample of animals from the population. The cross-sectional study with follow-up is convenient to use as we are able to estimate relevant proportions regarding disease and exposures in the population. Furthermore, by random selection of animals, we are able to evaluate a number of possible risk factors, instead of focusing on a single factor (exposure/non-exposure).

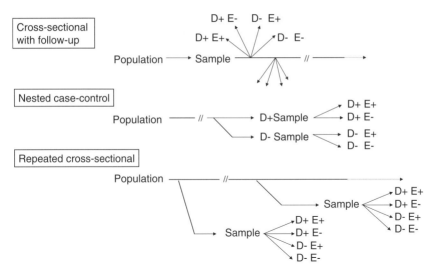

Figure 4.4. *Three examples of hybrid designs: a cross-sectional study with follow-up, a nested case–control study and a repeated cross-sectional study. (Exposure E+/E−, disease D+/D−.)*

EXAMPLE 4.4. The study of risk factors for endometritis in dairy cows was performed using a retrospective longitudinal study with a cross-sectional design with follow-up. The study is described in Bruun *et al.* (2002). Data were collected from the Danish Cattle Database during 1993–1994. The study included 2 144 herds and 102,060 cows. Herds were randomly selected from three regions in Denmark. All cows in the selected herds were included in the study. Examples of risk factors included are on herd level: herd size, housing and grazing and on cow level: parity, breed and whether the cow was treated by a veterinarian for diseases. The follow-up period was 1 year.

4.6.2 *Nested case–control study*

A nested case–control study (also called an ambi-directional design) combines a cohort study and a case–control study. In a nested case–control design, a single population (a cohort) is defined at onset, opposite to the usual case–control design. New cases of disease are selected as they develop.

Controls are simultaneously selected from the same population with respect to the exposure status (age, sex, breed, herd size, geographic area), see Figure 4.4. The main advantage of the nested case–control design compared to a case–control design is that the cases and controls are selected from the same population. Compared to the cohort design, the nested case–control design is also suitable for the study of rare diseases.

EXAMPLE 4.5. An example of a nested case–control design is a study of risk factors for development of very virulent infectious bursal disease (vvIBD, also called Gumboro) among broiler chickens. Risk factors to study were breed, hatchery, feed mill, age of parent birds and use of thinning. During 1998, 16 broiler chicken producers were affected with vvIBD.

For each affected producer, five control flocks (from five different producers) were randomly selected among producers within a geographical zone of 30 km. Data regarding exposure status for the controls were collected for the same month as the case flock was affected with vvIBD.

4.6.3 *Repeated cross-sectional study*

A repeated cross-sectional study, also called a repeated survey, is a sequence of two or more cross-sectional studies based on selection in the same population. At each sampling, we obtain information regarding disease and individual risk factors. We do not include the same animals, but we select a sample of animals from the same population at different points in time. Repeated surveys are used to assess overall health and changes across time.

EXAMPLE 4.6. The Danish bovine virus diarrhoea (BVD) surveillance programme is using repeated cross-sectional designs as a part of the surveillance. Every 3 months a bulk tank milk sample is taken in the dairy herds and tested for BVD. All lactating cows in the herd are included in this bulk tank milk sample. However, the population of cows in the herd is dynamic as some cows are culled and sold. Therefore, the same cows are not included in the bulk tank milk sample across time.

4.7 Further reading

For further reading regarding observational studies and for a detailed description of other designs see, e.g. Kleinbaum *et al.* (1982), Woodward (1999) and Thrusfield (1995).

5 EXPERIMENTAL STUDIES

Annette Kjær Ersbøll and Nils Toft

5.1 Introduction

An experimental study can be characterised as a study in which the animals to some extent are affected by intervention (e.g. treatments). In contrast to an observational study, we intervene in the experimental study by for example applying a treatment. We then observe the effect of the intervention on the outcome of interest. Therefore, experimental studies are also referred to as intervention studies. Except for the intervention, all units of the study are treated similarly. As a consequence the variation between experimental units, e.g. animals, can often be reduced compared to the variation between animals in observational studies. In an experimental study, homogeneous animals (e.g. litter mates) can be selected, hereby reducing the between animal variation. On the other hand, the more uniform conditions in experimental studies might not be valid for real life, meaning that it is not necessarily possible to draw conclusions of the effects for the population in general. As an example, experimental studies are often used in the initial phase of the evaluation of new drugs. If significant effects can be demonstrated under experimental conditions, further studies will follow under more natural conditions in order to demonstrate treatment effects under natural (less controlled) conditions. Many different designs are available for experimental studies. This chapter describes some of the commonly used designs in experimental studies including full factorial (parallel group and factorial), fractional factorial (Latin square) and cross-over designs.

5.2 Design of experimental studies

The observational studies presented in the previous chapter form a cornerstone of veterinary epidemiology. However, equally important to the advance of veterinary science are experiments. Experiments are conducted to compare the effect of various treatments on an experimental unit. Quite often our experimental units (or units of the study) are the individual animals, where the investigator must decide on allocation between treatments. Still, there are different possibilities as illustrated in the following examples:

1. A comparison of the effect of feeding different levels of copper to pregnant ewes. The underlying hypothesis is that the birth weight of the lambs is affected by the level of copper. The unit of study is the individual ewe and her lamb(s). The treatment is two different levels of copper given as a feed additive to the diet. The objective of the study is to test whether we can reject the null hypothesis of no difference in birth weights between the two groups of lambs in favour of the alternative hypothesis that there is a significant difference.
2. A prophylactic trial, i.e. a study of the preventive effect of a vaccine for *atrophic rhinitis* in pigs. The objective of the study is to evaluate the efficacy of the vaccine. Here, the unit of the study could be groups of pigs. The null hypothesis would be that there is no difference in the *atrophic rhinitis* prevalence between the groups of unvaccinated and vaccinated pigs.
3. A study of the effect of different eradication programmes for salmonellosis in pig herds. The objective of the study is to determine the optimal programme. The units of the study are pig herds with salmonella problems. The treatment is the allocation of the different eradication programmes to selected groups of herds.
4. A comparison in one dog suffering recurrent attacks of a chronic disease. The objective of the study is to evaluate the effect of different methods for easing discomfort. The unit of the study is now the successive occasions on which attacks occur. Hence, the choice of treatment is to be made for each occurrence of an outbreak.
5. Evaluation of the lethal half dose of a toxin (LD_{50}) is often performed using mice given different concentrations of the toxin. A dose–response curve is made and the lethal dose can be estimated. These experiments are performed in order to develop a limit value of the toxin for humans. These experiments are only performed in the laboratory.

The experiments described in the examples are taken within different contexts. Some of the above-mentioned examples involve elements that deem them clinical trials; we shall briefly discuss these issues later in the chapter. Others can be referred to as laboratory experiments and field trials. However, fundamentally there is no difference with respect to the primary concern of this chapter: the design of the experiments.

Another crucial question is how the treatments or interventions are to be allocated to the available units. The key issue here is to avoid any unintended difference between groups. If in Example 3 we would use only slaughter pigs producers for one group and sow herds for another group, it would be impossible to distinguish between the effect of the production form and the effect of the eradication programme. Likewise in Example 1, where the age structure in the two groups should be identical to remove the possible *bias* (see Chapter 11) introduced by the smaller birth weight of lambs from first-parity ewes compared to those of older ewes. To avoid the problems of such known and/or unknown systematic effects a widely-accepted solution is to include a random element in the allocation of units selected for different treatments (see Chapter 8).

While the experimental units should be formed to include an even distribution of relevant traits in the groups, there is also the possibility to select units that are more alike than usual in the population. An example could be to use litter mattes to reduce the variation among animals. The motivation is that the effect of the proposed treatment can be evaluated with fewer animals because of the lower variation among the animals (see Chapter 8 for details). However, the interpretation of the results can no longer be put in the context of the original target population of the study. On the other hand, if it is possible to demonstrate an effect of the treatment under experimental conditions, then this might be followed by further studies to investigate a possible effect under more realistic conditions.

The next sections will describe some commonly used study designs that each have their advantages and disadvantages, briefly summarised in Table 5.1. It is important to realise that the choice of study design depends on the objective of the study. Some study designs do not allow for exploring the interaction effects of different treatments or traits because of an incomplete design where not all combinations are included. The motivation is of course to reduce the size of the study in terms of study units. There may be several reasons for this, such as capacity constraints, budget restrictions or the time horizon of the study.

5.3 Full factorial designs

The group of *full factorial designs* or generally just factorial designs is very powerful and allows the researcher to investigate virtually any combination of factors and their potential interaction (see Chapter 11 for a discussion of interaction). In theory, there is no limit to what number of different factors one can investigate simultaneously, but in practice it is often only a moderate

Table 5.1. *Different designs used in experimental studies with advantages and disadvantages*

Design	Description	Advantages	Disadvantages
Factorial	One or more factors each with two or more levels	Possible interactions between factors can be investigated	More complicated and involves more treatment combinations compared to a parallel group design
Parallel group*	One factor with two or more levels	Simple	Only one factor in the study
Fractional factorial	A fraction of the combinations in the factorial design is applied	Reduced sample size compared to the complete factorial design. Depending on the design, some interactions can be investigated	Some interactions not possible to investigate.
Latin square†	Three factors each with the same number of levels	Reduced sample size compared to the complete factorial design	Not possible to investigate possible interactions between factors
Graeco-Latin square†	Four factors each with the same number of levels	Reduced sample size compared to the complete factorial design	Not possible to investigate interactions between factors
Split plot	A design where one factor is randomised within another factor	The subplot effect is tested with the same precision and power as in a complete randomised factorial design	The main-plot effect is tested with less precision than the subplot effect
Strip plot	A design where the levels of the factor are randomised in stripes	Practical problems might suggest a strip-plot design as the only one possible	The factors are tested with less precision than in a complete randomised factorial design
Cross-over	All study units receive all treatments in a randomised sequence	Reduce the effect of between study unit variation. Comparison of treatment effects within study units. Reduced sample size compared to the parallel group design	Problems if carry-over effect is present. Duration of the study is prolonged corresponding to the number of treatments to evaluate

*Special case of a factorial design.
†Special case of a fractional factorial design.

number of different factors with a restricted number of levels. Before we discuss the general factorial design in greater detail, we introduce the simplest possible factorial design, the parallel group design.

5.3.1 Parallel group design

The simplest experimental design is a parallel group design in which two or more different groups of experimental units, e.g. animals, are studied at the same time. The groups are supposed to be identical in all matters, except for the level of the factor being studied. Quite often the groups and the associated level of the factor are referred to as *treatments*. Thus, the study units are randomly allocated (divided) to one of two or more treatments. A parallel group design is often used in human and veterinary clinical trials for evaluation of new drugs. In the simplest case we have a parallel group design with two treatments A and B. Study units are randomly allocated to one of the two treatments. The general structure of a parallel group design is shown in Table 5.2. Even if the study units are randomly allocated to the different groups, the number of study units in each group is not necessarily equal. However, random allocation ensures that the study is *balanced* (see Chapter 8).

EXAMPLE 5.1. An example of a parallel group design is a study of the effect of Malaseb® shampoo on *Malassezia pachydermatis* in dogs with chronic dermatitis. The effect of the Malaseb® shampoo was compared to a standard (placebo) shampoo, expected to have no effect on *Malassezia pachydermatis* in dogs with chronic dermatitis. A group of dogs with chronic dermatitis was used in the study. The dogs were randomly allocated into two groups, one group of dogs was treated with the standard (placebo) shampoo and the other group of dogs was treated with the Malaseb® shampoo. Except for the shampoo, all dogs were treated in the same way. The dogs were washed three times during the study (a week) with the shampoo. The effect of the two shampoos was evaluated after 1 week by measuring the amount of *Malassezia pachydermatis* at specific areas on the dog. The design is illustrated in Table 5.3.

Table 5.2. *The general structure of a parallel group design with k different treatments (or factor levels)*

	Treatment (or factor level)				
	1	2	3	$\cdots$	k
Number of study units	n_1	n_2	n_3	$\cdots$	n_k

Table 5.3. *A parallel group design to study the effect of Malaseb®
shampoo compared to a standard (placebo) shampoo on Malassezia
pachydermatis in dogs. Dogs were randomly allocated to either the
Malaseb® shampoo or the standard (placebo) shampoo*

	Dogs that received Malaseb®	Dogs that received standard (placebo)
Name of dog	Mille	Trofast
	Nellie	Victor
	Fido	Felix
	Vaks	Luna
	Bastian	Walde
	.	Luffe
Number of study units	5	6

5.3.2 *Factorial design*

A parallel group design is a special case of a factorial design, sometimes also
called a one-way factorial design. If further factors are to be evaluated, a factorial design in which two or more factors are used in combination can be
applied. Each factor can have two or more levels. Using the three two-level
factors X, Y and Z for illustration, the two-way factorial design to study X
and Y is shown in Table 5.4(a), and the three-way factorial design to study all
three factors is given in Table 5.4(b).

These designs enable possible interactions (see Chapter 11 for a discussion
on interaction) to be evaluated. The factorial design is a very powerful design.
However, the cost of that strength is an explosion of the number of groups
required in the design. For the general factorial design with k factors and
l_i levels for the ith factor, the number of groups in a full factorial design is

$$l_1 \times l_2 \times \cdots \times l_k = \prod_{i=1}^{k} l_i,$$

i.e. the product of the number of levels for each of the factors. A sufficient
number of study units has to be selected for each group.

> **EXAMPLE 5.2.** An example of a factorial design is a study of the effect of two new diets
> on body condition. The hypothesis was that the new diets have an effect on body condi-
> tion compared to a standard diet. Further, the effect of exercise (little or extensive) was
> evaluated in combination with the diets. The design is shown in Table 5.5. The effect of com-
> bining diet and exercise was also of interest to evaluate in order to investigate an increased
> effect of diet with some degree of exercise. The total number of combinations is $3 \times 2 = 6$.

Two parallel group studies to evaluate the two factors separately would require only $3 + 2$ groups. However, this design would not allow us to examine if the effect of the diets changed with the degree of exercise.

Table 5.4. *(a) A two-way (two factors) factorial design of X and Y with four different combinations. (b) A three-way (three factors) factorial design of X, Y and Z using eight different combinations. (c) The three-way factorial design of (b) reduced to a fractional factorial design by using the interaction between X and Y. In this design the interaction between Z and X, or Z and Y can still be assessed*

(a) n_{ij} is the number of animals in the X_i, Y_j combination		Factor Y	
		Y_1	Y_2
Factor X	X_1	n_{11}	n_{12}
	X_2	n_{21}	n_{22}

(b) n_{ijk} is the number of animals in the X_i, Y_j, Z_k combination		Factor Z × factor Y			
		Z_1		Z_2	
		Y_1	Y_2	Y_1	Y_2
Factor X	X_1	n_{111}	n_{121}	n_{112}	n_{122}
	X_2	n_{211}	n_{221}	n_{212}	n_{222}

(c) n_{ij} is the number of animals in the X_i, Y_i, Z_j combination		Factor Z	
		Z_1	Z_2
Factor combination (X, Y)	(X_1, Y_1)	n_{11}	n_{12}
	(X_2, Y_2)	n_{21}	n_{22}

Table 5.5. *A study of the effect of two new diets on body condition evaluated using a factorial design with two factors. The two new diets are compared to a standard diet. The effect of exercise (little or extensive) was evaluated in combination with the diets*

		No. of animals in each combination	
		Little exercise	Extensive exercise
Diet	Standard	7	8
	New A	5	7
	New B	6	9

5.4 Fractional factorial designs

A fractional factorial design is a special case of a factorial design where only a fraction of all possible factor combinations is applied. The fraction of the combinations to apply is selected by using one or more of the interactions to divide the combinations into parts. Hereby, not all interactions are possible to evaluate. Consider the three-way factorial design in Table 5.4(b). A reduction of this design into a fractional three-way factorial design is given in Table 5.4(c). The number of combinations have been reduced from the original eight in the full design to only four, but at the cost of losing the possibility to evaluate the interaction between X and Y. For larger and more complicated designs, the sample size can be considerably reduced, e.g. by using only 2^{6-2} ($= 16$) combinations rather than all 2^6 ($= 64$) combinations in a design with six factors with two levels each.

5.4.1 Latin and Graeco-Latin square design

A Latin square design is a special case of a three-way fractional factorial design as we are evaluating three factors in combination. In a Latin square design three factors are always used. All factors must have the same number of levels. An example of a Latin square design with three factors, each having three levels is given in Table 5.6(a). As seen in Table 5.6(a), only nine combinations

Table 5.6. *(a) A Latin square design with three factors each with three levels. Factor 1 has the levels a, b and c; factor 2 has the levels x, y and z and factor 3 has the levels I, II and III. (b) A Graeco-Latin square design with four factors each with four levels. Factor 1: a, b, c and d; factor 2: 1, 2, 3 and 4; factor 3: I, II, III and IV and factor 4: α, β, γ and δ*

(a)		Factor 1		
		a	b	c
Factor 2	x	I	III	II
	y	II	I	III
	z	III	II	I

(b)		Factor 1			
		a	b	c	d
Factor 2	1	I γ	III δ	IV α	II β
	2	IV β	II α	I δ	III γ
	3	II δ	IV γ	III β	I α
	4	III α	I β	II γ	IV δ

Table 5.7. *A Latin square design to study the development of parasites in outdoor pigs. Three grazing systems (A, B and C) are combined with feed from three feed mills (x, y and z) and three feed additives (I, II and III)*

		Grazing system		
		a	b	c
Feed mill	x	I	III	II
	y	II	I	III
	z	III	II	I

are performed, that is one-third of the possible combinations. If a complete factorial design was performed with three factors each with three levels, we would in total have $3 \times 3 \times 3 = 27$ combinations. As not all combinations of the three factors are performed, the number of combinations is considerably reduced compared to the complete factorial design. The disadvantage of the reduced design is that it is not possible to evaluate interactions between the three factors. Since interactions are often very valuable, this is a limitation in relation to other experimental designs. However, if one is in the initial phase of evaluating the effect of new treatments or drugs, the Latin square design can be used for screening different factors without using a large number of animals. Despite this, a Latin square design is seldom used.

In a Graeco-Latin square design a fourth factor has been applied compared to the Latin square with three factors. An example is a study of four factors each with four levels, including 16 combinations out of a total of 256 possible combinations (see Table 5.6b).

EXAMPLE 5.3. The effect of grazing system, feed mill and feed additives on development of parasites in outdoor pigs was studied using a Latin square design. Three grazing systems were used (A, B and C) in combination with three feed mills (x, y and z) and three feed additives (I, II and III). In each combination, 10 pigs were randomly selected. The development of parasites was evaluated at slaughter. The design is shown in Table 5.7. When using a Latin square design, only nine of the $3 \times 3 \times 3 = 27$ combinations are used.

5.5 Split-plot and strip-plot designs

A split-plot design is a factorial design in which one factor is randomised within the levels of the other factor. This means that it is not possible to have complete randomisation. A split-plot design with two factors was used in a study by Thamsborg *et al.* (2001) evaluating the effects of nematodes on health and productivity of piglets. The two factors were: sow infection (no, low, high) and piglet infection (no, high). In this study 39 sows were randomly allocated to one of three infection levels of nematodes. The piglets in each litter were randomly allocated to one of two infection levels as well. The effect of the nematode infections on daily weight gain in piglets was evaluated. The effect of infections in sows and piglets could be investigated separately, as well as in combination. The combined effect of sow and piglet infections is the interaction between the sow infection and piglet infection. The design is illustrated in Table 5.8.

A strip-plot design is also a factorial design with limitations in the ran-domisation procedure. An example could be a study of the effect of grazing system (three levels) and infection level (two levels) on the weight gain of lambs. The study is performed in the field. An area is divided into six parts with two stripes in one direction and three stripes in the perpendicular direc-tion (see Figure 5.1a). If a factorial design with complete randomisation is used, the six combinations of grazing system and infection levels should be randomly distributed in the six plots. However, due to practical problems in

Table 5.8. *A split-plot design with two factors used to evaluate the effect of nematodes on health and productivity of piglets. The factors evaluated in the study were sow infections (no, low, high) and piglet infection (no, high). Sows were randomly allocated to one of the three sow infection levels. The individual piglets in their litter were randomly allocated to one of the two piglet infection levels. Sow infection is the main-plot effect and piglet infection is the subplot effect*

		Sow infection level		
		No	Low	High
Distribution of litters on sow infection levels				
Litter No.	1	X		
	2		X	
	3		X	
	4			X
	5			X
	6			X
	7	X		
	.	.	.	.
No. of piglets for each combination				
Piglet infection	No	57	63	66
level	High	59	62	67

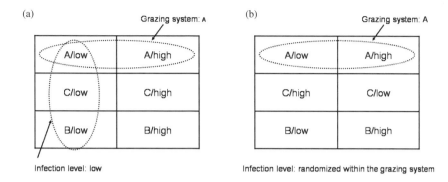

Figure 5.1. *(a) A strip-plot design used to evaluate the effect of grazing systems and infection levels on the weight gain of lambs. The factors evaluated in the study were grazing system with three levels (A, B and C) and infection level with two levels (low, high). Outline of the field divided into six plots. (b) The same study, but carried out in a split-plot design.*

the field, the same grazing systems were applied in the horizontal stripes. To compare the strip-plot design with the split-plot design, a split-plot design for the same problem is given in Figure 5.1(b).

5.6 Cross-over design

An alternative to the parallel group design is a cross-over design. In a cross-over design all animals are given all treatments in a pre-planned sequence. The study is conducted in a number of periods, corresponding to the number of different treatments. In the simplest case we have a study with two treatments, A and B, evaluated in two periods, illustrated in Table 5.9.

Table 5.9. *A cross-over design with two treatments A and B*

Animal number	Period	
	1	2
1	A	B
2	A	B
3	B	A
4	A	B
5	B	A
6	B	A
7	A	B
⋮	⋮	⋮

In a cross-over design, randomisation is used to allocate animals to a specific sequence (or order) of treatments. This means that some animals receive treatment A in the first period and some animals receive treatment B in the first period. In the second period the animals which received treatment A in the first period are now given treatment B and vice versa. Hereby, all animals receive all treatments once during the study. Between the periods, there should be a so-called wash-out period. The intention of the wash-out period is that the effect of the treatments should be eliminated (to a minimum) before a new treatment is applied. If the wash-out period is too short, the effect of the second treatment might be influenced by the remaining effect of the first treatment. This is called a carry-over effect or cross-over effect. However, if the wash-out period is too long, the conditions might change between the periods. The study is performed with a number of periods depending on the number of treatments. In a cross-over study with two treatments, the study should be performed in two periods with a wash-out period in between. The duration of the study is therefore longer compared to a parallel group design. The cross-over design has two main advantages. First of all, the comparison of treatments is performed within animals rather than between animals. Second, the required sample size for a cross-over design is smaller compared to the sample size for a parallel group design. The disadvantages include the assumption of no carry over of treatment effect between the two periods, so that the results in the second period are not affected by the treatment in the first period, e.g. if the animal is cured by treatment A, then applying treatment B afterwards is meaningless.

EXAMPLE 5.4. Horses often need sedation during, e.g. scanning in order to be calm and hereby get a reliable scanning result. However, the sedation might have an effect on the outcome of the investigation. Therefore, a study was performed in order to evaluate the effect of different types of medical sedation on the function of the heart in horses. A cross-over design was used in order to reduce the impact of the between horse variation as the within horse variation is used for testing the treatment effect. The three drugs used were romifidin, detomidin and acepromazin. The effect of the drugs on six horses was evaluated by echocardiography. The horses were randomly allocated to a sequence of treatments (see Table 5.10).

5.7 Clinical trials, laboratory experiments and field trials

Although we have focused on different designs of experiments, we must note that before selecting the actual design of the experiment there are some other considerations to be made. This includes specific features related to the type of study. Here we briefly outline some different types of experimental studies.

Table 5.10. *A cross-over design to study the effect of sedation by medicine on the function of the heart in horses. The three drugs used were romifidin, detomidin and azepromazin. The effect of the drugs on the six horses was evaluated by echocardiography*

Treatment sequence	Period		
	1	2	3
1: A-B-C	A	B	C
2: A-C-B	A	C	B
3: B-C-A	B	C	A
4: B-A-C	B	A	C
5: C-A-B	C	A	B
6: C-B-A	C	B	A

5.7.1 *Laboratory experiments*

A laboratory experiment is an experiment performed *in the laboratory* under very well-controlled conditions. The aim is to evaluate the effect of treatments, often using rodents or other small animals, e.g. mice, rats, rabbits and dogs. Here the word laboratory means research conditions and can be cages with rats. The experiments are performed under controlled conditions so it is possible to limit the variation between animals to a minimum. The variation can be reduced by using the same breed and litter mates, and having similar facilities for all animals such as feed, cages, etc. When the variation between animals is reduced, the efficacy of treatments is obtained more easily. However, animals in laboratory experiments do not necessarily represent the population.

EXAMPLE 5.5. Use of anaesthesia for rats has an impact on the heart rate. In order to evaluate how much impact different types of anaesthesia have on the heart rate, an experiment was performed. Ten similar rats were used in a study to compare two different types of anaesthesia and placebo (saline water). The placebo treatment was included in the experiment in order to assess the effects of handling the rats on the heart rate. A cross-over design was used for the experiment. In a randomised order all rats were given the two different types of anaesthesia and the control treatment. The heart rate was recorded 10 min before injection of the treatment and until an hour after injection. The effects of the two types of anaesthesia were compared to each other and to the placebo (control) treatment.

5.7.2 *Clinical trials*

A clinical trial is an experiment designed to compare the effect of one or more drugs or treatments on humans or animals. Traditionally, the term clinical has implied that the study was carried out on patients, i.e. humans or animals already suffering from the disease or condition in question. However, today vaccine studies and other trials involving preventive measures are also referred to as clinical trials.

Our distinction between experiment and clinical trial lies in the objective of the study where a clinical trial is a special case of an experiment. If the experiment is concerned with treatment or prevention of disease, then we refer to the study as a clinical trial, whereas studies involving other traits of the animal in general are called experiments.

Animals involved in clinical trials often experience discomfort caused by illness. For animal welfare reasons, it has been deemed necessary to perform closer monitoring of such experiments. Hence, a clinical trial must be carefully planned and a protocol describing the study must be made. The protocol should be approved by ethical authorities before conducting the experiment. This is mainly to ensure that the correct design with a minimal number of animals required to address the study question is selected. Also, a clear termination criteria should be established to prevent unnecessary suffering.

Often the patients are recruited over a period of time as they are diagnosed with the disease and hence, the number of subjects increases gradually. This often limits the choice of study design to the more simple ones. In trials involving animals, the option of experimental infection exists, allowing more control over the subjects selected for the experiment. As the ultimate objective of the clinical trial is to gain information on the target population this selection process might limit the possible generalisation of the results obtained from the experiment.

5.7.3 Field trials

A field trial is an experiment performed in the field. In order to assess the efficacy of a treatment (e.g. a new vaccine against *Actinobacillus pleuropneumoniae*) a trial on animals *in the field* is needed. By animals in the field we mean animals naturally exposed to infection in the environment where the animals usually are kept. The field trial is performed under conditions typical for the animals, which the new treatment is developed for. The animals are, e.g. pigs in Danish pig herds, where the farmer agrees to participate in the trial. Field trials are often used to validate the findings of laboratory experiments and clinical trials.

> **EXAMPLE 5.6.** When a new prophylactic or therapeutic drug is ready for sale it has been evaluated during a number of different experiments. An example is a new vaccine against *Actinobacillus pleuropneumoniae* for pigs. The first experiments will usually be laboratory

trials evaluating the toxicity and an acceptable single drug dosage. In the next step, the new drug is evaluated in initial clinical trials investigating the treatment effect. Hereafter, full-scale clinical trials are performed. Finally, the new drug is evaluated under field conditions in a field trial.

5.8 Further reading

Classic textbooks on experimental design include Cochran and Cox (1992), Cox (1992) and Hicks (1982). Cross-over trials are given special attention in Senn (1993). For further introduction to clinical trials see, e.g. Pocock (1983), Fleiss (1986) and Armitage *et al.* (2002). For a Bayesian perspective towards the analysis of clinical trials see, e.g. Spiegelhalter *et al.* (2000).

6 MEASURES OF DISEASE FREQUENCY

Nils Toft, Jens Frederik Agger, Hans Houe
and Jeanett Bruun

6.1 Introduction

Information regarding disease frequency is fundamental to epidemiologists. For example, when assessing the importance of a disease, information regarding the number of diseased animals as well as the transition from healthy to diseased is required. The combined effect of these two properties of a disease can provide essential information regarding the importance of the disease in the population.

In general, we will have more benefit from knowledge of disease frequency in relative terms, i.e. as a percentage of diseased animals rather than the absolute number of diseased animals. Still, for practical purposes the total count of cases is relevant to consider, for example, for the purpose of allocating manpower to veterinary services in a national eradication programme, to determine the cost of eradication programmes or to establish the requirements for capacity at destruction facilities, etc. needed in stamping out diseases such as foot and mouth disease.

In this chapter, we shall present the commonly used measures of disease frequency. Basically, these measures are divided into two categories: prevalence which is a measure of presence of disease at a specific point in time, and incidence, which measures the occurrence of new cases through time.

6.2 Proportions and rates

Before discussing prevalence and incidence as measures of disease frequency, we must establish some common terms to use as measures.

Consider as the first of these the *proportion* of diseased animals in a population. A proportion is a fraction where the numerator is included in the denominator, i.e.:

$$\text{proportion} = \frac{d}{d+h}$$

where d is the number of diseased and h the number of healthy animals so that the total population n is $n = d + h$. The proportion of diseased animals (or animals possessing some other trait of interest) can be seen as the probability or risk of being diseased in the study population. The proportion is a dimensionless number between 0 and 1, but often we express the proportion as a percentage, i.e. multiply the proportion by 100.

A more complex measure is the *rate*, which expresses the potential for change in one quantity per unit of change in another quantity. An example is the speed of a car, which is expressed as distance per time unit, e.g, kilometres per hour. In this chapter we usually express rates as cases per animal time, e.g. diarrhoea per calf day.

6.3 Prevalence

By *prevalence* (p) of a disease or condition we mean the proportion of the population which at a given point in time has the disease. So, prevalence is a here-and-now measure of disease:

$$p = \frac{\#\text{ diseased animals at time } t}{\#\text{ animals in sample at time } t}$$

where # denotes 'number of'. Essentially, the prevalence of a disease can be interpreted as the probability that an animal selected at random from the population has the disease in question at time t. As the prevalence is a proportion, the derivation of a confidence interval is straightforward under the common assumption that the prevalence is normal distributed. Hence, the $(1 - \alpha)100\%$ confidence interval of the proportion (prevalence (p)) may be given as:

$$p \pm Z_{1-\alpha/2}\sqrt{\frac{p(1-p)}{n}}$$

where n is the number of animals in the sample at time t and $Z_{1-\alpha/2}$ is the value of the standard normal distribution corresponding to a two-sided confidence level of $1 - \alpha/2$. This means that $Z_{1-0.05/2} = Z_{0.975} = 1.96$ is the Z-value where 2.5% of the probability mass lies to the right of Z and 2.5% lies to the left of $-Z$.

Often we allow the prevalence to be based on a sample accumulated over a short time period, e.g. a week's samples in a slaughter house rather than just the samples taken in one day. The point here is that time is *at slaughter*.

Table 6.1. *Example of registrations and resulting prevalence of high somatic cell count (SCC > 400,000 per millilitre) for six consecutive control milkings in a herd (see Example 6.1)*

Month	High SCC	Total testings	Prevalence of high SCC
1	12	120	0.10
2	12	110	0.11
3	15	125	0.12
4	13	122	0.11
5	8	110	0.07
6	10	115	0.09

If it is known that there is substantial seasonal variation in disease prevalence, then sometimes the prevalence is calculated as the proportion of cases in the samples taken over an entire year, but the point-in-time is *at testing*. However, better approaches to reduce seasonal variation exist and should be used (see, e.g. West and Harrison (1997)).

The *lifetime prevalence* is a term sometimes used to describe the probability that an animal at some point in life had a specific disease. We discourage the use of this term, as the above probability is better described by incidence risk, as introduced in the next section.

EXAMPLE 6.1. In a dairy herd, the milk is controlled on a monthly basis. The measurement consists of a sample of milk from each cow taken at the morning milking on one specific day during that month. These samples are analysed for different elements. One of these is the somatic cell count (SCC) of the milk. A large value of the SCC is an indication of mastitis. Cows with high SCC cause an increase in the bulk tank SCC, which is used for pricing the milk at the dairy. Hence, farmers often choose to milk cows with increased SCC separately and discard the milk or use it for calves. In Table 6.1, the prevalences of cows with high SCC (SCC > 400,000 per millilitre) are given for six consecutive milkings.

We should be careful not to interpret the change in prevalences too much. For instance, the 12 cows in the first 2 months might be the same 12 cows in both months or 24 different cows. This has quite an impact on the inference about how SCC develops.

As Example 6.1 illustrates, the prevalence is a poor measure of how disease develops in a population through a period of time. For such inference we need incidence measures.

6.4 Incidence

Incidence is a measure of the new cases that occur within a given time period. It can be represented by the count of new cases; however, we are often more interested in expressing the incidence as a relative measure with respect to the population at risk. We will present two different types of incidence measure in this section: the *incidence risk* and the *incidence rate*.

6.4.1 *Incidence risk*

A risk is the probability that an event occurs, hence the incidence risk is the probability that a disease-free animal develops a disease over a specified period, given that the animal does not leave during that period. We can define the incidence risk (I_{risk}) as:

$$I_{risk} = \frac{\text{\# new infected or diseased animals in the study period}}{\text{\# animals at risk at the start of the study period}}$$

Note that the term 'infected' can be substituted for any other condition of interest, e.g., disease, pregnancy, culling. It is important to realise that only animals that actually are capable of getting the disease (i.e. the animals at risk) are included in the denominator. Thus, prior to the start of the study care should be taken to determine if the animals have the disease, if they are immune to it or whether they are not at risk due to other traits, e.g. bulls are not at risk of mastitis. The above definition of I_{risk} and its interpretation assumes that no animals leave or enter the study during the study period, i.e. we have a closed (or static) population. This assumption makes the interpretation of the incidence risk straightforward. Unfortunately, direct estimation of the incidence risk using the above definition is impossible in most studies, because of premature withdrawal or late entering of animals. Rather than adjust the definition of incidence risk to allow direct estimation in dynamic populations, we proceed to introduce the incidence rate and elaborate to some extent on the connection between the incidence rate and the incidence risk. Using this rigid definition of I_{risk} has the advantage that the calculation of confidence intervals can be carried out in the same way as for the prevalence, i.e. using the assumption of a normal distributed incidence risk. Thus, the $(1 - \alpha)100\%$ confidence interval for the incidence risk (I_{risk}) when calculated directly using the above formula is given as:

$$I_{risk} \pm Z_{1-\alpha/2}\sqrt{\frac{I_{risk}(1 - I_{risk})}{n}}$$

where n is the number of animals at risk at the start of the study period. Whenever the incidence risk is derived using some of the other methods discussed later in this chapter, the confidence interval is more complicated to calculate and is considered to be beyond the scope of this book.

6.4.2 *Incidence rate*

The incidence risk is a measure of an animal's probability of contracting disease, and as such it relates to the individual animal. The incidence rate is a measure of the intensity of change of healthy animals into infected or diseased animals, hence it relates to the population. The incidence rate can be seen as a measure of the speed at which healthy animals become diseased. Since the incidence rate is a measure of change, we need a unit to measure this change. Thus, we need to express the rate in terms of cases per animal time unit, such as cases per animal day or animal year. It is obvious that the rate may assume any number by adjusting the unit of measure. Often we express the incidence rate for diseases in dairy cows as cases per 100 cow years. This way the incidence rate can express how many cases to expect in a year in a herd with an average of 100 milking cows. Formally, we may define the incidence rate (I_{rate}) as:

$$I_{rate} = \frac{\text{\# new infected or diseased animals in the study period}}{\text{time at risk}}$$

The problem here lies in determining the 'time at risk'. Strictly speaking we should refer to the time at risk, as animal time at risk, since we are using a unit that combines time with animals. The time at risk for one animal, is the number of time units (e.g. days) from entering the study to one of the following: (1) disease occurs; (2) the animal is withdrawn (e.g. is sold or dies); or (3) the study ends. The time at risk for the entire group is the sum of these individual animal time units.

$$\text{time at risk} = \sum_{i=1}^{n} t_i$$

where t_i is the time at risk for the ith animal. To actually carry out this calculation we need rather detailed information regarding the animals in the sense of exact dates for inclusion and exclusion. In an experimental study, this information should be available, but in observational studies we are often faced with less detailed information; however, computer records usually have these details.

It is possible to produce reasonably good estimates of the time at risk by assuming that animals leave and enter the study uniformly throughout the study period. If animals leave and enter at all times then on average they will leave and enter at exactly the middle of the study period. Hence, animals that leave or enter the study will be present for half of the study period; this gives us an approximation of the time at risk:

$$\text{time at risk}_{est} = \left(\text{\# animals at risk at start} + \frac{\text{\# new animals}}{2}\right.$$

$$\left. - \frac{\text{\# withdrawals}}{2} - \frac{\text{\# diseased}}{2}\right) \times \text{time period}$$

$$= \frac{\text{\# animals at risk at start} + \text{\# animals at risk at end}}{2}$$

$$\times \text{time period}$$

The assumption behind this usually becomes 'more' true as the sample size of the study increases. Note that we assume that disease occurs throughout the entire study period, i.e. on average in the middle of the study. This assumption is fundamental in the calculation of the incidence rate, since we implicitly assume that the incidence rate is constant during the study period.

The following example shows how the time at risk might differ between the exact and approximate calculations:

EXAMPLE 6.2. At the beginning of the year, six stallions were at a stud farm. During the year, five were sold and three purchased, leaving four stallions at the end of the year. None of the stallions were diseased during the study.

$$\text{Time at risk} = \left(6 + \frac{3}{2} - \frac{5}{2}\right) \times 365 \text{ horse days}$$

$$= \left(\frac{6+4}{2}\right) \times 365 \text{ horse days}$$

$$= 5 \times 365 \text{ horse days}$$

$$= 1825 \text{ horse days}$$

Now we use the exact information from the stud farm:

1/1 ——————————— 31/12	365	
1/1 —— 2/3	60	
1/1 ——— 1/5	120	
1/1 ——— 16/4	105	
1/1 ——————————— 22/10	294	= 1856 horse days
1/1 ——————————— 22/10	294	
15/1 ——————————— 31/12	350	
1/6 ——————————— 31/12	214	
7/11 —— 31/12	54	

The exact number of days at risk is 1856 horse days, the estimated number was 1825 horse days. So there is a difference of 31 horse days between the two methods; however, this difference may easily become larger if there is a more pronounced seasonal pattern in sales and purchase. So, whenever possible we should use exact information to calculate the time at risk.

Calculation of confidence intervals for the incidence rate is possible, but far from simple when compared to the confidence intervals for the incidence risk or the prevalence. Under certain assumptions it is, however, possible to derive an approximation of the confidence interval. Suppose that the new cases really do occur randomly and independently, then it is a reasonable assumption that they follow a Poisson distribution. If we further assume that the time at risk is more or less constant, i.e. animals enter and leave the population uniformly, then we can find approximate confidence limits for the number of new cases during the study period. Define C as the number of new cases during the study period, i.e. the numerator of the fraction, defining the incidence rate. Then, the upper limit (C_U) and the lower limit (C_L) for the $(1 - \alpha)100\%$ confidence interval of C are given as:

$$C_L = \left(\frac{Z_{1-\alpha/2}}{2} - \sqrt{C} \right)^2$$

$$C_U = \left(\frac{Z_{1-\alpha/2}}{2} + \sqrt{C+1} \right)^2$$

which gives the $(1-\alpha)100\%$ confidence interval of the incidence rate by dividing these limits by the time at risk. However, according to Woodward (1999) this approximation requires that $C > 100$, i.e. the number of new cases during the study period must exceed 100. Hence, the approximation is only good for studies of rather large populations since a high number of cases in a small population probably indicates that the cases are not independent as in, e.g. infectious diseases such as swine influenza.

6.4.3   The relationship between incidence rate and incidence risk

To estimate the incidence risk or incidence rate in a study it is a fundamental assumption that the measure is constant throughout the period used for estimation. Under this assumption we can also derive a relationship between the incidence rate and the incidence risk. The incidence rate (I_{rate}) is a measure of the speed of the transformation from disease free to diseased. So, if we assume that this rate is constant for the time period of our study, then at time t we are left with:

$$N_t = N_0 \, e^{-I_{\text{rate}} \times t} \tag{6.1}$$

disease-free animals, with N_0 being the initial number of disease-free animals, i.e. at time $t = 0$. Equation 6.1 resembles the formula for decay of a radioactive substance. Essentially, the interpretation is the same: the initial number of healthy animals, N_0, decays at a constant rate I_{rate}.

From Equation 6.1 we deduce that the probability of being healthy (disease free) at time t is N_t/N_0 which implies that the incidence risk at time t is:

$$I_{\text{risk}} = 1 - N_t/N_0 = 1 - e^{-I_{\text{rate}} \times t} \tag{6.2}$$

Using Equation 6.2, it is possible to calculate back and forth between the two measures, i.e. given the incidence risk at time t, we can calculate the incidence rate:

$$I_{\text{rate}} = \frac{-\ln(1 - I_{\text{risk}})}{t}$$

EXAMPLE 6.3. Assume that we follow a litter of 10 piglets from birth to weaning 4 weeks later (a nursing period). Assume that all piglets are still alive at the end of the study period. During these 4 weeks, four piglets developed diarrhoea. In this situation we can calculate the incidence risk directly:

$$I_{\text{risk}} = \frac{4}{10} = 0.4$$

e.g. there is a 40% chance that a piglet being alive for 4 weeks develops diarrhoea. To calculate the incidence rate we must calculate the time at risk. We have 10 piglets at risk at the start of the study and six are still at risk at the end of the study:

$$\text{time at risk}_{\text{est}} = \frac{10 + 6}{2} \times 4 \text{ pig weeks} = 32 \text{ pig weeks}$$

Thus, the incidence rate becomes:

$$I_{\text{rate}} = \frac{4}{32} = 0.125 \text{ diarrhoea case per pig week}$$

Suppose we prefer to express this number in terms of cases per pig day, then we divide by 7 days per week, i.e.

$$I_{\text{rate}} = \frac{0.125}{7} \frac{\text{case/pig week}}{\text{day(s)/week}} = 0.018 \text{ case per pig day}$$

If we on the other hand prefer to talk about the number of diarrhoea cases per litter per nursing period, then we may express the incidence rate in terms of cases per 10 piglet nursing periods, i.e. we multiply $I_{\text{rate}} = 0.125$ by 4 to get cases per nursing period (4 weeks) and then multiply by 10 to get an estimate per 10 piglets.

$$I_{\text{rate}} = 0.125 \text{ case/pig week} \times 4 \text{ weeks/nursing period} \times 10 \text{ pigs/litter}$$

$$= 0.125 \times 4 \times 10 \frac{\text{case} \times \text{weeks} \times \text{pigs}}{\text{pig week} \times \text{nursing period} \times \text{litter}}$$

This gives $I_{rate} = 5$ cases per litter nursing periods, which we prefer to express as cases per 10 piglet nursing periods to avoid problems with variation in litter size. Now we can calculate the incidence risk from the estimate of incidence rate using Equation 6.2. The thing to consider when using an estimate of the incidence rate is what time unit it is associated with. For $I_{rate} = 0.125$ case per pig week, we have weeks as the time unit, hence $t = 4$. To calculate the incidence risk for the nursing period:

$$I_{risk} = 1 - e^{-0.125 \times 4} = 0.39 \approx 0.4$$

Should we decide to use $I_{rate} = 0.018$ case per pig day, we have $t = 28$, hence:

$$I_{risk} = 1 - e^{-0.018 \times 28} = 0.39 \approx 0.4$$

Finally, if we use the measure $I_{rate} = 5$ cases per 10 piglet nursing periods, then the time unit of interest is only one-tenth of that, i.e. $t = 0.1$

$$I_{risk} = 1 - e^{-5 \times 0.1} = 0.39 \approx 0.4$$

Hence, t is the time at risk for the individual animal in the animal time at risk unit that we are currently using.

6.4.4 Extending the time period

As it has been emphasised, we assume that the incidence risk or rate is constant throughout the period in which we estimate it. Basically, the way we estimate the rate or risk produces an average of the risk or rate through the period. An average is only a reasonable estimate of the true parameter as long as the parameter is reasonably constant. However, quite often we are well aware that there is increased risk of disease during certain stages of life or the production cycle of an animal. Thus, it might be appropriate to calculate measures for certain specific periods. Afterwards, on the other hand, it might be relevant to have an idea of the incidence risk or rate for a longer period.

To combine the incidence rate of different periods, we add the incidence rates of the individual periods. The important element here is to only add rates of the same unit, e.g. convert all rates regarding dairy cows to cow days. If the incidence rate for the ith period is $I_{rate}(i)$ and the incidence rate for the entire period is I_{rate}, then:

$$I_{rate} = \sum_{i=1}^{n} I_{rate}(i) \tag{6.3}$$

where n is the total number of periods. This formula also states that to convert a rate in cases per cow month to cases per 100 cow years, we multiply the rate by 1200, just like the calculations in Example 6.3.

The same idea cannot be applied to the incidence risk, because the incidence risk of disease in the individual periods is conditional on the animals being disease free at the onset of the period. Thus, the easiest way to determine the risk of disease after n periods is through the probability of not being diseased. Having determined this probability, the incidence risk is one minus the probability of not being diseased at any time period. For any one time period, the probability of avoiding disease is $(1 - I_{risk}(i))$, hence the probability to completely avoid disease is the product of these terms. This gives us the following formula for estimating the incidence risk (I_{risk}) through n periods (where $\prod$ denotes a product, just as $\sum$ denotes a sum):

$$I_{risk} = 1 - \prod_{i=1}^{n}(1 - I_{risk}(i)) \qquad (6.4)$$

If the incidence risk is constant throughout all the periods, then the formula can be written as:

$$I_{risk} = 1 - (1 - I_{risk}^{*})^{n} \qquad (6.5)$$

where n is the number of time periods, and I_{risk}^{*} is the (constant) incidence risk of the individual periods.

EXAMPLE 6.4. In Houe and Meyling (1991) an example of backwards use of Equation 6.5 is given. The study utilises the fact that presence of antibodies against BVDV is lifelong: the presence of antibodies indicates that the cow has had the disease, absence of antibodies indicates that the cow has not had the disease. This implies that the sero-prevalence (i.e. prevalence of antibodies) of a sample of cows at a certain age is a measure of the incidence risk of BVDV infection through the life of a cow until that age. The study assumes that the annual incidence risk is constant, hence Equation 6.5 can be used to derive I_{risk}^{*}, the annual incidence risk, using the sero-prevalence as an estimate of the incidence risk I_{risk}. Rearranging terms and taking logarithms on both sides of Equation 6.5 yields:

$$I_{risk} = 1 - (1 - I_{risk}^{*})^{n} \Leftrightarrow \ln(1 - I_{risk}) = n \times \ln(1 - I_{risk}^{*})$$

$$\Leftrightarrow I_{risk}^{*} = 1 - e^{\frac{\ln(1-I_{risk})}{n}}$$

Using this result we may calculate the cohort-specific annual incidence risk (under the assumption of constant incidence risk) for 1–2 year old cows using $n = 1.5$, 2–3 year old cows using $n = 2.5$, etc. Results from Houe and Meyling (1991) give a seroprevalence (i.e. incidence risk throughout life) of 0.48 for the former and 0.65 for the latter group. This implies that the annual incidence risk ($I_{risk}(1)$) for the cohort of cows between age 1 and 2 years is:

$$I_{risk}(1) = 1 - e^{\frac{\ln(1-0.48)}{1.5}} = 0.35$$

which compares quite well to the same estimate for the cohort of cows aged 2–3 years:

$$I_{risk}(1) = 1 - e^{\frac{\ln(1-0.65)}{2.5}} = 0.34$$

6.4.5 *Dynamic populations*

The formulas from the previous section give us an idea how to handle dynamic populations, where animals constantly leave and enter the study. For the time unit where information is added, we calculate the time at risk. Using the estimate of time at risk, we calculate the incidence rate and subsequently the incidence risk using Equation 6.2. The only challenge is to adopt a systematic approach, such as the one proposed in Example 6.5.

We use an approach where the incidence risk is calculated indirectly from the incidence rate. This way we can ensure that there is consistency between the definitions and the estimation of the parameters. It is possible to adopt other methods and we suggest that the reader consult Kleinbaum *et al.* (1982) for a discussion.

EXAMPLE 6.5.   On a mink farm, newly purchased animals are inserted in a separate section. In connection with transport, change of feed and housing, problems with pneumonia and deaths occur (see Table 6.2a). It is assumed that mink that get diseased and survive have acquired resistance that will protect from reinfection for at least a month. For each of the 4 weeks as well as for the entire period we want to estimate the incidence rate as well as incidence risk.

To keep track of the animals we use Table 6.2(b), where we have recorded entries and exits. This way we can calculate the time at risk using the number of animals at risk at the start and end of the period.

Observe that the dead animals given in Table 6.2(a) already are counted as diseased. Note also, that the information pertaining to number of mink alive at the start of each week is not used except for the first week. In subsequent weeks, we use the number at risk at the end of week 1 as the number at risk at the start of week 2, etc. Here, we can assume that diseased animals will not lose their resistance during the study period (4 weeks); however, this assumption depends on the circumstances regarding the disease and should always be scrutinised prior to the calculations, i.e. mastitis in dairy cows might be recurrent right after the end of treatment.

Using the time at risk we can estimate the incidence rate (I_{rate}), and subsequently the incidence risk (I_{risk}) for the individual weeks (Table 6.2c).

Note that we interpret the incidence risk for, say, week 3 as the probability that a mink which is still disease free at the start of week 3 will become diseased during week 3. For the entire period we can calculate the incidence rate as the sum of incidence rates for each of the 4 weeks:

$$I_{rate} = 0.0717 + 0.1528 + 0.1457 + 0.0741 = 0.4443 \text{ case per 4 mink weeks}$$

The incidence risk for the entire period can now be calculated as:

$$I_{risk} = 1 - e^{-0.4443 \times 1} = 0.3587$$

As an alternative to this, we can use Equation 6.4 and the incidence risk for the individual weeks.

$$I_{risk} = 1 - (1 - 0.0692)(1 - 0.1417)(1 - 0.1356)(1 - 0.0714) = 0.3588$$

We have chosen to use more digits to present the results here in this example than we usually would deem appropriate. This was done to illustrate that there is little effect of using different approaches for calculation.

As a final element of this example, consider the lazy approach where we calculate the incidence rate for the entire period using the time at risk for the entire period estimated as:

$$\text{time at risk}_{\text{est}} = \left(\# \text{ animals at risk at start} \right.$$

$$\left. + \frac{\# \text{ new animals}}{2} - \frac{\# \text{ diseased}}{2} \right) \times \text{ time period}$$

$$= 112 + \frac{36 + 46}{2} - \frac{9 + 22 + 23 + 10}{2} \times 4 \text{ mink weeks}$$

$$= 121 \text{ (4 mink weeks)}$$

which gives us an incidence rate of:

$$I_{\text{rate}} = \frac{64}{121} = 0.529 \text{ case per 4 mink weeks}$$

This estimate differs substantially from the estimate calculated as the sum of the individual weeks estimates. This is in accordance with what we anticipate, since the incidence rates for the individual weeks clearly differ. In addition, mink are only added for the first 2 weeks, and disease occurs more frequently during the 2 middle weeks, hence the assumption of homogeneous distribution of cases, withdrawals and newcomers fails.

Table 6.2. *The data and calculations used in Example 6.5*

(a)

Week	No. alive on first day of the week	No. of new minks added during the week	No. of new cases (diseased)	No. of deaths among the diseased
1	112	36	9	0
2	148	46	23	1
3	193	0	22	1
4	192	0	10	0

(b)

Week	At risk start + new minks − diseased = at risk end							Time at risk (mink weeks)
1	112	+	36	−	9	=	139	$(112 + 139)/2 = 125.5$
2	139	+	46	−	23	=	162	$(139 + 162)/2 = 150.5$
3	162	+	0	−	22	=	140	$(162 + 140)/2 = 151$
4	140	+	0	−	10	=	130	$(140 + 130)/2 = 135$

(c)

Week	I_{rate} (cases per mink week)	$I_{risk} = 1 - e^{-I_{rate} \times t}$
1	$9/125.5 = 0.0717$	$1 - e^{-0.717} = 0.0692$
2	$23/150.5 = 0.1528$	$1 - e^{-0.1528} = 0.1417$
3	$22/151 = 0.1457$	$1 - e^{-0.1457} = 0.1356$
4	$10/135 = 0.0741$	$1 - e^{-0.0741} = 0.0714$

6.4.6 Incidence rate or incidence risk?

We have established that the incidence rate is a measure of what is essentially a population-specific property, whereas the incidence risk is a measure of the individual's chance of developing disease.

Thus, to make individual prediction for animals, we need the risk measure, but for causal inference the rate is just as good. Figure 6.1 summarises how to select the appropriate incidence measure based on the properties of the population. Starting at the left of the figure, we distinguish between closed and dynamic populations. For a closed population with no withdrawal or addition, we accept the direct calculation of the incidence risk; however, in most cases we propose to work through the incidence rate (second and third column in Figure 6.1). If the exact time at risk can be calculated then we suggest using animal-specific information to get exact information regarding the time at risk; otherwise, an estimate may be calculated using the method applied throughout this chapter. Having calculated the empirical measure we can derive the theoretical measure as a rate or risk depending on our objective of the study (columns 4 and 5).

6.4.7 Prevalence and incidence

Prevalence was defined earlier as the proportion of diseased animals at a given point in time. The objective of a cross-sectional study is often to find an estimate of the prevalence. Thus, sampling from the population on a single

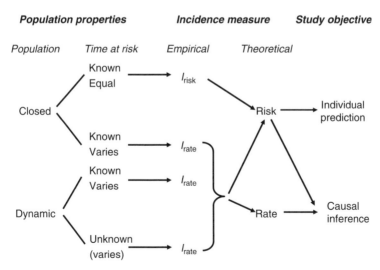

Figure 6.1. *Outline of the elements involved in selecting an appropriate incidence measure with respect to population properties. Adopted and modified from Kleinbaum et al. (1982).*

day makes it more likely to find chronic diseases than diseases with a short duration.

For a chronic disease such as paratuberculosis in cattle we will ultimately see a reduction in prevalence if we are able to reduce the incidence rate. On the other hand, improvements in therapy for fatal diseases such as cancer in cats, may decrease the mortality, but increase the prevalence, since life is prolonged for animals that otherwise die quickly (e.g. the duration of the disease is increased).

Following this discussion we realise that the prevalence (p) depends on the incidence rate (I_{rate}) and the duration (D) of the disease, i.e.:

$$p \propto I_{rate} \times D \quad (\propto \text{ means proportional to})$$

This implies that a change in prevalence can be due to (1) a change in incidence rate, (2) a change in the average duration of the disease or (3) a change in both.

The exact relationship is rather complex; however, under *steady-state* conditions we may assume that:

$$\frac{p}{1-p} = I_{rate} \times D \tag{6.6}$$

which implies that

$$p = \frac{I_{rate} \times D}{I_{rate} \times D + 1} \tag{6.7}$$

For rare diseases (e.g. $p < 0.05$) Equation 6.6 reduces to:

$$p \approx I_{rate} \times D \tag{6.8}$$

By steady-state conditions we refer to a situation where: (1) the population is at equilibrium, i.e. stable in size and demographics and (2) prevalence and incidence rate are constant, i.e. the number of new cases within a period is equal to the number of terminated cases.

A common use for these relations is when trying to estimate the duration of chronic diseases. Thus, Equation 6.6 is usually rewritten to express the duration in terms of prevalence and incidence rate:

$$D = \frac{p}{I_{rate} \times (1-p)}$$

For a more in-depth discussion of these issues, please consult Kleinbaum *et al.* (1982).

EXAMPLE 6.6. Suppose that a disease affecting dairy cattle is reported to have an incidence rate $I_{rate} = 8$ (cases/100 cow years) and a duration of $D = 2$ months. Then, we can estimate the prevalence using Equation 6.7; however, we must transform the incidence rate and duration of the disease to have the same time unit, i.e. years. Hence, using $I_{rate} = 0.08$ (cases/cow year)

---

and $D = 1/6 = 0.167$ years we find the prevalence:

$$p = \frac{I_{rate} \times D}{I_{rate} \times D + 1} = \frac{0.01336}{0.01336 + 1} = 0.0132 = 1.32\%$$

or using the approximation (which is okay, since the disease seems rare) in Equation 6.8 we find the prevalence to be:

$$p \approx I_{rate} \times D = 0.08 \times 0.167 = 0.0134 = 1.34\%$$

Here, we see that the approximation is very close to the exact value. When using either formula only 1.3% should be reported, the last digit is only given for illustration.

6.5 Other measures

So far we have implicitly assumed that our concern regarded some disease. Hence, our associated measures have been defined in these terms. However, the mathematical properties of a proportion, a risk and a rate are of course not affected by the properties of the trait under study. Hence, the elements regarding prevalence and incidence of the previous sections may be implemented directly for other measures.

What we have discussed so far are often called *morbidity* measures, i.e. measures of disease. *Mortality* measures are analogous to morbidity measures where the relevant outcome is death rather than new cases of the disease. We define *mortality risk* (M_{risk})

$$M_{risk} = \frac{\# \text{ animals that die during study period}}{\# \text{ animals in the population at start of study}}$$

and *mortality rate* (M_{rate}) as

$$M_{rate} = \frac{\# \text{ animals that die during the study period}}{\text{time at risk of dying}}$$

The mortality rate is sometimes referred to as *death rate* or *crude mortality rate*. If we are only concerned with cases and deaths regarding a specific disease, we might use the *cause-specific* measure defined above, but using only cases and deaths attributed to the specific disease.

Another measure regarding death is the *case fatality* (CF) or *lethality* which is used to describe the proportion of animals that have a specific disease and die from that disease:

$$CF = \frac{\# \text{ deaths due to disease in the time period}}{\# \text{ new cases in time period}}$$

This measure is sometimes incorrectly referred to as the case fatality rate in literature. The case fatality is the probability that an animal that is diseased eventually dies from the disease. There might be animals that survive the disease. The proportion of surviving animals among the diseased is called the *survival* (S):

$$S = \frac{(\text{\# new cases} - \text{\# deaths due to disease}) \text{ in time period}}{\text{\# new cases in time period}}$$

Obviously we have CF + S = 1, since survival and case fatality are complements of each other: either the animal is alive at the end of a period or it is dead, there is no in-between.

The two last measures are part of a special group of measures known as *proportional measures*. In general a *proportional risk* (PR) of a certain feature (such as death or disease due to a specific cause) can be defined as:

$$PR = \frac{\dfrac{\text{\# new cases due to a specific cause in time period}}{\text{\# animals in the population at start of study}}}{\dfrac{\text{\# new cases due to a general cause in time period}}{\text{\# animals in the population at start of study}}}$$

$$= \frac{\text{\# new cases due to a specific cause in time period}}{\text{\# new cases due to general causes in time period}}$$

i.e. the number of cases due to the specific cause divided by the total number of cases. When using such measures, the numerator and denominator of the fraction should have something in common, e.g. the proportion of mastitis cases due to *Staphyloccus agalactiae* to the total number of mastitis cases, rather than the total number of cases of disease in general. However, as always the appropriate use is determined by the underlying questions that one seeks to have answered when calculating the proportional risks. Note, that numerator and denominator of the PR may change almost independently; this often leads to incorrect inference about changes in proportional risks.

EXAMPLE 6.7. On 1 September 2000 disease is discovered in a fish tank. The disease results in either recovery or death. The tank is observed for a year. There are no new fish introduced during that period and all fish are accounted for at the end of the year.

Fish in the tank 1 September 2000	75
Clinically ill 1 September 2000	15
No. developing disease between 1 September 2000 and 1 September 2001	12
No. dying from disease from 1 September 2000 to 1 September 2001	9

From these numbers we can calculate a number of different measures. Note, that we estimate time at risk using the number at risk at the start and end of the time period, since no detailed information regarding timing of the individual cases and death is available.

Prevalence on 1 September 2000	$= 15/75$	$= 0.20$
Incidence rate (cases per fish year)	$= 12/([60+48]/2)$	$= 0.22$
Incidence risk* (1 September 2000 to 1 September 2001)	$= 1 - e^{-0.22 \times 1}$	$= 0.20$
Mortality rate (deaths per animal year)	$= 9/([75+66]/2)$	$= 0.13$
Mortality risk (1 September 2000 to 1 September 2001)	$= 1 - e^{-0.13 \times 1}$	$= 0.12$
Case fatality (1 September 2000 to 1 September 2001)	$= 9/(12+15)$	$= 0.33$
Survival (1 September 2000 to 1 September 2001)	$= (27-9)/27 = 1-0.33$	$= 0.67$

*Since no losses occur except from the disease, we may calculate $I_{risk} = 12/60 = 0.2$ directly.

6.6   Further reading

Kleinbaum *et al.* (1982) give a thorough discussion of prevalence, incidence and the association between them. Rothman and Greenland (1998) also cover measures of disease frequency intensively. Dohoo *et al.* (2003) cover standardisation of risks and rates as well as an introduction to several other measures of disease frequency.

7 MEASURES OF ASSOCIATION AND EFFECT

Nils Toft, Jens Frederik Agger and Jeanett Bruun

7.1 Introduction

Often our concern in an epidemiological study is to assess the chance that an animal that possesses certain traits also has a specific disease. These traits might be intrinsic risk factors such as a specific sex, age or weight or extrinsic risk factors such as housing or management related issues (see Chapter 3). The chance that a healthy animal exposed to a risk factor becomes diseased is defined as the risk of disease. While the risk is a useful summary of the relationship between disease and the risk factor, it is not sufficient to assess the importance of the risk factor. A high risk of developing disease in a group exposed to a certain factor does not implicate the factor as a possible risk factor unless a similar group of animals left unexposed to the factor show a lower risk of developing disease.

In this chapter we present some measures frequently used to determine the association between risk factor and disease as well as methods to assess the effect, i.e. the importance of the risk factor to the study population and target population.

7.2 The 2 × 2 table

To keep things simple we will for the remainder of this chapter focus on situations where data can be presented in a 2 × 2 table as displayed in Table 7.1. Quite often data of this kind will be obtained from an observational study, i.e. from a cross-sectional, a cohort or a case–control study. Let us here briefly remind ourselves how data are obtained in these different study types.

Table 7.1. *The 2 × 2 table for calculating measures of association and effect*

Risk factor status	Disease status		Total
	Disease	No disease	
Exposed	a	b	$a + b$
Not exposed	c	d	$c + d$
Total	$a + c$	$b + d$	n

In a cross-sectional study our primary interest is an estimate of the prevalence. We obtain a sample from the population under study by randomly selecting n animals (i.e. without regard to exposure or disease status) and afterwards assigning them to one of the four categories defined by Table 7.1 ((1) disease + exposed; (2) no disease + exposed; (3) disease + not exposed; and (4) no disease + not exposed). As we do not follow the animals over a time period, we cannot estimate the incidence risk; however, we can estimate the risk of disease (which is the prevalence among animals in the group) for the exposed ($a/(a + b)$) and the unexposed ($c/(c + d)$) group. This risk is sometimes referred to as the *prevalence risk*. Essentially, it is just the measure of prevalence already introduced in Chapter 6. However, here we add the term *risk* to acknowledge that our focus is the prevalence among animals exposed or unexposed to a certain *risk factor*.

In a cohort study we sample two initially disease-free groups of animals, one group exposed to the suspected risk factor and one group left unexposed. These groups are then followed over time and we can estimate the risk of developing disease (i.e. the incidence risk) for each group using $a/(a + b)$ for the exposed and $c/(c + d)$ for the unexposed. Thus, for a cohort study we have defined the groups row-wise, so we are allowed to make calculations and interpretations row-wise.

In a case–control study we sample column-wise. That is, we have selected a group of diseased (cases) and a group of non-diseased (controls) animals and then subsequently divided them into subgroups with respect to exposure status. This implies that we cannot justify calculating the same kind of risk as in the previous study: having selected column-wise, we cannot calculate measures row-wise, since there is no justification to assume that the proportion of diseased animals in the sample is the same as in the general population. It is, however, possible to calculate the risk of exposure to the risk factor for the diseased ($a/(a + c)$) and not diseased ($b/(b + d)$), but these measures are often of very little direct interest. The risk of exposure may also be calculated in a cross-sectional study, but there is little reason to do so. For case–control studies we abandon risk as a measure and turn to something else, i.e. odds. Before turning to this alternative we shall, however, give the risk measure some more attention.

7.3 Measures of association

7.3.1 *Risk and relative risk*

In this chapter we use a definition of risk that differs a bit from the one used to define incidence risk in Chapter 6. We define risk (r) as:

$$r = \frac{\text{\# animals with condition (i.e. disease or exposure)}}{\text{\# animals in population (or exposure group)}} \tag{7.1}$$

We will, in general, distinguish between incidence risk, prevalence risk and exposure risk, as mentioned in the previous section. As we assume that data are presented in a 2×2 table (Table 7.1) the above definition is valid for all three cases. However, the methods for calculating incidence risk presented in Chapter 6 should still be used whenever data permit.

There is no reason why one should not combine the exposed and unexposed groups of a cohort study and calculate the total risk of disease within the sample as $(a + c)/n$ (but be aware that this does not necessarily reflect the risk of disease in the target population). Still, as already mentioned the risk itself is an inadequate measure of the association between disease and exposure status. The risk needs to be compared to the risk in a similar group which has been unexposed. To make this comparison, the *relative risk* RR is defined:

$$\text{RR} = \frac{\frac{a}{a+b}}{\frac{c}{c+d}} = \frac{a(c+d)}{c(a+b)}, \tag{7.2}$$

i.e. the risk in the exposed group relative to the risk in the unexposed group. By definition it only makes sense to calculate the relative risk in a cohort or cross-sectional study, because risk is an inappropriate measure in a case–control study, as we have sampled column-wise. Whenever the value of RR is above 1, there is increased risk of disease for the exposed group, whereas a value below 1 means that exposure to the factor is protective.

By definition, the risk (r) is a probability (proportion), hence the standard error (se) according to general statistical rules (e.g. assuming that the proportion is normal distributed) is given as:

$$\text{se}(r) = \sqrt{\frac{r(1-r)}{n_r}} \tag{7.3}$$

Table 7.2. *Hypothetical data from a study regarding the association between feline hip dysplasia and the exercise options of cats. The letters in the subscripts refer to the notation in Table 7.1*

	Hip dysplasia		Total cats
	+	−	
Indoor	$50_{(a)}$	$150_{(b)}$	200
Outdoor	$20_{(c)}$	$780_{(d)}$	800
Total cats	70	930	1000

and the $(1 - \alpha)100\%$ confidence interval as:

$$r \pm Z_{1-\alpha/2}\text{se}(r), \tag{7.4}$$

where we use $Z_{1-0.05/2} = 1.96$ to calculate the 95% confidence intervals. In Equation 7.3, we have chosen to write n with a subscript n_r to indicate that the number of animals underlying the estimate depends on the estimate itself (e.g. for the risk of the exposed group, $n_r = a + b$, but for the entire sample population $n_r = a + b + c + d = n$).

The confidence interval for the relative risk is somewhat more complicated to compute. The relative risk can be regarded as the ratio between two approximative normal distributions. This is in itself not a normal distribution. However, it has been shown that the particular ratio defined as the relative risk, when log-transformed follows a normal distribution. On the logarithmic scale Katz *et al.* (1978) showed that the standard error of the relative risk is:

$$\text{se}(\ln \text{RR}) = \sqrt{\frac{1}{a} - \frac{1}{a+b} + \frac{1}{c} - \frac{1}{c+d}} \tag{7.5}$$

Using Equation 7.5 it is straightforward to establish a confidence interval for the log-transformed variable using Equation 7.4, which in turn leads to upper (U_{RR}) and lower (L_{RR}) confidence limits for the relative risk itself:

$$U_{\text{RR}} = \exp(\ln \text{RR} + Z_{1-\alpha/2}\text{se}(\ln \text{RR})) \tag{7.6}$$

$$L_{\text{RR}} = \exp(\ln \text{RR} - Z_{1-\alpha/2}\text{se}(\ln \text{RR})) \tag{7.7}$$

EXAMPLE 7.1. Lack of exercise might be a risk factor in feline hip dysplasia (HD). In Table 7.2 we present data from a hypothetical study regarding the association between HD in cats and their choice of exercise options, i.e. are the cats allowed outdoors or are they kept indoors.

We will use this example throughout the chapter; we will vary the study design accordingly to be able to apply the different measures. For now we consider that the data have been obtained in a cohort study, where the (initially healthy) cats are followed through a period of 5 years.

In such as study we can calculate the incidence risk for each group as well as the relative risk. The incidence risk (I_{risk}) of HD for the exposed (indoor) and unexposed (outdoor) is:

$$I_{risk}^I = \frac{50}{200} = 0.25, \qquad I_{risk}^O = \frac{20}{800} = 0.025$$

The relative risk (RR) is:

$$RR = \frac{\frac{a}{a+b}}{\frac{c}{c+d}} = \frac{I_{risk}^I}{I_{risk}^O} = \frac{0.25}{0.025} = 10$$

This implies that the incidence risk of HD (i.e. the risk that an initially healthy cat develops HD during a 5 year period) among cats kept indoors, is 10 times higher than among cats allowed outdoors. However, had the data in Table 7.2 originated from a cross-sectional study, then RR = 10 should be interpreted as a 10 times higher risk of finding a cat with HD among cats kept indoors, compared to cats allowed outdoors.

To calculate the confidence interval for the relative risk, we use Equation 7.5 to calculate the standard error of the log-transformed relative risk:

$$se(\ln RR) = \sqrt{\frac{1}{a} - \frac{1}{a+b} + \frac{1}{c} - \frac{1}{c+d}} = \sqrt{\frac{1}{50} - \frac{1}{200} + \frac{1}{20} - \frac{1}{800}} = 0.25$$

Applying this to Equations 7.6 and 7.7 we obtain the following 95% confidence interval for the relative risk:

$$U_{RR} = \exp(\ln RR + Z_{1-0.05/2}se(\ln RR)) = \exp(\ln 10 + 1.96 \times 0.25) = 16.4$$

$$L_{RR} = \exp(\ln RR - Z_{1-0.05/2}se(\ln RR)) = \exp(\ln 10 - 1.96 \times 0.25) = 6.1$$

i.e. a 95% CI: [6.1; 16.4].

7.3.2 Odds and odds ratio

A compulsive gambler knows that the risk, i.e. probability, is not the only measure of chance. There is an alternative called the *odds*:

$$odds = \frac{\text{\# animals with disease (or exposure)}}{\text{\# animals without disease (or unexposed)}} \qquad (7.8)$$

If P is the probability of disease (or exposure), then there is the following connection between odds and P:

$$odds = \frac{P}{1 - P}$$

The interpretation of odds is somewhat less intuitive than that of a risk.

The motivation to apply a measure such as odds lies not in the odds themselves but more in the ratio between two different odds, the *odds ratio*. For a cohort study, the odds ratio (OR_{CO}) for disease is estimated by the ratio between the odds of the exposed group and the odds of the unexposed group as:

$$OR_{CO} = \frac{\frac{a}{b}}{\frac{c}{d}} = \frac{ad}{bc}, \tag{7.9}$$

i.e. the odds of disease in the exposed group relative to the odds of disease in the unexposed group.

For a case–control study, however, the odds are defined in the columns as the ratio between exposed and unexposed for the diseased group and non-diseased group respectively. Hence, the odds ratio for a case–control study (OR_{CC}) is defined as:

$$OR_{CC} = \frac{\frac{a}{c}}{\frac{b}{d}} = \frac{ad}{bc}, \tag{7.10}$$

which is the odds of being exposed to the risk factor in the group of diseased animals relative to the odds of being exposed in the group of non-diseased animals.

Note that even though the odds ratios of the case–control and the cohort study are defined using different odds, the odds ratios are calculated in the same way. In a cross-sectional study both interpretations of the odds ratio are possible, but usually Equation 7.9 is preferred. Thus, it is possible to compare the results of different study designs using the odds ratios. Hence, from now on we will refer to the odds ratio as simply OR and omit the subscripts.

Although it is possible to calculate OR for all kinds of studies it is still very important to realise that there is a difference in the interpretation of OR for case–control studies compared to cohort and cross-sectional studies. The reason is that we cannot make inference row-wise in a case–control study, because the data were sampled column-wise. So in a cohort study, OR = 3 means that the odds of getting disease is three times greater for the group exposed to the factor in question compared to the unexposed group. For the case–control study, OR = 3 implies that odds of having been exposed to the factor is three times greater for the diseased group than for the non-diseased group of animals. Hence, to interpret the OR of a case–control study in terms of exposure being a risk factor, you need to be sure of the causality between exposure and outcome.

Another reason for adopting odds ratio is a matter of convenience in calculation (e.g. in logistic regression or analysis, see Chapter 13). Still, whenever possible, i.e. in cohort or cross-sectional studies, one should always calculate the relative risk because of the more intuitive interpretation of parameters expressed in terms of probabilities.

The odds themselves are rarely quoted in a study, because they are of limited interest. Thus, we will ignore the calculation of confidence intervals for these and only focus on the approach for the odds ratio. Woolf (1955) showed that a logarithmic transformation would yield a better approximation to a normal distribution with a standard error:

$$se(\ln OR) = \sqrt{\frac{1}{a} + \frac{1}{b} + \frac{1}{c} + \frac{1}{d}} \qquad (7.11)$$

Confidence limits for the OR itself are derived analogously to the relative risk (Equation 7.6):

$$U_{OR} = \exp(\ln OR + Z_{1-\alpha/2}se(\ln OR)) \qquad (7.12)$$

$$L_{OR} = \exp(\ln OR - Z_{1-\alpha/2}se(\ln OR)) \qquad (7.13)$$

EXAMPLE 7.2. Consider the table from Example 7.1 (Table 7.2). The odds ratio for these data is:

$$OR = \frac{ad}{bc} = \frac{50 \times 780}{150 \times 20} = 13$$

The standard error of the log-transformed OR (Equation 7.11) is:

$$se(\ln OR) = \sqrt{\frac{1}{50} + \frac{1}{150} + \frac{1}{20} + \frac{1}{780}} = 0.28$$

which gives a 95% confidence interval (Equations 7.12 and 7.13):

$$U_{OR} = \exp(\ln OR + Z_{1-0.05/2}se(\ln OR)) = \exp(\ln 13 + 1.96 \times 0.28) = 22.5$$

$$L_{OR} = \exp(\ln OR - Z_{1-0.05/2}se(\ln OR)) = \exp(\ln 13 - 1.96 \times 0.28) = 7.5$$

i.e. a 95% CI: [7.5; 22.5].

If we still assume that data are from a cohort study (and ignore that we normally would not calculate OR in such a case) we can interpret OR = 13 as odds being 13 times greater for developing HD among cats kept indoors compared to cats allowed outside.

However, if we assume that the data are from a case–control study, then we should interpret OR = 13 as odds of being kept indoors being 13 times greater among cats with HD than among those that do not develop HD. It is important to keep this distinction in mind when interpreting odds ratios.

The calculations in Examples 7.1 and 7.2 are good illustrations of the use of OR as an approximation of RR whenever the disease in question is rare. Referring to Table 7.1, the numbers defined by a and c must be small, because the prevalence $((a + c)/n)$ is low. Hence, it follows that:

$$a + b \approx b \qquad (7.14)$$

$$c + d \approx d \qquad (7.15)$$

Table 7.3. *Data for Example 7.3 to illustrate the need for the disease to be rare in both case and control groups when approximating the relative risk by the odds ratio*

Risk factor status	Disease status		Total
	Disease	No disease	
Exposed	3	3	6
Not exposed	5	989	994
Total	8	992	1000

where $\approx$ means approximately equal to. Combining Equations 7.9 and 7.2 gives:

$$\text{OR} = \frac{ad}{bc} \approx \frac{a(c+d)}{(a+b)c} = \text{RR} \tag{7.16}$$

However, the assumption of rare must be true for both the exposed and the unexposed group as the next example shows:

EXAMPLE 7.3. Consider the data in Table 7.3. Here, we have a case where disease is present in only eight out of 1000 cases. But the RR and OR, respectively, are:

$$\text{RR} = \frac{\frac{3}{6}}{\frac{5}{994}} = 99$$

$$\text{OR} = \frac{3 \times 989}{3 \times 5} = 197,$$

i.e. the OR is nearly twice as big as RR because there is a relatively high occurrence of disease within the exposed group even though the overall occurrence is rare. Note that the data in Table 7.3 are an example of a poor study design with only six exposed and eight cases in a total of 1000 study units.

7.4 Measures of effect

Through relative risk or odds ratio it is possible to establish the relative importance or association of the risk factor to the disease. However, this does not tell us the overall importance of that risk factor. To achieve this we must have a measure that combines the relative risk with the proportional occurrence of the risk factor (i.e. the prevalence of the risk factor). One possible measure is the *attributable risk*. The intuitive motivation is that there is a risk of developing disease even if the animal is left unexposed. The difference in the risk of developing disease between the exposed group and the unexposed group is the *attributable risk* (AR):

$$AR = \frac{a}{a+b} - \frac{c}{c+d} \tag{7.17}$$

Note that this is an absolute measure. It might be easier to use the relative equivalent, i.e. the fraction (proportion) of the total risk in the exposed group that refers to the subjects being exposed. This measure is called the *attributable fraction* (AF):

$$AF = \frac{\frac{a}{a+b} - \frac{c}{c+d}}{\frac{a}{a+b}} = \frac{AR}{\frac{a}{a+b}} = \frac{RR - 1}{RR} \tag{7.18}$$

The last part of the formula suggests that an approximation can be used in case–control studies. The result is the *estimated attributable fraction* (AF_{Est}):

$$AF_{Est} = \frac{OR - 1}{OR} \tag{7.19}$$

The precautions regarding the validity of the formula are essentially the same as the one underlying the substitution of odds ratio for relative risk, i.e. if OR is a poor estimate of RR, then AF_{Est} is a poor estimate of AF. In a case where it is possible to calculate AF directly, we should do so.

It is possible to calculate confidence intervals for AF, but the formula is rather tedious and is omitted. The interested reader is instead referred to Woodward (1999) for details.

EXAMPLE 7.4. Turn again to the data from Example 7.1 (Table 7.2) and assume that the data originate from a cohort study. Then Equation 7.17 gives the attributable risk (AR):

$$AR = \frac{a}{a+b} - \frac{c}{c+d} = \frac{50}{200} - \frac{20}{800} = 0.225,$$

i.e. the risk among indoor cats which may be attributed to them being indoors is 0.225 out of a total risk of 0.25. The attributable fraction (AF) is given from Equation 7.18 as:

$$AF = \frac{RR - 1}{RR} = \frac{10 - 1}{10} = 0.9,$$

thus 90% of the HD among indoor cats is due to their being kept indoors (and hence deprived of proper exercise).

The estimated attributable fraction (AF_{Est}) which should only be used in a case–control study is given here for comparison:

$$AF_{Est} = \frac{OR - 1}{OR} = \frac{13 - 1}{13} = 0.92,$$

which is only slightly different from the true AF.

In a cross-sectional study or whenever the sample is representative of the target population it is possible to estimate, not only the effect, but also the importance of the risk factor in the population. This is achieved by comparing the risk in the population to the risk in the unexposed group using the *population attributable risk* (PAR):

$$\text{PAR} = \frac{a+c}{n} - \frac{c}{c+d} = \frac{a+b}{n}\text{AR} \qquad (7.20)$$

which is completely analogous to the AR defined in Equation 7.17. PAR denotes the risk in the population that can be attributed to the risk factor. Again it might be easier to interpret the importance when expressed as a fraction of the total risk. Hence, we introduce the *population attributable fraction* (PAF):

$$\text{PAF} = \frac{\frac{a+c}{n} - \frac{c}{c+d}}{\frac{a+c}{n}} \qquad (7.21)$$

i.e. the proportion of cases in the population that are due to the risk factor. It is possible to estimate PAF using the population odds ratio (not defined here, see Table 7.6). However, we omit these calculations because the assumptions underlying this approximation are rarely fulfilled.

EXAMPLE 7.5. Assume for the time being that the data in Example 7.1 (Table 7.2) are from a cross-sectional study. This allows us to calculate the measures of effect defined as population attributable risk (PAR) and population attributable fraction (PAF) (Equations 7.20 and 7.21):

$$\text{PAR} = \frac{a+c}{n} - \frac{c}{c+d} = \frac{70}{1000} - \frac{20}{800} = 0.045 \qquad (7.22)$$

$$\text{PAF} = \frac{\frac{a+c}{n} - \frac{c}{c+d}}{\frac{a+c}{n}} = \frac{\frac{70}{1000} - \frac{20}{800}}{\frac{70}{1000}} = 0.64. \qquad (7.23)$$

Hence, the risk of HD in the population that may be attributed to indoor cats is 0.045. Hence, we would expect the total risk of HD in the population ($70/1000 = 0.07$) to drop 0.045 if all cats had access to outdoor exercise. (Note that this suggests that the overall risk would fall to the outdoor level (0.025).) The PAF of 0.64 implies that 64% of the HD cases in the population are due to some cats being housed indoors.

7.5 Summary of measures

To conclude this chapter we briefly summarise the measures of association, with respect to strength, effect and importance with the emphasis on the appropriate use in different types of study. For cross-sectional studies the

Table 7.4. *The applicable measures of association, effect and importance in a cross-sectional study*

Summations

		D		Total
		+	−	
E	+	a	b	$a+b$
	−	c	d	$c+d$
Total		$a+c$	$b+d$	n

D = diseased
E = exposed

Measure of association

Relative risk	$RR = \dfrac{\frac{a}{a+b}}{\frac{c}{c+d}}$	The relative risk is a measure of the *prevalence* risk
Odds ratio	$OR = \dfrac{ad}{bc}$	Interpret in rows, but use RR whenever possible
Population relative risk*	$RR_{pop} = \dfrac{\frac{a+c}{n}}{\frac{c}{c+d}}$	Note that the risks are not independent, as c and d are used in both risks
Population odds ratio*	$OR_{pop} = \dfrac{d(a+c)}{c(b+d)}$	Again, use RR_{pop} whenever possible

Measure of effect

Attributable risk	$AR = \dfrac{a}{a+b} - \dfrac{c}{c+d}$	This is an absolute measure of effect
Attributable fraction	$AF = \dfrac{AR}{\frac{a}{a+b}}$ $= \dfrac{RR-1}{RR}$	This is a relative measure of effect

Measure of importance

Population attributable risk	$PAR = \dfrac{a+c}{n} - \dfrac{c}{c+d}$ $= \dfrac{a+b}{n}AR$	This is an absolute measure of importance
Population attributable fraction	$PAF = \dfrac{\frac{a+c}{n} - \frac{c}{c+d}}{\frac{a+c}{n}}$	This is a relative measure of importance

*Not mentioned in this chapter.

summary is given in Table 7.4, for cohort studies in Table 7.5, and for case–control studies in Table 7.6. Some elements in the tables that have been excluded from the previous presentation, are included in the summary for completeness.

Table 7.5. *The applicable measures of association, effect and importance in a cohort study*

Summations

		D		Total
		+	−	
E	+	a	b	$a+b$
	−	c	d	$c+d$
Total		$a+c$	$b+d$	n

D = diseased
E = exposed

Measure of association

Relative risk	$RR = \dfrac{\frac{a}{a+b}}{\frac{c}{c+d}}$	The relative risk is a measure of the *incidence* risk
Odds ratio	$OR = \dfrac{ad}{bc}$	Interpret in rows, but use RR whenever possible
Population relative risk*	$RR_{pop} = \dfrac{\frac{a+c}{n}}{\frac{c}{c+d}}$	Use only when the cohorts are sampled so the ratio between exposed and un-exposed is representative of the target population

Measure of effect

Attributable risk	$AR = \dfrac{a}{a+b} - \dfrac{c}{c+d}$	This is an absolute measure of effect
Attributable fraction	$AF = \dfrac{AR}{\frac{a}{a+b}}$ $= \dfrac{RR-1}{RR}$	This is a relative measure of effect

Measure of importance

Population attributable risk	$PAR = \dfrac{a+c}{n} - \dfrac{c}{c+d}$ $= \dfrac{a+b}{n}AR$	An absolute measure of importance. Use only when the prevalence of disease in the sample is representative of the population prevalence
Population attributable fraction	$PAF = \dfrac{\frac{a+c}{n} - \frac{c}{c+d}}{\frac{a+c}{n}}$	A relative measure of importance. Use only when the prevalence of disease in the sample is representative of the population prevalence

*Not mentioned in this chapter.

There are, however, also measures that we have chosen to ignore both in the presentation and in the tables. One such measure is the *incidence rate ratio*, i.e. the ratio between the incidence rates in the exposed and unexposed groups (see Chapter 6 for a definition of incidence rate). The use of an incidence rate

Table 7.6. *The applicable measures of association, effect and importance in a case–control study*

Summations

		D +	D −	
E	+	a	b	
	−	c	d	
Total		$a + c$	$b + d$	n

$D =$ diseased
$E =$ exposed

Measure of association

Odds ratio	$OR = \dfrac{ad}{bc}$	Interpret in columns
Population odds ratio	$OR_{pop} = \dfrac{d(a + c)}{c(b + d)}$	Use only when the controls are sampled so the ratio between exposed and unexposed is representative of the target population

Measure of effect

Estimated attributable fraction	$AF_{Est} = \dfrac{OR - 1}{OR}$	Use when OR is a good approximation of RR, i.e. when the disease is rare in both the exposed and unexposed groups

Measure of importance

Estimated population attributable fraction*	$PAF_{Est} = \dfrac{OR_{pop} - 1}{OR_{pop}}$	Use only when OR_{pop} may be calculated

*Not mentioned in this chapter.

ratio is essentially that of a relative risk, but in terms of rates. This makes it somewhat less straightforward to interpret. Furthermore, the associated statistical tests for significance and calculation of confidence intervals are rather difficult compared to the relative risk. Other such measures might exist, but, in general, we recommend that you rely on the measures presented here. For a more thorough discussion and presentation of alternatives see, e.g. Kleinbaum *et al.* (1982).

Whenever there is serious doubt about the study design, one can always use the odds ratio. However, as we have emphasised in the text, the interpretation might differ depending on the study design used. As a starting point, each of the Tables 7.4–7.6 presents the 2 × 2 table with the summations, i.e. whether the study design allows column-wise, row-wise or both kinds of summation.

8 SAMPLE SIZE AND SAMPLING METHODS

Nils Toft, Hans Houe and Søren Saxmose Nielsen

8.1 Introduction

A central question in any epidemiological study is how many subjects to include in the study, i.e. what *sample size* to use. In connection with the sample size, the question of *how* to sample the subjects arises. Both of these questions are more naturally answered given that the question *'why* sample?' is addressed first. Hence, before using the formulas derived in this chapter, one should have a very clear idea of what will be a relevant result of the study regarding the object and the objective of the study (see Chapter 2), that is, e.g. to clearly define how big the difference between an exposed and an unexposed group should be to be deemed biologically important. Furthermore, the choice of objective might somehow influence how the sample may be obtained in order to ensure that the conclusions drawn from the study are in accordance with the objective.

It seems obvious that determining the sample size is a crucial part of any research project. Too large a sample means wasted time, money and resources. Too small a sample means that important results may be left undiscovered because the study lacks precision and power. For ethical reasons one should never use more animals than necessary in an experimental study, but conducting a study with a low power is a waste of animals that will suffer without contributing to science.

In veterinary epidemiology there has traditionally been a distinction between three different situations: (1) sampling for a survey; (2) sampling to detect presence of disease; and (3) sampling to detect a difference between groups. From a theoretical point of view, these three situations have very little in common. Some of the formulas derived in this chapter will be highly dependent on the underlying set of assumptions. Furthermore, the formulas generally cover only the most simple situations, i.e. sample size formulas for comparing two groups, rather than k groups. Despite these obvious limitations in the general applicability of the formulas presented here, we intend to not only present formulas covering a wide range of situations within the three general situations defined above, but also outline the basic concepts in the theory underlying each of the formulas. We believe that understanding the motivation for the formulas in the simplest cases will also provide useful insight for the reader who wishes to progress to the more complicated scenarios not covered in this book.

In general, it is an assumption underlying the derivation of sample size formulas, that the sampling units (or study units or the units of the study) are sampled so that all units in the study population have the same probability of being sampled, and the actual sample units are selected at random. However, in practice there are several methodologies for selecting a sample for a study, not all of which allow for such simple random selection of the study units. At the end of this chapter there will be a short discussion of some traditional sampling methods and how these might effect the necessary sample size.

8.2 Sampling for a survey

Suppose that the variable of interest, i.e. the weight of chickens, the frequency of lameness in dairy cows, etc., is unknown and that the study being planned is aimed at determining an initial estimate. Traditionally, we distinguish between a situation where it is reasonable to assume that the variable of interest follows a normal distribution (i.e. is a continuous trait such as weight) and the case where the proportion of affected animals (e.g. a prevalence) is the focus of investigation. The motivation for this distinction becomes obvious once the formulas are derived.

8.2.1 *Sample size to estimate a mean*

Consider the situation where the parameter of interest is a measurable quantity, e.g. the weight of white mice or the daily weight gain of pigs. It is often reasonable to assume that such quantities follow a normal distribution with mean (μ) and standard deviation (σ). The confidence interval of the mean of a normal distribution, where the standard deviation is assumed to *be known* is given by:

$$\hat{\mu} \pm Z_{1-\alpha/2}\frac{\sigma}{\sqrt{n}},\tag{8.1}$$

where $\hat{\mu}$ is the sample mean, n is the number of samples taken, σ is the known standard deviation and $Z_{1-\alpha/2}$ is the value of the standard normal distribution corresponding to a two-sided confidence level of $1 - \alpha/2$. This means that $Z_{1-0.05/2} = Z_{0.975} = 1.96$ is the Z-value where 2.5% of the probability mass lies to the right of Z and 2.5% lies to the left of $-Z$.

In Equation 8.1 the product at the righthand side of $\pm$ decides the width of the confidence interval. Assume that we want to fix this width at a certain size, say, L. Then L can be interpreted as the *maximum allowable error*, or said differently: L describes how much we can allow the final result to deviate from our initial guess. Equating the two terms

$$L = Z_{1-\alpha/2}\frac{\sigma}{\sqrt{n}},$$

and rearranging, it follows that the sample size to estimate a mean from a population with known standard deviation is given as:

$$n = \frac{Z_{1-\alpha/2}^2\sigma^2}{L^2} \tag{8.2}$$

EXAMPLE 8.1. Suppose you want to estimate the daily weight gain of slaughter pigs. From the literature you find out that a reasonable guess of a standard deviation (σ) is about 200 g/day. You require a confidence level of 95%, i.e. $Z_{1-\alpha/2} = 1.96$ and you will be content to know the average daily gain within ± 50 g/day ($L = 50$). Then the appropriate sample size is:

$$n = \frac{Z_{1-\alpha/2}^2\sigma^2}{L^2} = \frac{1.96^2 \times 200^2}{50^2} = 61.46 \approx 62.$$

In this kind of calculation you always round up.

If we believe that a standard deviation of 200 g/day might be too small we can redo the calculation with $\sigma = 250$ g/day:

$$n = \frac{1.96^2 \times 250^2}{50^2} = 96.04 \approx 97.$$

If we keep the original $\sigma = 200$ g/day, but reduce L to 20 g/day then:

$$n = \frac{1.96^2 \times 200^2}{20^2} = 384.14 \approx 385.$$

Finally, consider the original case, but the required level of confidence is lowered to 90%, i.e. $Z_{1-\alpha/2} = 1.64$:

$$n = \frac{1.64^2 \times 200^2}{50^2} = 43.03 \approx 44.$$

Example 8.1 illustrates the features of Equation 8.2. When the maximum allowable error (L) of our estimate is reduced the sample size increases. If we are sampling from a population with more variation, i.e. higher σ, then we need a larger sample size to obtain a confidence interval of the same width.

From Equation 8.2 we see that to calculate the adequate sample size for a study where the objective is to estimate the mean of a continuous trait such as daily weight gain of slaughter pigs, we do not need to have an idea in advance of the level of the mean, but it is important to have an idea of the variation of the trait, i.e. the standard deviation. The standard deviation is a property of the population that we are sampling from, it is in general not something that we can influence. This leaves us with only the confidence level and the maximum allowable error to adjust when aiming for a reduction of the required sample size. It is generally not advisable to deviate from the usual 95% confidence interval. Hence, the only choice is to accept that the maximum allowable error might be substantially larger than we originally intended, if the original choice of L proves to require too large a sample size. As Equation 8.2 is derived directly from Equation 8.1 which is based on an assumption of a normal distribution of μ, the sample size formula is of course invalid if this assumption is seriously compromised.

So far we have implicitly assumed that we are sampling from a population of infinite size. The motivation for this assumption is that the normal distribution has no limits. In theory it is possible to obtain values of any size, but with very low probability for values more than 2–3 times the standard deviation away from the mean. In a finite population there are known upper and lower limits, e.g. there is an animal with the largest value and one with the lowest. However, the assumption of a normal distribution does not account for that and as a consequence overestimates the effect of the standard deviation. To correct for this in the determination of the sample size, one should use:

$$n_a = \frac{n}{1 + \frac{n}{N}} = \frac{1}{\frac{1}{n} + \frac{1}{N}} \tag{8.3}$$

where n is the sample size calculated in Equation 8.2, N is the size of the population and n_a is the new *adjusted sample size*. As a rule of thumb the correction for final size should be carried out whenever $n/N > 0.1$. However, the correction can be made to reduce sample size, whenever there is a known population size. Thus, for expensive or time-consuming tests one can always apply the reduction factor if there is a finite size of the study population.

EXAMPLE 8.2. Assume that the previous example was concerned with estimating the average daily gain in a unit of 200 pigs. The sample size of 62 should be adjusted to:

$$n_a = \frac{1}{\frac{1}{n} + \frac{1}{N}} = \frac{1}{\frac{1}{62} + \frac{1}{200}} = 47.3 \approx 48$$

The formula used here might not be the most easy to interpret but it is certainly the easiest to carry out on a calculator. Should our interest be in a single pen with only 16 pigs, then

---

the required samples size reduces to 13. The required sample size will always reduce to a sample size below or equal to the total study population. But the sample will include a larger and larger proportion of the total population as the size of the study population decreases.

8.2.2 Sample size to estimate a proportion

Often we are concerned with estimating the prevalence of a certain feature, e.g. disease or presence of antibodies. Essentially, this is a question of determining the proportion of animals in a population that possesses a certain property, e.g. disease, sex or any other dichotomous trait.

Derivation of the sample size formula is analogous to the sample size for a mean. The starting point is the confidence interval for a proportion (p):

$$p \pm Z_{1-\alpha/2}\sqrt{\frac{p(1-p)}{n}} \tag{8.4}$$

where p is the proportion of interest. Again, if L is the maximum allowable error, then equating and rearranging gives the sample size to estimate a proportion:

$$n = \frac{Z_{1-\alpha/2}^2 p(1-p)}{L^2} \tag{8.5}$$

Note that the formula requires a guess of the size of the proportion being estimated. From Equation 8.5 it is seen that in the absence of such a guess, choosing $p = 0.5$ will give a sample size that is always adequate, because n is maximised when $p(1-p)$ is maximised which occurs at $p = 0.5$. Hence, $p = 0.5$ covers the worst case situation with respect to sample size, but at the cost of increasing the sample size. As for the case with a continuous trait, reducing the sample size to estimate a proportion can be done by allowing a larger error, i.e. increase L, but in general $Z_{1-\alpha/2}$ should be kept at 1.96 to reflect that calculations are based on a 95% confidence interval.

This sample size should also be corrected to allow for a finite population using Equation 8.3 in case the ratio between sample size (n) and population size (N) is large enough, i.e. $n/N > 0.1$.

EXAMPLE 8.3. Assume that you would like to know the prevalence of a certain microorganism in slaughter pigs. You are really uncertain about the true level, so you assume that the organism is present in 50% of the slaughter pigs ($p = 0.5$). You would like to know the prevalence within 10% points, i.e. between 45 and 55% for a prevalence of 50%. This corresponds to $L = 0.05$. Using a confidence level of 95% requires a sample size of:

$$n = \frac{Z_{1-\alpha/2}^2 p(1-p)}{L^2} = \frac{1.96^2 \times 0.5 \times (1-0.5)}{0.05^2} = 384.14 \approx 385$$

Should we desire a more narrow interval, say $L = 0.01$, then:

$$n = \frac{Z_{1-\alpha/2}^2 p(1-p)}{L^2} = \frac{1.96^2 \times 0.5 \times (1-0.5)}{0.01^2} = 9604$$

Now suppose that you are content with the original $L = 0.05$, but after careful examination of the available literature decide that a good guess of the prevalence is $p = 0.1$, then the sample size becomes:

$$n = \frac{Z_{1-\alpha/2}^2 p(1-p)}{L^2} = \frac{1.96^2 \times 0.1 \times (1-0.1)}{0.05^2} = 138.29 \approx 139$$

If the population in question was a section with 200 pigs, then the required sample sizes would be reduced to 132, 196 and 82 for the three situations above using Equation 8.3.

Assume that the study was performed by sampling from 385 pigs and found 46 positive samples, i.e. a prevalence of $46/385 = 0.12$. Now let us check what the error (L) of this estimate is. We can calculate the confidence interval:

$$p \pm Z_{1-\alpha/2}\sqrt{\frac{p(1-p)}{n}} = 0.12 \pm 1.96\sqrt{\frac{0.12(1-0.12)}{385}} = 0.12 \pm 0.032$$

i.e. between 8.8 and 15.2%. As expected, we find that for an estimate of prevalence in this range using 385 samples, $L = 0.032 < 0.05$ which was stated as the maximum allowable error.

8.3 Sampling to detect disease

Often the prevalence of a disease within a group of animals is more or less defined by the nature of the disease in question. Hence, a more interesting question is whether or not the disease is present in a herd, a flock or a geographic region (e.g. an island). We would very much prefer not to examine every animal in a herd or flock, but merely test a small sample. Still, to be 100% sure that a herd is disease free, we are required to examine virtually every animal within that herd.

Say that we are content to know with, e.g. 95% probability that the herd is disease free. Furthermore, we acknowledge that if disease is present in a herd, then it is usually present in more than one animal. Under these conditions the question becomes less hard to answer. What we seek to answer is: what is the necessary sample size to observe a probability P of finding at least one diseased animal in a population of size N, given that the prevalence of the disease is p?

Define $D = p \times N$, i.e. D is the number of diseased animals in the population, if the disease is actually present in the population. Assume that disease is present, and that we sample one animal from the population. The probability that this animal is diseased is D/N and the probability that the animal is not diseased is $1 - D/N = (N - D)/N$. Assume that we sample two animals.

The probability that both animals are negative then becomes:

$$\frac{N-D}{N} \times \frac{N-D-1}{N-1},$$

where the second term of the product is the probability that the second sample is negative conditional on the first sample being negative. If the first sample is negative, then one of the $N-D$ negative (or non-diseased) animals has already been sampled among the N animals, hence only $N-D-1$ negative animals remain among $N-1$ animals. The probability that both animals are negative in the sample is less than the probability that one animal in a sample of one is negative. Adding more animals to the sample will further decrease the probability that the sample contains only negative animals. Finally, for a sample of $N-D+1$ the probability of not selecting a positive animal becomes 0. We have sampled more animals than the number of negatives in the population, hence at least one positive must have been included. Define P as the probability of observing at least one diseased animal, then for a sample of n animals we have:

$$1-P = \frac{N-D}{N} \times \frac{N-D-1}{N-1} \times \cdots \times \frac{N-D-(n-1)}{N-(n-1)}$$

Thus to be 95% sure to observe at least one diseased animal, we simply increase n until the product is so small that $1-P < 0.05$, i.e. $P > 95\%$. Although this approach might give us the required sample size, we would much prefer to have an expression which gives us the sample size directly, i.e. isolate n. It is not straightforward to isolate n in the above expression, but fortunately a very good approximation to n can be found using:

$$n = \left(1 - (1-P)^{1/D}\right)\left(N - \frac{D-1}{2}\right) \tag{8.6}$$

where P is the probability of observing at least one diseased animal, N is the total number of animals in the population and D is the expected number of diseased animals, i.e. $D = p \times N$, where p is the assumed prevalence of disease within the herd. This prevalence must of course be based on the knowledge regarding the biology of the disease in question. For example, the decision to sample 60 eggs from each flock of laying hens for use in a salmonella control campaign seems to be based on the assumption that if present, the salmonella prevalence will be around 5%.

To determine the maximum possible number of cases present in a population of size N given that all n samples tested negative, more or less the same formula can be used:

$$D = \left(1 - (1 - P)^{1/n}\right)\left(N - \frac{n-1}{2}\right) \tag{8.7}$$

Both formulas assume that the test used for detection of disease have perfect sensitivity and specificity (see Chapter 9). In case this is not true, then the usual approach is to assume that no false-positives will pass through the additional examination of test positives, hence the specificity might be assumed to be 100% despite the shortcomings of the test itself. This assumption is crucial in the above discussion and derivation. If it cannot be justified that the specificity of the test is 100%, then a positive animal no longer necessarily implies that disease is present. It might just be a false-positive of the test, hence more sophisticated approaches for determining the appropriate sample size are needed. To allow for a sensitivity below 100% one simply reduces the prevalence by multiplying with the sensitivity (Se) of the test. This implies that the number of detectable cases becomes $D = Se \times p \times N$, since the apparent prevalence (the number of cases that the test detects) becomes $Se \times p$, when all test positives are truly diseased (for an elaboration of the difference between the true and apparent prevalences, see Chapter 9).

EXAMPLE 8.4. Assume that the prevalence of salmonella among broilers is 5% if the bacteria are present. We want to be 95% sure ($P = 0.95$) of detecting salmonella if it is present in the flock. In a house of $N = 10,000$ broilers there are $D = 0.05 \times 10,000 = 500$ detectable cases. The required sample size is:

$$n = \left(1 - (1 - P)^{1/D}\right)\left(N - \frac{D-1}{2}\right)$$

$$= \left(1 - (1 - 0.95)^{1/500}\right)\left(10,000 - \frac{500-1}{2}\right) = 58.25 \approx 59 \text{ broilers.}$$

Suppose that we actually test 100 broilers, which all turn out to be negative, then we can at most have:

$$D = \left(1 - (1 - P)^{1/n}\right)\left(N - \frac{n-1}{2}\right)$$

$$= \left(1 - (1 - 0.95)^{1/100}\right)\left(10,000 - \frac{100-1}{2}\right) = 294 \text{ cases,}$$

which corresponds to a prevalence of maximum 2.94%. So it is important to base the assumed prevalence on a solid biological foundation. Simply producing a 'good' guess might lead to a situation where results are seriously misinterpreted.

Now let us suppose that the test used for detection of salmonella in broilers is not perfect. Assume that a positive test result means that the sample actually is infected with salmonella (i.e. the specificity of the test is 100%); however, on average the test only detects 95 out of 100 truly infected samples (i.e. the sensitivity of the test is 95%). As discussed

---

above, this implies that we can no longer expect to have $D = 0.05 \times 10{,}000 = 500$ detectable cases as the test only finds 95% of the cases. Hence, we have $D = 0.95 \times 0.05 \times 10{,}000 = 475$ detectable cases, which requires a sample size of:

$$n = \left(1 - (1 - P)^{1/D}\right)\left(N - \frac{D-1}{2}\right)$$

$$= \left(1 - (1 - 0.95)^{1/475}\right)\left(10{,}000 - \frac{475-1}{2}\right) = 61.38 \approx 62 \text{ broilers}$$

to be 95% sure of detecting at least one positive. If the test has a sensitivity of 50% rather than the 95% used above, then the required sample size increases to 118 broilers.

Let us use the values from the example to explore how the required sample size to detect disease behaves when the assumptions are challenged a bit. We have produced two plots based on Equation 8.6. In Figure 8.1(a) it is illustrated how the assumption of prevalence determines the number of samples required to establish 95% certainty of disease detection in a population of 1000 animals. Starting with about 260 for $p = 0.01$ we end up with only one animal needed if $p = 1$ (since every animal is infected, only one is required). In Figure 8.1(b) we vary the population size from 1 to 1000 for an expected prevalence of $p = 0.05$ and $P = 0.95$. Note how the slope of the curve gradually reduces to 0. This implies that no matter how big a population we are sampling from, there is an upper limit on the number of samples required. In our case it is about 60.

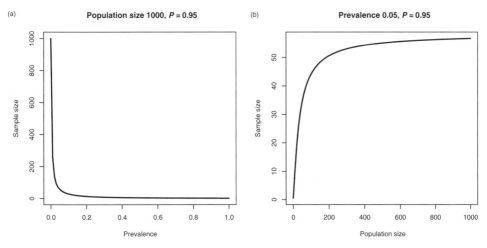

Figure 8.1. *Illustration of (a) the association between prevalence and sample size required to detect disease with 95% probability in a population of N = 1000 and (b) the association between population size and sample size required to detect disease with 95% probability in a population with prevalence p = 0.05.*

8.4 Sampling to detect a difference between groups

So far the problem has been to either establish a level for some variable, e.g. the prevalence in a region, or to detect the presence of disease. However, quite often our goal is either to explore whether a change has occurred or to compare the outcome between two different groups in an observational or experimental study. In general, we might need fewer animals for this kind of analysis compared to a survey. However, the formulas tend to get a bit more complicated. The objective is to detect a deviation (from a given value) or difference (between two groups) if it is present, while simultaneously ensuring that only real differences are found significant.

We will base our formulas on those presented in Woodward (1999) using the *power calculation method* (although it is called the power calculation method, both type I and type II errors are included in the calculation). Here, we will briefly outline the elements underlying this concept, but we refer the motivated reader to Woodward (1999).

8.4.1 *The power of a hypothesis test*

In Chapter 13.2 we give a general introduction to hypothesis testing, but we need to outline some elements here in order to proceed. The key to understanding the motivation for the sample size calculations derived in the remainder of this chapter lies in accepting a basic concept in hypothesis testing: *the decision to accept or reject the null hypothesis might be wrong.*

If we reject the null hypothesis and conclude a significant effect, when there is no true difference we are making a type I error (see Table 8.1). The type I error is denoted by α and is called the *significance level*, often set to 0.05 (5%). The *confidence* of a test is the probability that the null hypothesis is accepted when it is correct.

Alternatively, if we accept the null hypothesis and conclude a non-significant effect when there truly is a difference, we are making a type II

Table 8.1. *The type I and type II errors in hypothesis testing*

		True condition	
		H_0 true	H_0 false
H_0 hypothesis	Accepted (not rejected)	Correct decision $1 - \alpha$: Confidence	Type II error: β
	Rejected	Type I error: α α, significance level	Correct decision $1 - \beta$: Power

error (Table 8.1). The type II error is usually denoted β and $1 - \beta$ is called the power of the test ($1 - \beta$ is often set to 80%). Hence the *power* of a hypothesis test is the probability that the null hypothesis is rejected when it is false.

Having determined the significance level and power that we wish to achieve for a hypothesis test we can establish the corresponding sample size formulas. However, deriving the specific formulas depends on the context and becomes quite hard for more complicated hypotheses. Consider for illustrative purposes the case where we wish to test a mean value against a one-sided alternative, i.e.:

$$H_0: \quad \mu \leq \mu_0$$

$$H_1: \quad \mu > \mu_0$$

If we assume that the standard deviation σ of the population is known, then to test this hypothesis we must calculate the test statistic (Z):

$$Z = \frac{\bar{x} - \mu_0}{\sigma / \sqrt{n}},$$

which should be compared to a standard normal distribution, i.e. we reject H_0, whenever $Z > 1.64$ for a 5% significance level in a one-sided test situation. In general we reject H_0 at the $(1 - \alpha) \times 100\%$ confidence level, whenever $Z > Z_{1-\alpha}$.

The definition of power simply means that:

$$\text{Power} = \Pr\{Z > Z_{1-\alpha} \mid H_1 \text{ true}\}$$

i.e. the probability that Z exceeds $Z_{1-\alpha}$ given that the alternative hypothesis H_1 is true (equals the probability that the null hypothesis is rejected when it is false). The vertical line in the formula denotes the term 'given that'. Suppose that we change our alternative hypothesis from $\mu > \mu_0$ to $\mu = \mu_1$, i.e. a specific alternative to μ_0. Under this new H_1: $\mu = \mu_1$ the definition of power becomes:

$$\text{Power} = \Pr\{Z > Z_{1-\alpha} \mid \mu = \mu_1\} \tag{8.8}$$

Standardising with respect to the mean μ_1 and rewriting to once again compare to a standard normal distribution Equation 8.8 implies that:

$$\text{Power} = \Pr\left\{Z < \frac{\mu_1 - \mu_0}{\sigma / \sqrt{n}} - Z_{1-\alpha}\right\} \tag{8.9}$$

In Figure 8.2 we have illustrated the concept of the significance (or confidence level) and the power of a test. From Figure 8.2 and Equation 8.8 it can be deduced that a sample size based on the power calculation method will increase whenever (1) the standard deviation (σ) increases (this will widen the shape of the distributions), (2) the confidence level increases (this will cause a

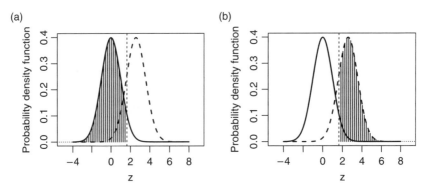

Figure 8.2. *Distributions of test statistic value Z, the left-hand distribution (solid line) represents the null hypothesis and the right-hand distribution (dashed line) the alternative hypothesis. In (a) the confidence (shaded area) of the test under the assumption that H_0 is true is shown. In (b) the power (shaded area) of the test (the probability of accepting H_1 when it is true) is shown.*

right shift in point Z, unless the sample size is increased to reduce the standard error of the sample distribution, (3) the power increases (which has the same effect as an increase in confidence level, only on the alternative distribution), and finally (4) the difference between the null hypothesis and the alternative decreases (i.e. the difference between μ_0 and μ_1 decreases).

8.4.2 *Sample size to test a difference between means*

If we wish to determine whether there is a *difference* between two means we have to define the size of this difference. Is a gap of, say 2, really a difference? This depends on what is measured. A gap in daily milk yield of 2 kg energy corrected milk (ECM), i.e. from 20 to 22 can be interesting. However, a difference between 10,000 kg ECM and 10,002 kg ECM in the annual milk yield of dairy cows is not important. Determining what is considered a relevant difference is thus crucial to further planning of the study.

Define d as the expected difference between the mean of two groups of animals, regarding some specific continuous trait of interest. Our hypothesis to be tested may be written as:

$$H_0: \quad \mu_1 = \mu_2$$

$$H_1: \quad \mu_2 - \mu_1 = d \neq 0$$

We will assume that the standard deviation σ is identical in the two groups, and furthermore we will require a significance level, α, and a power $1 - \beta$. The appropriate sample size to select from each group can be derived from

Equation 8.8 as:

$$n = \frac{2(Z_\beta + Z_{1-\alpha})^2 \sigma^2}{d^2} \tag{8.10}$$

If we wish to test against a two-sided alternative, i.e. we are uncertain about the true direction of a difference, then $Z_{1-\alpha}$ should be replaced by $Z_{1-\alpha/2}$, i.e.:

$$n = \frac{2(Z_\beta + Z_{1-\alpha/2})^2 \sigma^2}{d^2} \tag{8.11}$$

for a two-sided test.

A closer examination of the elements of Equations 8.10 and 8.11 tells us how to reduce the sample size of a study: (1) reduce the confidence level (which reduces $Z_{1-\alpha}$ or $Z_{1-\alpha/2}$); (2) reduce the power (which reduces Z_β); (3) reduce the standard deviation (σ); and finally (4) increase the difference, d, that has been suggested as important. While it is possible to adjust conditions (1), (2) and (4) without too much difficulty, the standard deviation in condition (3) should be regarded as a property of the target population of the study. The standard deviation simply reflects the variation within the target population. However, it is still possible to aim for a lower standard deviation between the sampled individuals and thus reduce the required sample size by this approach. This is often done in early phases of an experimental study by, e.g. selecting litter mates, which are supposed to have less genetic variation than the total population.

Using Equation 8.10 or the two-sided alternative (Equation 8.11) as a starting point, the *minimum detectable difference* (δ) can be derived:

$$\delta = \sqrt{\frac{2}{n}}(Z_\beta + Z_{1-\alpha})\sigma \tag{8.12}$$

for a one-sided test and

$$\delta = \sqrt{\frac{2}{n}}(Z_\beta + Z_{1-\alpha/2})\sigma \tag{8.13}$$

for a two-sided test. Here δ is the minimum difference the test can determine between two groups, if the sample size in each group is n and the power and significance levels are $1 - \beta$ and α, respectively.

EXAMPLE 8.5. A manufacturer of a feed additive claims that there is a gain of at least 2 kg ECM per day from each cow using their supplement opposed to the one produced by the competitors. From the literature you obtain an estimate of the standard deviation in daily milk yield of $\sigma = 2.92$ kg ECM per day. If we require a power of 80% and a significance of 5% of the result in a two-sided test, then $Z_\beta = 0.84$ and $Z_{1-\alpha} = 1.96$. The required sample

---

size is calculated from Equation 8.11 as:

$$n = \frac{2(Z_\beta + Z_{1-\alpha/2})^2\sigma^2}{d^2} = \frac{2(0.84 + 1.96)^2 2.92^2}{2^2} = 33.4 \approx 34$$

Hence we require 34 cows fed on the acclaimed feed additive and 34 fed on a competitor's brand. As factors such as the stage of lactation and the parity also influence the daily milk yield of cows, the cows used in the study should probably be sampled very carefully in order to ensure that an observed difference is due to the feed additives and not other traits such as stage of lactation.

Suppose that for some reason we can only test each brand with 15 cows. From Equation 8.13 we see that:

$$\delta = \sqrt{\frac{2}{n}}(Z_\beta + Z_{1-\alpha/2})\sigma = \sqrt{\frac{2}{15}}(0.84 + 1.96)2.92 = 2.99$$

So we can only detect a significant difference in daily milk yield in ECM, if the difference exceeds 2.99 kg ECM per day. An alternative in such a situation would be to decrease the power and increase the significance level of the test to reduce the certainty that we can establish the claimed difference of 2 kg ECM per day.

It is possible to extend Equations 8.10 and 8.11 to allow for different sample sizes in the two groups. However, we refer to Woodward (1999) for details.

Sometimes we have a study with data in two groups, that are not independent. If they are paired (for example, measurements before and after some medical intervention), then the appropriate way to proceed is by analysing the difference between measurements on individual subjects.

Thus, we reduce the situation to a one-group scenario, with measurements being the difference between original measurements. This implies that we should adopt Equation 8.2 from Section 8.2.1 rather than the formulas derived here.

Note that L will be the difference defined to be interesting (since no difference between the measurements will result in a mean of 0) based on the objective of the study. The standard deviation that is used here reflects the variation of *the difference* which must be assessed prior to the study.

8.4.3   *Sample size to test a relative risk*

Assume now that we are interested in outcomes expressed as proportions. The two-sample problem is then to compare two proportions. However, rather than test the difference we will test the ratio between the proportions, i.e. the relative risk (RR $= p_1/p_2$, where $p_1 = \Pr\{D+ \mid E+\}$ and $p_2 = \Pr\{D+ \mid E-\}$) as discussed in Chapter 7. Hence, the null hypothesis to be tested against an alternative is:

$$H_0: \quad RR = \frac{p_1}{p_2} = 1 \tag{8.14}$$

$$H_1: \quad RR = \frac{p_1}{p_2} \neq 1 \tag{8.15}$$

If we focus only on situations with equal-sized groups, then the pooled risk (p_c) (i.e. the common risk of the entire population) is estimated as:

$$p_c = \frac{p_1 + p_2}{2} = \frac{p(RR + 1)}{2}$$

where $p = p_2$ is the risk in the unexposed group. Using the power calculation method, the required sample *in each group* turns out to be:

$$n = \frac{\left[Z_{1-\alpha/2}\sqrt{2p_c(1 - p_c)} + Z_\beta\sqrt{RR \times p(1 - RR \times p) + p(1 - p)}\right]^2}{(RR - 1)^2 \times p^2} \tag{8.16}$$

To do a one-sided test $Z_{1-\alpha/2}$ is replaced by $Z_{1-\alpha}$. Observe that n depends on p_2, the risk in the unexposed group. Often this proportion will have to be estimated from past experience or other sources. The sample size also depends on how large a relative risk is considered important. The following example illustrates this.

EXAMPLE 8.6. A cohort study of milking systems and teat lesions is being planned. The aim is to establish whether or not there is a difference in the proportion of teat lesions between cows milked in automatic milking systems (AMS) and manual systems (i.e. where suction cups are placed by a person). It is decided that a relative risk of 1.3 against AMS is relevant. The study period is set to be 12 months. Previous studies have indicated that there is an annual risk of teat lesions in traditional systems of 15% per teat. We seek a significance level of 5% and a power of 80% in a two-sided test. The estimate of the common proportion is:

$$p_c = \frac{p(RR + 1)}{2} = \frac{0.15(1.3 + 1)}{2} = 0.1725$$

The required sample size in each group is:

$$n = \frac{\left[Z_{1-\alpha/2}\sqrt{2p_c(1 - p_c)} + Z_\beta\sqrt{RR \times p \times (1 - RR \times p) + p(1 - p)}\right]^2}{(RR - 1)^2 \times p^2}$$

$$= \frac{\left[1.96\sqrt{2 \times 0.1725(1 - 0.1725)} + 0.84\sqrt{1.3 \times 0.15(1 - 1.3 \times 0.15) + 0.15(1 - 0.15)}\right]^2}{(1.3 - 1)^2 \times 0.15^2}$$

$$= 1104.1 \approx 1105$$

Hence we must include 1105 teats from cows milked in AMS and 1105 teats from cows milked in manual systems in the study. Strictly speaking, they should be selected randomly among all teats, but one might use all four teats of a selected cow for convenience.

However, suppose we think that RR must be at least 2.3 for the difference to be important, then we require only:

$$n = \frac{\left[Z_{1-\alpha/2}\sqrt{2p_c(1-p_c)} + Z_\beta\sqrt{RR \times p(1 - RR \times p) + p(1-p)}\right]^2}{(RR - 1)^2 \times p^2}$$

$$= \frac{\left[1.96\sqrt{2 \times 0.2475(1 - 0.2475)} + 0.84\sqrt{2.3 \times 0.15(1 - 2.3 \times 0.15) + 0.15(1 - 0.15)}\right]^2}{(2.3 - 1)^2 \times 0.15^2}$$

$$= 75.6 \approx 76$$

teats in each group.

8.4.4 Sample sizes in case–control studies

Recall from Chapter 7 that in a case–control study it is not possible to compare
the risk of disease between the exposed and the unexposed. Thus, we cannot
test the desired hypothesis against the alternative in the form of Equation 8.14.
What we can do is to test:

$$H_0^*: \quad \lambda = 1 \tag{8.17}$$

$$H_1^*: \quad \lambda \neq 1 \tag{8.18}$$

where $\lambda = p_1^*/p_2^*$ with $p_1^* = \Pr\{E + |D+\}$ and $p_2^* = \Pr\{E + |D-\}$. Unfortunately,
we are not interested in studying exposure but disease. This means that we
must try to express the components of H_0^* and H_1^* in terms of something that
we are interested in. It turns out that we can use $p_e = \Pr\{E+\}$, the prevalence
of the risk factor and the relative risk $RR = p_1/p_2$. Using Bayes Theorem
we find:

$$p_1^* = \Pr\{E + |D+\}$$

$$= \frac{\Pr\{D + |E+\}\Pr\{E+\}}{\Pr\{D + |E+\}\Pr\{E+\} + \Pr\{D + |E-\}(1 - \Pr\{E+\})}$$

$$= \frac{p_1 \times p_e}{p_1 \times p_e + p_2 \times (1 - p_e)}$$

$$= \frac{p_1/p_2 \times p_e}{p_1/p_2 \times p_e + (1 - p_e)}$$

$$= \frac{RR \times p_e}{1 + (RR - 1) \times p_e}$$

and by assuming that the chance of exposure in general is equal to the chance of exposure among non-diseased we get:

$$p_2^* = \Pr\{E+ |D-\} \approx \Pr\{E+\} = p_e$$

Note that we cannot estimate the relative risk from a case–control study. Still it seems fair to only estimate the odds ratio in cases where the relative risk is above a level that we find relevant. The approximated formula (expressed using RR and p_e) for the sample size (of each group) for a case–control study where we assume equal-sized groups then becomes:

$$n = \frac{(1 + (RR - 1)p_e)^2}{p_e^2(p_e - 1)^2(RR - 1)^2}$$

$$\times \left[Z_{1-\alpha/2}\sqrt{2p_c^*(1 - p_c^*)} + Z_\beta\sqrt{\frac{RRp_e(1 - p_e)}{(1 + (RR - 1)p_e)^2} + p_e(1 - p_e)} \right]^2 \quad (8.19)$$

where

$$p_c^* = \frac{p_1^* + p_2^*}{2} = \frac{p_e}{2}\left(\frac{RR}{1 + (RR - 1)p_e} + 1\right) \quad (8.20)$$

Equation 8.19 gives the required sample size for a two-sided test. To get the formula for a one-sided test, replace $Z_{1-\alpha/2}$ by $Z_{1-\alpha}$.

EXAMPLE 8.7. Suppose that we did a case–control study rather than the cohort study from Example 8.6. We are looking for a change in the relative risk (which is reasonably approximated by the odds ratio) of RR = 2.3 and the proportion of AMS (the exposure) is found to be 10% ($p_e = 0.1$). Assume the same significance level and power as before (5 and 80%), and that we seek the sample size for a two-sided test. Substituting into Equation 8.20

$$p_c^* = \frac{0.1}{2}\left(\frac{2.3}{1 + (2.3 - 1)0.1} + 1\right) = 0.15$$

Then, by Equation 8.19, the sample size required for each group (of cases and controls, respectively) is:

$$n = \frac{(1 + (2.3 - 1)0.1)^2}{0.1^2(0.1 - 1)^2(2.3 - 1)^2} \left[1.96\sqrt{2 \times 0.15(1 - 0.15)} \right.$$

$$\left. + 0.84\sqrt{\frac{2.3 \times 0.1(1 - 0.1)}{(1 + (2.3 - 1)0.1)^2} + 0.1(1 - 0.1)} \right]^2 = 185.8 \approx 186$$

8.5 Sampling and allocation methods

The remainder of this chapter addresses the other element of sampling: *how* to sample the units for the study. A similar problem arises in experimental studies, where the question is not so much how to sample the units, but how to allocate the subjects available for the study to the different groups. While many of the elements in the next sections are discussed in the context of sampling for observational studies, most of the elements relate to allocation issues as well. However, we address specific elements of allocation of sampling units in experimental studies at the end of the chapter.

The formulas for sample sizes derived in this chapter all assumed that all sampling units (animals, herds, etc.) were sampled randomly using simple (or completely) random sampling which will be defined shortly. However, in practice it is often difficult or impossible to obtain a random sample. A proper random sample of animals from the Danish cattle population for blood testing would mean that we would have to drive to a large number of herds at many different places. Obtaining a truly random sample is therefore often expensive and time-consuming. Further, the owner of some of the randomly selected herds may not want to participate in the study. When planning a study it is therefore important to consider different alternatives to random sampling or modifications of random sampling that still give good representation of the population.

8.5.1 *Simple random sampling*

In simple random sampling, all animals in the study population are listed (i.e. numbered), and the desired sample is drawn using a formal random process. The random selection can be done using the principle from lottery. All animal numbers are written on separate pieces of paper and put in a 'hat' and the desired sample is drawn blindly. Often it is easier to use random number tables available in statistical textbooks or have a computer generate random numbers. Assume you have 938 animals in the study population and want a random sample of 100 animals. First you list all animals from 1 to 938. Then you look up in a random number table, by selecting an arbitrary starting place and a direction, and the numbers are written down selecting three digits at a time. You just reject numbers higher than 938. You may also want to reject numbers selected more than once, e.g. in a prevalence survey it would not make sense to test the same animal twice. This continues until 100 different numbers between 1 and 938 have been selected. Obviously, the approach of using a computer program to generate a sequence of 100 random numbers between 1 and 938 has more appeal since this can be done in, e.g. a spreadsheet with considerably less effort. A common mistake is to assume that just jumbling down 100 numbers on a piece of paper will generate a random sequence. We encourage you to try this yourself and see how non-random your sample will be.

8.5.2 Systematic random sampling

In systematic random sampling the animals are sampled at equal intervals of sampling units, e.g. every tenth animal is desired for a survey. The first animal is randomly selected among the first 10 animals, for example, number 7. Hereafter number 17, 27, 37, etc. are selected. If all animals on the list are sorted according to age the procedure will ensure that the sample contains animals from all age groups. Systematic random sampling also has the advantage that it can be performed without having a list of all animals. You can simply start sampling by taking, e.g. every tenth animal at a slaughter line.

8.5.3 Stratified random sampling

There is often a desire to ensure that different strata (i.e. different levels of a (risk) factor) in the study population are represented. It may be relevant that different breeds or age groups are represented in the sample. Using 100 herds as study population we can ensure that a certain percentage of herds or cattle consists of Jersey breed, etc. Afterwards, we can select animals randomly within each stratum. This may have the advantage that we can increase the sample size in strata where the variation is known to be higher.

8.5.4 Cluster sampling

Cluster sampling selects groups (clusters) of animals. However, the study unit is still the individual animal and by definition all animals in the cluster are sampled. Typical clusters consist of herds or litters or pens, i.e. animals that are physically located together. The technique therefore has practical advantages. Usually the same treatment is applied to the entire cluster. Thus, the estimates are often less precise than random or systematic sampling because of higher variation between than within groups. Dohoo *et al.* (2003) suggests the following formula to adjust the sample size when cluster sampling is applied:

$$n_C = n(1 + \rho_{IC}(c - 1)) \qquad (8.21)$$

where n_C is the adjusted sample size, n is the original sample size estimate determined by one of the methods given in this chapter, ρ_{IC} is the intracluster correlation coefficient (see Chapter 13 for a definition of correlation coefficients) and c is the size of the cluster, i.e. the average litter or pen size.

From Equation 8.21 it can be seen that the adjusted sample size is always larger than the original estimated sample size when ρ_{IC} is assumed to be positive. The intra-cluster correlation measures the degree to which the observations within a cluster are similar. Thus, the higher the intra-cluster correlation coefficient, the higher the adjusted sample size needs to be. The same applies to the cluster size, the larger the cluster, the higher the increase in sample size.

8.5.5 Multistage sampling

In multistage sampling the selection occurs at more than one level. The difference from cluster sampling is that not all animals within the cluster are sampled. Sampling of 100 dairy herds among all dairy herds in Denmark followed by selection of 10 animals in each herd is a multistage sampling where the herds are the primary sampling units and animals within the herd are the secondary sampling units. Sampling 100 sow herds followed by selection of five litters per herd and three piglets per litter would be a three-stage sampling with herd as primary unit, litter as secondary unit and piglets as tertiary sampling unit.

8.5.6 Non-probability sampling

In practice, it is often much easier to select animals about which you have some prior knowledge. You may know the owners of the animals and that they are very collaborative. It may also be convenient to select herds that participate in other studies because some data are already available or you may prefer herds that are located close to where you live. Such sampling is called convenience sampling. The samples may have considerable problems with bias. For example, farmers that have some expectation of presence of an infectious disease may be more willing to participate in a prevalence survey involving testing of all animals simply because they get a free test of the animals. Therefore, the survey will overestimate the prevalence. In other situations, the farmers may not be interested in having their disease status confirmed which will underestimate the prevalence.

If we want to perform a risk factor study where one of the risk factors seldom occurs, we may deliberately choose animals known to have been exposed to the factor together with control animals without exposure. Similarly we may want to select animals known to have a certain disease. This type of sampling is called purposive sampling.

8.5.7 Combinations of sampling methods

In many practical situations the methods of sampling are combined in different ways. The example below outlines the elements in the sampling carried out in a survey for BVDV antibodies among young stock (Houe, 1994).

EXAMPLE 8.8. A survey for BVDV antibodies among young stock selected 500 animals among 50 herds using the following approach (Houe, 1994) (Figure 8.3). For convenience, the primary sampling unit was restricted to three counties in Jutland. As secondary sampling unit, only veterinary practices servicing more than 20 dairy herds were selected. Among these, 10 practices were randomly selected. In each practice, five herds (the tertiary sampling unit) were selected by random sampling. Finally, 10 heifers between the ages of 8 and 18 months (the quaternary sampling unit) were selected in each herd. The animals were selected using systematic random sampling based on the following method. In each herd, the heifers from the 8–18 month age group were listed according to age and every $N/10$ animal was selected with N being the number of animals in the age group 8–18 months in the herd. Initially, a starting point between 1 and $N/10$ was sampled. The total sampling procedure thus has elements of convenience sampling, simple random sampling, systematic random sampling and multistage sampling.

The procedure in Example 8.8 had several advantages, many of which of course were related to the purpose of the study. The hypothesis was that in herds with animals that were persistently infected, PI (i.e. virus carriers), the infection pressure would be very high and thus almost all animals would be antibody positive. In herds without PI animals the infection would either be absent or there would be a very low infection pressure. The idea was that rather than testing all animals in the herds, it would be sufficient initially just to test a few young stock for antibodies. Then, whole-herd screening would only be necessary where there were many antibody carriers among young stock. The reason to test animals in the age group 8–18 months was that older animals could be antibody positive due to infection having occurred a long time ago (not revealing the present situation). Calves younger than 8 months could be antibody positive due to colostrum.

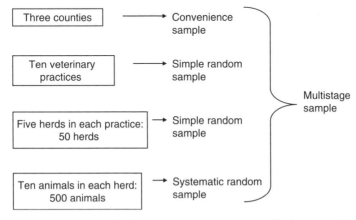

Figure 8.3. *Sampling strategy for developing a BVDV screening test for detection of herds containing PI animals.*

The calculation of sample size in the individual herd was based on an earlier finding where herds with PI animals typically had more than 80% antibody carriers, whereas herds without such animals typically had less than 10% antibody carriers. Using the sample size formula for estimating a proportion (Equation 8.5):

$$n = \frac{Z^2_{1-\alpha/2}\, p(1-p)}{L^2}$$

with a maximum allowable error of 30% ($L = 0.3$) to ensure that the herd was a high-prevalence versus a low-prevalence herd gives the following sample sizes for the two situations:

High-prevalence herd:

$$N = \frac{1.96^2 \times 0.8 \times 0.2}{0.3^2} = \text{seven animals}$$

Low-prevalence herd:

$$N = \frac{1.96^2 \times 0.1 \times 0.9}{0.3^2} = \text{four animals}$$

As it could not be known *a priori* whether a herd belonged to the high- or the low-prevalence category the sample size should have been 7. For convenience 10 was selected as the sample size.

8.5.8 *Block randomisation*

A key point in allocation of sample units to a study, whether it is an experimental study or an observational study is to ensure a reasonable balance of the groups, i.e. to have approximately the same number of animals assigned to the specific treatments or cohorts. Quite often the number of units available for experimental studies is restricted, hence it becomes more important to ensure balance in the study when assigning the units to the different groups.

One possibility is to adopt a block randomisation, where we assure that every block of n animals is balanced.

EXAMPLE 8.9. Suppose we have an experimental study with a parallel group design, i.e. two groups receiving different treatments (A and B). We would like to ensure that for every $n = 12$ animals we have balance in the design. For randomisation one could simply toss a coin; however, we prefer to draw random numbers between 0 and 9. Even numbers means treatment A and odd numbers treatment B. Using a sequence of 12 digits (124526128298) results in the sequence BAABAABAABBB, where the last three Bs are assigned to ensure balance between groups, even though the sequence suggested two more treatment A assignments.

8.6 Further reading

The power calculation method and more general formulas are covered intensively in Woodward (1999). Alternative derivations of sample size formulas are given in, e.g. Snedecor and Cochran (1967).

9 EVALUATING DIAGNOSTIC TESTS

Søren Saxmose Nielsen, Hans Houe, Annette Kjær Ersbøll and Nils Toft

9.1 Introduction

A key role for the veterinary practitioner is to make a diagnosis. Unless some pathognomonic signs, i.e. features unique to a disease, are seen, some technical tools are necessary to help making the final diagnosis. These technical tools are called diagnostic tests (diagnosis (Greek): dia – through; gnosis – knowledge). Also, the clinical examination by itself can actually be seen as a diagnostic test. For convenience, a *diagnosis* is often separated into different entities, depending on the diagnostician. The clinician usually makes a clinical diagnosis based on clinical signs. A pathologist bases the diagnosis on pathological lesions, whereas microbiologists may prefer an aetiological diagnosis where a specific aetiological agent has been detected. The definition of diagnosis must refer to the study outcome rather than to one's profession (see Chapter 2 for a definition of study outcomes and Chapter 3 for disease clarification). A key element in preventive veterinary medicine is to determine the disease status in populations, either to establish a prognosis for disease development or to do screening for pathogens or pathological conditions. The technical tools used for these purposes are prognostic tests and screening tests, respectively. In some contexts, all three tests are referred to as diagnostic tests and in this chapter the term *test* is used to include all three concepts. However, *diagnostic*, *prognostic* and *screening* tests are basically three different tests, a difference that relates to their purpose. This chapter will deal with the various types of tests, calculation of test performance and the evaluation of tests. The performance measures are calculated similarly, but their interpretations are different. For tests with more than two outcomes their performance and use are discussed. In some disease situations, more tests are preferred and simple calculations for multiple testing are shown.

9.2 Types of tests

Diagnostic tests include a wide range of technical and non-technical methods that may aid in obtaining a final diagnosis. Basic diagnostic tests include auscultation of the heart and lungs, evaluation of hair coat, etc., all of which may be person dependent and contain some degree of subjectivity. More objective tests include laboratory and other technical tests, which are based on strict protocols. Common to all these tests is that they measure whether something is normal or deviates from normal. In the ideal situation, 'normal' is the absence of an indicator that something is 'wrong', e.g. absence of pathogenic bacteria such as *Salmonella* spp. in samples from an animal. In other situations, 'normal' is when something is in a certain range, e.g. body temperature is $37.5 \pm 0.5°C$. When normal is defined in such a manner, further knowledge about criteria for normality for subgroups of animals is required. For example, body temperature differs with different animal species and younger animals usually have higher normal temperature than older animals. Therefore, ideally, using the body temperature of an animal for diagnostic purposes would be based on two measurements (or more): the temperature when the animal is not suspected to have disease and the temperature when the animal is suspected to have a disease. A cut-off value to determine 'disease' is necessary to distinguish between the two stages. How the evaluation of a test is performed depends on the definition of what disease is being measured (see Chapter 2 for definition of disease). The disease or disorder can have one or more levels (e.g. healthy, mildly affected, severely affected, dead) and also the test can have two or more levels. The latter can be referred to as the test outcome. In Table 9.1, a list of test outcomes and examples is given (see also Chapter 3). The simplest and frequent outcomes used are dichotomous and continuous, and the remainder of the chapter will focus on these two types of outcome. However, other types can be considered as derivatives of the same methodology and such techniques can be adapted similarly.

9.3 Performance measures: sensitivity, specificity and predictive values

How well does a test perform? We call this description validity of a test. What inferences can be drawn on the test result? This is described by predictive

Table 9.1. *Test outcomes and examples*

Outcome	Levels	Example
Dichotomous	Two levels	Presence or absence of bacteria in a bacteriological culture
Nominal	Three or more independent levels with no distinct order	Colour of bacterial colony: white, grey, yellow
Ordinal	Three or more levels with a distinct order but with no numerical distance	Number of bacteria in bacteriological culture: 1, none; 2, few; 3, many; 4, countless
Continuous	Innumerable levels only dependent on the unit of measurement	Distance (e.g. mm) between colonies in bacteriological culture

Table 9.2. *A 2 × 2 cross-classification table of test results versus gold standard*

Test result	Disease status (gold standard)		
	$D+$	$D-$	Total
$T+$	a	b	$a+b$
$T-$	c	d	$c+d$
Total	$a+c$	$b+d$	n

values. The validity can include elements of both systematic and random errors. The validity describes how close the test result is relative to an objective diagnostic standard of the disease or a reference group. This reference group is often referred to as the *gold standard*. The gold standard is perceived as being the *true state* of disease. As an example, complete bone fractures of the humerus can usually be identified by a pathological examination. However, a full pathological examination often requires that the animal is dead. Therefore, X-ray machines are used as diagnostic tests to aid in the diagnosis. Evaluation of the X-ray machine requires a gold standard. A full pathological examination of the humerus would be an excellent choice in this situation. The validity of all new tests should usually be evaluated against this gold standard if a unique gold standard exists for a given disease. However, often some conditions do not readily have a unique gold standard and different approaches must be chosen. This could be the case in diseases where there is a gap between disease and infection, i.e. infection will not necessarily lead to disease. When a reliable gold standard does exist, the validity can be assessed against this standard. The evaluation usually centres on cross-classification of test results and disease results in a 2 × 2 table as shown in Table 9.2. This chapter only deals with gold

Table 9.3. *Terms, formulae and definitions of test performance. The formulae for the confidence intervals (CI) are approximate*

Term	Definition	Mathematical formula
Analytical sensitivity	Number or amount of analytes (things being measured) required to trigger a positive test; that is, the ability of an assay to detect analytes if present in a sample	Formula not defined. Example: minimum concentration that needs to be present in an assay for a positive result to occur
Analytical specificity	Ability of an assay to identify correctly or distinguish between similar analytes	Formula not defined. Example: cross-reactive antibodies, i.e. antibodies that are very similar to those that we want to detect
Diagnostic sensitivity (Se)	Probability that a truly positive (D+) animal will be classified as positive using the test (T+)	$Se = Pr\{T+ \mid D+\} = \dfrac{a}{a+c}$ $CI_{Se}: Se \pm Z_{1-\alpha/2}\sqrt{\dfrac{Se(1-Se)}{a+c}}$
Diagnostic specificity (Sp)	Probability that a truly negative (D−) animal will be classified as negative using the test (T−)	$Sp = Pr\{T- \mid D-\} = \dfrac{d}{b+d}$ $CI_{Sp}: Sp \pm Z_{1-\alpha/2}\sqrt{\dfrac{Sp(1-Sp)}{b+d}}$

standard methods. Methods for evaluation of diagnostic tests in the absence of a gold standard can be found elsewhere (Hui and Walter, 1980; Enøe *et al.*, 2000; Nielsen *et al.*, 2002).

Sensitivity (Se) and specificity (Sp) are test characteristics used in the description of the validity of tests. These two terms can be further divided into *diagnostic sensitivity* and *analytical sensitivity*, *diagnostic specificity* and *analytical specificity*. The definitions are given in Table 9.3. Analytical sensitivities and specificities are subsets of the diagnostic sensitivities and specificities, respectively. Analytical sensitivity refers to the detection limit. For example, if a test for detection of nematode eggs in faeces requires the presence of a minimum of 50 eggs per gram (EPG) faeces in order to be detected at all, the analytical sensitivity is 50 EPG. It is important to recognise the existence of this parameter, but we will not deal with it further in this textbook, as it mathematically is included in diagnostic sensitivity. Analytical specificity is a term that refers to differences in the composition of the analyte. For example, *Mycobacterium avium* has three subspecies: *M. a. avium*, *M. a. paratuberculosis* and *M. a. silvaticum*. There are some differences in the composition of these three bacterial subspecies and this difference is reflected in the analytical specificity. If a test to be used to detect only *M. a. paratuberculosis*, and *M. a. silvaticum* is also wrongly detected, these will be lowering of the analytical specificity, i.e. the test is not specific for paratuberculosis. In epidemiological studies, the terms usually used are diagnostic sensitivity and specificity, but it should be acknowledged that these depend on their analytical counterparts.

Diagnostic sensitivity and specificity are basic features of a test and it must be considered a requirement that people using the test results have an idea of these performance measures for the disease entity they need to draw inferences on. If not, they should somehow be estimated. The diagnostic sensitivity (Se) is defined as: The probability that a truly diseased animal tests positive ($Pr\{T+ \mid D+\}$). The diagnostic specificity (Sp) is defined as: The probability that a truly non-diseased animal tests negative ($Pr\{T- \mid D-\}$). The above definitions may also be expressed as the proportion of truly diseased (non-diseased) animals that tests positive (negative). By definition, Se and Sp are constant for all prevalences, in practice they may change. However, it also means that if the test has been evaluated to determine the validity at one disease stage, the test is not equally valid for another disease stage. The sensitivity will usually be affected by the stage of disease whereas the specificity will remain constant, as specificity is unrelated to the presence of disease. Example are chronic diseases like paratuberculosis, where the sensitivity of most tests is increased as the disease progresses.

The predictive values of diagnostic tests express the probability that a given test result is actually expressing the true state of disease. The positive predictive value (PPV) is thus the probability that a positive test result is reflecting the presence of disease ($Pr\{D+ \mid T+\}$). The negative predictive value (NPV) is the probability that a negative test result is really from a non-diseased animal ($Pr\{D- \mid T-\}$). The definitions are given in Table 9.4. They are very dependent on the prevalence of the disease or disorder that the test is measuring. Therefore, care should be taken when interpreting these values. They are also dependent on Se and Sp, in that predictive values are conditional estimates. A link between Se ($Pr\{T+ \mid D+\}$), Sp ($Pr\{T- \mid D-\}$) and true prevalence ($Pr\{D+\}$, see later) can be obtained through Bayes' Theorem, which for dichotomous variables can be written as

$$Pr\{B \mid A\} = \frac{Pr\{A \mid B\} \times Pr\{B\}}{Pr\{A \mid B\} \times Pr\{B\} + Pr\{A \mid B^c\} \times Pr\{B^c\}}$$

Table 9.4. *Terms, formulae and definitions of predictive properties. The formulae given for confidence intervals (CI) are approximate*

Term	Definition	Mathematical formula
Positive predictive value (PPV)	Probability that an animal tested positive (T+) is truly positive (D+)	$$\text{PPV} = \Pr\{D+ \mid T+\} = \frac{a}{a+b}$$ $$\text{CI}_{\text{PPV}}: \text{PPV} \pm Z_{1-\alpha/2}\sqrt{\frac{\text{PPV}(1-\text{PPV})}{a+b}}$$
Negative predictive value (NPV)	Probability that an animal tested negative (T−) is truly negative (D−)	$$\text{NPV} = \Pr\{D- \mid T-\} = \frac{d}{c+d}$$ $$\text{CI}_{\text{NPV}}: \text{NPV} \pm Z_{1-\alpha/2}\sqrt{\frac{\text{NPV}(1-\text{NPV})}{c+d}}$$
Likelihood ratio of a positive test (LR+)	The ratio between the likelihood of a positive test result in an animal with disease and the likelihood of a positive test result in an animal without disease	$$\text{LR+} = \frac{\Pr\{T+ \mid D+\}}{\Pr\{T+ \mid D-\}}$$ $$= \frac{\Pr\{D+ \mid T+\}}{\Pr\{D- \mid T+\}} \times \frac{\Pr\{D-\}}{\Pr\{D+\}}$$ $$= \frac{\text{PPV}}{1-\text{PPV}} \times \frac{1-\text{TP}}{\text{TP}}$$ $$= \frac{\text{Se}}{1-\text{Sp}} = \frac{a(b+d)}{(a+c)b}$$
Likelihood ratio of a negative test (LR−)	The ratio between the likelihood of a negative test result in an animal with disease and the likelihood of a negative test result in an animal without disease	$$\text{LR-} = \frac{\Pr\{T- \mid D+\}}{\Pr\{T- \mid D-\}}$$ $$= \frac{\Pr\{D+ \mid T-\}}{\Pr\{D- \mid T-\}} \times \frac{\Pr\{D-\}}{\Pr\{D+\}}$$ $$= \frac{1-\text{NPV}}{\text{NPV}} \times \frac{1-\text{TP}}{\text{TP}}$$ $$= \frac{1-\text{Se}}{\text{Sp}} = \frac{c(b+d)}{(a+c)d}$$
True prevalence (TP)	The proportion of truly diseased animals in the population	$$\text{TP} = \Pr\{D+\} = \frac{a+c}{n}$$ $$= \frac{\text{AP} + \text{Sp} - 1}{\text{Sp} + \text{Se} - 1}$$
Apparent prevalence (AP)	The proportion of test positive animals	$$\text{AP} = \Pr\{T+\} = \frac{a+b}{n}$$ $$= \text{Se} \times \text{TP} + (1-\text{Sp}) \times (1-\text{TP})$$

where B^c denotes the complementary outcome of B, i.e. if $B = D+$ then $B^c = D-$. Thus,

$$PPV = Pr\{D+ \mid T+\}$$

$$= \frac{Pr\{T+ \mid D+\} \times Pr\{D+\}}{Pr\{T+ \mid D+\} \times Pr\{D+\} + Pr\{T+ \mid D-\} \times Pr\{D-\}}$$

$$= \frac{TP \times Se}{TP \times Se + (1 - TP) \times (1 - Sp)}$$

and

$$NPV = Pr\{D- \mid T-\}$$

$$= \frac{Pr\{T- \mid D-\} \times Pr\{D-\}}{Pr\{T- \mid D-\} \times Pr\{D-\} + Pr\{T- \mid D+\} \times Pr\{D+\}}$$

$$= \frac{(1 - TP) \times Sp}{TP \times (1 - Se) + (1 - TP)Sp}$$

where TP is the true prevalence $(= Pr\{D+\})$. An alternative to calculation of predictive values is the likelihood ratios of positive and negative test results (see definitions in Table 9.4). These values are attempts to correct for the prevalence. The likelihood ratio of a positive test result (LR+) expresses the likelihood ($\sim$probability) of having a positive test result in an animal with disease relative to the likelihood of having a positive test result in an animal without disease. Thus, the LR+ provides an indication of the value of a positive test result irrespective of the prevalence. Yet, a high LR+ would indicate that disease is very likely to be present when a positive test result is seen. A low LR− indicates that disease is not very likely when a negative test result is seen.

EXAMPLE 9.1. The dependence of predictive values on prevalence can be derived using Bayes Theorem:

$$PPV = \frac{a}{a + b} = \frac{TP \times Se}{TP \times Se + (1 - TP) \times (1 - Sp)}$$

and

$$NPV = \frac{d}{c + d} = \frac{(1 - TP) \times Sp}{TP \times (1 - Se) + (1 - TP)Sp}$$

Given Se $= 0.9$ and Sp $= 0.9$, PPV and NPV can be calculated at different prevalences (TP) as shown in Figure 9.1. In this example, we have a relatively valid test. At a low prevalence, the PPV is low because it is 'difficult' to find cases. However, at high prevalences, it is fairly easy to detect true positive cases. Thus, the PPV is high. The opposite situation is the case with NPV. It is difficult to find negative cases in a population with a high prevalence. Therefore, the NPV is low at high prevalences and high at low prevalences.

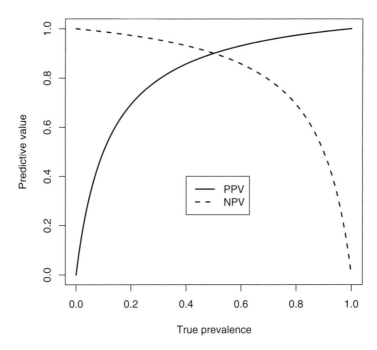

Figure 9.1. *Relations between predictive values and true prevalence at* (Se = 0.9 *and* Sp = 0.9).

EXAMPLE 9.2. Paratuberculosis is a chronic disease in cattle and other ruminants. The causal agent is *Mycobacterium avium* subsp. *paratuberculosis*. In the end-stage of the disease, a major clinical feature is chronic or intermittent diarrhoea. Pathologically, a characteristic thickening of the gut wall in the terminal ileum is usually seen. A test to detect and confirm the condition is cultivation of the mycobacteria from faecal samples on Löwenstein–Jensen medium (faecal culture (FC)). The laboratory performing the FC wants to determine the diagnostic validity among adult cows with permanent or intermittent diarrhoea (determined by the herd veterinarian) and the characteristic thickening of the gut wall (as determined by a pathologist). A study was carried out including 2598 cows and faecal culture was performed. The results are as shown in Table 9.5. The diagnostic sensitivity of the faecal culture was: Se = 60/92 = 0.65 with a 95% CI of Se, [0.54–0.75]. The diagnostic specificity of the faecal culture as a measure of paratuberculosis associated diarrhoea and gut wall thickening was: Sp = 2456/2506 = 0.98 with 95% CI of Sp, [0.97–0.99]. The PPV was 60/110 = 0.55 (95% CI, [0.45–0.64]) and the NPV was 2456/2488 = 0.99 (95% CI, [0.98–0.99]). The likelihood ratio of a positive test: LR+ = 0.65/(1 − 0.98) = 32.5. The likelihood ratio of a negative test: LR− = (1 − 0.65)/0.98 = 0.36. Here, the data were collected in a cross-sectional study; therefore, used in a similar population we can draw inferences on the predictive values. Thus, if a test result is negative, there is a 99% chance that the cow is really not having a condition with diarrhoea and the characteristic thickened gut wall. However, this conclusion only applies when the prevalence is: TP = 92/2598 = 0.035 as is the case here. An alternative would be using the likelihood ratios, where the relatively high LR+ indicates that in general we can have faith in positive test results whereas the low LR− reflects that negative test results are fair predictors of absence of disease though a lower LR− could have been preferred.

Table 9.5. *Evaluation of faecal culture to detect clinical paratuberculosis with permanent or intermittent diarrhoea and characteristic gut wall thickening*

Faecal culture	Diarrhoea and gut wall thickening		
	D+	D−	Total
T+	60	50	110
T−	32	2456	2488
Total	92	2506	2598

Table 9.6. *Evaluation of faecal culture to detect paratuberculosis infection including both clinical and subclinical paratuberculosis*

Faecal culture	Infection		
	D+	D−	Total
T+	63	47	110
T−	189	2299	2488
Total	252	2346	2598

EXAMPLE 9.3. A second objective of the test evaluation in Example 9.2 was to determine the sensitivity and specificity of the faecal culture when used for cows with either clinical or subclinical infection. Here, subclinical is defined as presence of an immunological response measured using an antibody ELISA. The resulting classification in the study is the distribution shown in Table 9.6.

The diagnostic sensitivity, specificity and predictive values of faecal culture are now: Se = 63/252 = 0.25 (95% CI, [0.20–0.31]); Sp = 2299/2346 = 0.98 (95% CI, [0.97–0.99]); PPV = 63/110 = 0.57 (95% CI, [0.47–0.67]); NPV = 2299/2488 = 0.92 (95% CI, [0.91–0.93]); TP = 252/2598 = 0.097 (95% CI, [0.086–0.108]). The predictive values are only interpretable at a prevalence of 9.7%. Notice that the diagnostic sensitivity and specificity of the faecal culture are not the same as those in Example 9.2, because the disease definition has been changed.

9.4 True and apparent prevalences

The prevalence is defined as the proportion of cases with the disease or disorder in a specific population at a specific time point. Usually, the term *prevalence* is used to describe the proportion of diseased among those investigated: $TP = (a + c)/n$. The *true prevalence* (TP) expresses the true number of cases

Table 9.7. *The cell probabilities of the 2 × 2 table (Table 9.2) expressed using Se, Sp and TP*

Test result	Disease status (gold standard)		Total
	D+	D−	
T+	Se × TP	(1 − Sp) × (1 − TP)	Se × TP + (1 − Sp) × (1 − TP)
T−	(1 − Se) × TP	Sp × (1 − TP)	(1 − Se) × TP + Sp × (1 − TP)
Total	TP	1 − TP	n

among those investigated. However, in many cases the test used in the investigation is not 100% sensitive and 100% specific. Therefore, a frequently used approach is to express an *apparent prevalence* (AP), which is the equivalent to the *test prevalence*. In the 2 × 2 cross-classification table (Table 9.2) this is: $AP = (a + b)/n$. If the diagnostic sensitivity and specificity of the test are known, the true prevalence can be estimated from the apparent prevalence:

$$AP = Se \times TP + (1 − Sp) \times (1 − TP) \quad \Leftrightarrow \quad TP = \frac{AP + Sp − 1}{Sp + Se − 1}$$

If we know the estimates of Se, Sp and TP, the cell probabilities of the cells a, b, c and d in the 2 × 2 table from Table 9.2 can be calculated as shown in Table 9.7. To obtain the expected cell counts (i.e. a, b, c and d) one must simply multiply these probabilities by the sample size (n).

9.5 Performance measures for tests with continuous outcome

Tests with ordinal or continuous outcomes are often classified into *positive* and *negative* or into more groups. However, this requires that the test with the continuous response can make a clear-cut separation of the results into diseased and non-diseased groups. The *separator* is usually referred to as the *cut-off value*.

9.5.1 Cut-off values

If the test has a perfect sensitivity and a perfect specificity, the test results are divided into two separate distributions. Thus, selection of a cut-off value is fairly easy just by choosing a value in between the two distributions. Most often the diagnostic sensitivity and specificity are not 100% and the situation is more likely to be as shown in Figure 9.2. At which optical density (OD) value should the antibody ELISA be separated into positive and negative to provide optimal information? There is no unique answer to this. Selection of the cut-off point depends on the purpose of the test. If a 100% specific test is required,

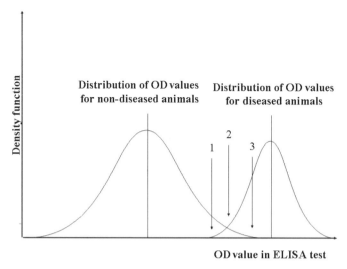

Figure 9.2. *Theoretical distribution of optical density (OD) values for diseased and non-diseased animals in an antibody ELISA test.*

cut-off point 3 should be chosen (we want to ascertain that a positive result is really true-positive). If a 100% sensitive test is required (e.g. with foot and mouth disease), cut-off point 1 should be chosen (we want to ascertain that all infected animals are detected). A frequently used approach is choosing point 2 where both the sensitivity and the specificity are optimised. However, no point can generally be said to be more correct than others. Various tools to help in deciding a cut-off are available. Two of these tools, differential positive rate (DPR) and receiver operating characteristic (ROC) analysis, will be introduced below.

9.5.2 *Differential positive rate*

The cut-off value can be optimised using the DPR, which is calculated as:

$$DPR = Se + Sp - 1$$

DPR is also known as Youden's index. Plotting the DPR at each cut-off reveals the point where sensitivity and specificity are optimised simultaneously. Notice that *differential positive rate* is not a rate, but a proportion. However, in other literature, DPR is used and we stick to this designation. The optimal cut-off point using DPR is the cut-off point where DPR is at its maximum, corresponding to cut-off point 2 in Figure 9.2.

9.5.3 *ROC analysis*

ROC analysis is a technique that can be used to evaluate the validity of a test with a continuous outcome and to provide estimates similar to diagnostic sensitivities and specificities of dichotomous tests. An ROC analysis begins with producing an ROC curve. First, the sensitivity and the specificity are calculated at all possible cut-off values. The ROC curve is created by plotting sensitivity as a function of (1 − Specificity) (Figure 9.3a). Simultaneous plots of sensitivity and specificity at different cut-off values (Figure 9.3b) can be used to find the cut-off point where sensitivity and specificity are optimised. The cut-off value where the two lines intersect puts equal weighting on sensitivity and specificity, which is not always desirable and reasonable. It is the same point where DPR is at its maximum.

For cut-off selection, the ROC curve and the plot in Figure 9.3b are tools for determining optimal cut-off points. However, optimal values differ for different situations. Sometimes a high sensitivity is necessary. It is of outmost importance that tests to detect foot and mouth disease are very sensitive in order not to overlook just a single case of this infectious disease. Such a mistake could mean that a lot of farms and animals are identified as not infected until a sensitive test detects infection. On the other hand, it is also important that the test that confirms an outbreak of foot and mouth disease is specific, so that a country is not classified as having the disease without true presence of the disease.

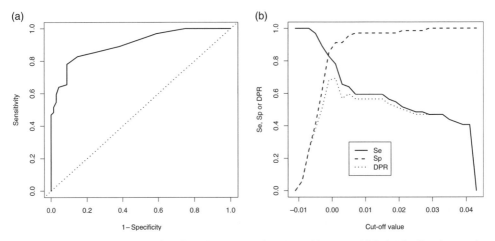

Figure 9.3. *(a) ROC-curve, a plot of sensitivity as a function of (1 − specificity). The line from point (0,0) to (1,1) shows a test with* AUC = 0.5. *(b) Plot of Sensitivity (Se), Specificity (Sp) and differential positive rate (DPR) at different cut-off values.*

Table 9.8. *Common reasons for lack of sensitivity and specificity in laboratory tests*

Reduced sensitivity	Reduced specificity
Natural or induced tolerance to infections	Antigenic relations between infectious agents
Timing: the agent/immune response is not yet established	Cross-reacting immune reactions with other infectious agents
Poor growth in bacteriological media	Non-specific laboratory reactions
Maternal antibodies removes infectious agent	Immune reactions caused by vaccination
Only intermittent shedding of infectious agent	Passive immunisation from colostrums uptake
Laboratory errors	Laboratory errors
High analytical sensitivity	

In general, the purpose of the testing determines whether a high sensitivity, a high specificity or both should be approached. High sensitivity is required if one desire to detect all possible cases. High specificity is required to confirm a suspect case or in the situation that the effect of a false-positive case has severe consequences. For different diseases and different tests, there are different reasons for lack of sensitivity and lack of specificity. This should be considered when the sensitivity and specificity are selected from the ROC analysis as in other situations. Common reasons are given in Table 9.8.

The ROC curve also provides information of the overall validity of the test. A test where the area under curve (AUC) is 0.5 (dashed line in Figure 9.3a) is worthless: You might as well flip a coin. A test with an AUC of 1.0 is perfect. However, you seldom obtain such perfect tests. In the ROC curve in Figure 9.3(a), the AUC is 0.9. This means that a randomly selected diseased animal will have a higher test value than a randomly selected non-diseased animal, 90% of the time. One application of ROC analyses could, therefore, be to compare different tests and their AUC. In general, the test with the higher AUC is the better. However, under some conditions (and at some cut-off values), the one with the smaller AUC may actually perform better. For test of differences between AUC we refer to Jensen and Poulsen (1992).

EXAMPLE 9.4. The cows in Example 9.3 were also tested using an antibody ELISA to detect antibodies to paratuberculosis (detecting whether an immune response had occurred or not). We wish to see if the ELISA results can be divided into two distinct populations: one with bacteria-shedding cows and one with non-shedding cows. Therefore, the cows were plotted as shown in Figure 9.4. Unfortunately, the ELISA does not appear to be able to separate the cows into shedding (FC positive) and non shedding (FC negative) animals. Has the ELISA any value at all for this separation?

The distribution of the data shows no indication that this ELISA provides any diagnostic information. However, when the cut-off is approximately zero, the sensitivity and the specificity are optimised simultaneously (Figure 9.5b). Also, the AUC is 0.72 and testing whether this is significantly different from 0.5 shows that this is the case (Figure 9.5a). The test actually has some value, but care should be used when interpreting it.

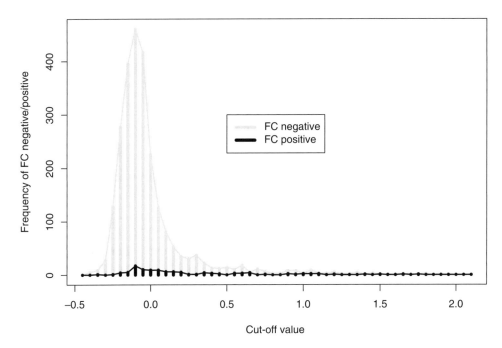

Figure 9.4. *Distribution of ELISA results for faecal culture positive and faecal culture negative cows.*

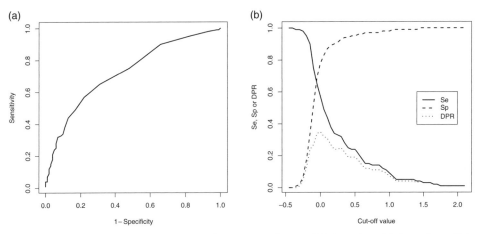

Figure 9.5. *(a) ROC curve for Example 9.4. The AUC equals 0.72. (b) Plots of sensitivity and specificity at different cut-off values in Example 9.4.*

9.6 Multiple testing

Rather than just performing one test, more tests are usually carried out to obtain more valid diagnoses. For example, it is common to determine the pulse, the temperature and the respiratory frequency when doing a clinical examination. Thus, three tests are carried out to when making a diagnosis. More can be added, and for each test added, some information on the condition is obtained. However, independent tests provide more information than dependent tests. For instance, a test for rectal temperature is expected to be highly correlated to oral temperature. Hence, very little information is obtained through such extra testing (which is also why both tests are rarely carried out). The less dependent two tests are, the more information they provide. In the following, we assume that the tests are independent. For more information on dependency of tests and how to deal with it, the reader is referred to Gardner *et al.* (2000). What is the diagnostic sensitivity and specificity when two tests are used together? Basically, tests can be interpreted in two ways: *parallel testing* and *serial testing*. Parallel testing covers situations where more tests are carried out simultaneously and only if all test results are negative is the overall result considered negative. If just one test is positive, the condition is thought to be present. The effect of this strategy is to increase the diagnostic sensitivity of the combined test. However, a negative effect of this strategy is that the diagnostic specificity of the combined test is decreased. Usually, parallel testing is carried out to rule out that a disease condition is present. The parallel diagnostic sensitivity (Se_{par}) and parallel diagnostic specificity (Sp_{par}) of two tests are:

$$Se_{par} = 1 - (1 - Se_1) \times (1 - Se_2); \qquad Sp_{par} = Sp_1 \times Sp_2$$

assuming conditional independence.

Serial testing is the situation where multiple tests are carried out and all results are required to be positive for the condition to be present. The effect of serial testing is an increase in diagnostic specificity and a concomitant drop in diagnostic sensitivity. Usually, serial testing is carried out to confirm that a condition is present. Serial diagnostic sensitivity (Se_{ser}) and serial diagnostic specificity (Sp_{ser}) are calculated as:

$$Se_{ser} = Se_1 \times Se_2; \qquad Sp_{ser} = 1 - (1 - Sp_1) \times (1 - Sp_2)$$

EXAMPLE 9.5. In another study on paratuberculosis, the sensitivity and specificity of a faecal culture test and an antibody ELISA for detection of clinical disease were estimated. For faecal culture:

$$Se_{FC} = 0.67 \quad \text{and} \quad Sp_{FC} = 0.98$$

For the antibody ELISA:

$$Se_{ELISA} = 0.88 \quad \text{and} \quad Sp_{ELISA} = 0.96$$

What are the sensitivities and specificities and the tests when combined in serial and parallel?

$$Se_{par} = 1 - (1 - 0.88)(1 - 0.67) = 0.96; \quad Sp_{par} = 0.96 \times 0.98 = 0.94$$

and

$$Se_{ser} = 0.88 \times 0.67 = 0.59; \quad Sp_{ser} = 1 - (1 - 0.96)(1 - 0.98) = 0.99$$

Thus, when the two tests are interpreted in parallel, the combined sensitivity is greater than the individual sensitivities whereas the specificity is decreased. When interpreted in serial, the overall sensitivity is fairly low. However, most positive results are true (the specificity is almost 100%). Both interpretations require that the tests are conditionally independent meaning that the result of one test is not dependent on whether the result of the other test is positive or negative. The two tests mentioned here are considered to be conditionally independent.

Many tests used in veterinary medicine are used without prior knowledge of their sensitivity, specificity and predictive values. They are combined in multiple settings, and conclusions (= diagnoses) and decisions (= treatments or control actions) are drawn based on the results. In many situations, knowledge on the performance of the tests is desirable prior to applying the tests. If such performance tests are not carried out, tests may be applied without actually adding further information about the condition. Thus, there are expenses added through the diagnostic procedure without a simultaneous gain in information. Actually, a test result can provide the decision maker with false information where no information might have induced greater certainty. Great care should be taken when making diagnoses or using tests in screening and surveillance programs for infectious diseases. Decisions should be based on appropriate information rather than non-informative information that might as well have been achieved by flipping a coin.

9.7 Sensitivity and specificity at the herd level

At the herd level, we are (like the situation at the animal level) interested in correct classification of herds into truly positive and truly negative herds. The term positive can relate to any parameter of interest in the situation (diseased, infected, antibody positive etc.). The performance of a diagnostic test at the herd level (herd test) has implications for certification of herds (e.g. specific pathogen free (SPF) pig herds) and for the efficiency of control and eradication programmes. The herd tests also have importance for any epidemiological study that includes categorisation of herds such as, for example, many risk factor studies. Although we use the term herd, the concepts and formulae in this section can be used for any group of animals (litter, pen, section, etc.). The term *herd test* is used for the evaluation of a test result based on a sample from more than one individual animal. The herd test can be based on either test of samples from individual animals or it can be based on a pooled sample from the animals. Thus, a herd test can, for example, consist of a number of blood samples of individual animals or it can be a bulk tank milk sample from all lactating cows. The definitions of herd sensitivity (HSe) and herd specificity (HSp) are similar to the definitions at the individual level:

HSe The probability that a truly positive herd will be classified as positive using the herd test.

HSp The probability that a truly negative herd will be classified as negative using the herd test.

HSe and HSp can then be calculated using an appropriate gold standard as for individual animals. For many purposes, especially concerning disease eradication, a herd is said to be positive if there is just one positive animal in the herd. Thus, if only one cow has antibodies against infectious bovine rhinotracheitis (IBR), the herd as such is said to be infected or positive, although all other animals are truly antibody negative. This means that a positive herd test only gives a status for the herd and not the individual animals, as there can be both positive and negative animals present in a herd. We just know that there is at least one positive animal. On the other hand, a negative herd test automatically gives a negative status for individual animals. Therefore, a negative herd test is very useful. For example, animals that are traded can be given a test certificate without being tested. In some situations, it may be relevant to consider a *critical number* of truly positive animals where the herd is said to be positive. However, in this context we will only consider the situation where a herd is considered positive if there is at least one positive animal (the critical number in this situation is 1). When the herd test is based on testing a number of individual animals, HSe and HSp can be calculated from the sensitivity and specificity for the test on the individual animal. HSe and HSp depend not only on the individual Se and Sp, but also on the number of animals in the herd tested and the true within herd prevalence. In order to calculate HSe (the probability that a positive herd gives a positive herd test result) when testing n animals, consider the question: What is the probability that all n animals are negative? The apparent prevalence (AP) determines the probability of one animal testing positive; hence, the probability of one animal being tested negative is $1 - AP$, the probability of all n animals being negative is: $(1 - AP)^n$. Hence, $1 - (1 - AP)^n$ becomes the probability that at least one animal is positive. Thus,

$$HSe = 1 - (1 - AP)^n$$

AP is given in Table 9.4. HSp is the probability that the n animals in the sample in a truly negative herd are tested negative. As the probability for each truly negative animal to be tested negative is the specificity for the test at the animal level, the formula for calculating HSp becomes:

$$HSp = Sp^n$$

From the formulae it can be seen that when we increase the number of animals in the sample size, the HSe will increase whereas HSp will decrease. Further, HSe will increase along with the true prevalence in the population whereas HSp is not affected by the true prevalence. When one animal is required to be positive in a sample in order for a herd to be classified as positive, this is referred to as a critical value equal to 1. For critical values greater than one, the reader is referred to Christensen and Gardner (2000). In many control and eradication programmes, the herds may be classified into more than two categories. The Danish BVD program has thus operated with the three categories: free, infected and unknown. In the Danish Salmonella program in pig herds the herds are classified as levels 1–3 for low, moderate and high seroprevalence, respectively.

EXAMPLE 9.6. Consider a test for detection of antibodies against IBR with a sensitivity of 0.99 and specificity of 0.98 at the individual animal level. What would be the herd level sensitivity and specificity of the test if 10% of the animals in the herd are assumed to be infected and 10 animals are sampled. Using the expression from Table 9.4 the AP can be found from the true prevalence (TP = 0.10):

$$AP = Se \times TP + (1 - Sp) \times (1 - TP) = 0.99 \times 0.1 + (1 - 0.98) \times (1 - 0.1) = 0.117$$

hence
$$HSe = 1 - (1 - AP)^n = 1 - (1 - 0.117)^{10} = 0.71$$

and
$$HSp = Sp^n = 0.98^{10} = 0.82$$

If 20 animals are sampled instead of 10, the HSe and HSp become 0.92 and 0.67, respectively. Thus, when we increase the sample size, we increase HSe, but decrease HSp.

If the prevalence in an infected herd is 20% rather than 10%, then the apparent prevalence is:

$$AP = Se \times TP + (1 - Sp) \times (1 - TP) = 0.99 \times 0.2 + (1 - 0.98) \times (1 - 0.2) = 0.214$$

hence for a sample of 10 animals, HSe and HSp becomes:

$$HSe = 1 - (1 - AP)^n = 1 - (1 - 0.214)^{10} = 0.91$$

and
$$HSp = Sp^n = 0.98^{10} = 0.81$$

If 20 animals are sampled HSe becomes 0.99 and HSp becomes 0.67. Thus, when the true prevalence in the herd increases, then the HSe increase, but the HSp is unchanged.

9.8 Further reading

A general introduction to diagnostic tests is found in Kraemer (1992). More special issues are covered in, e.g. Gardner and Greiner (2000) and Coste and Pouchot (2003). For more insight into ROC analysis and decision analysis on these results, other literature should be consulted, e.g. Jensen and Poulsen (1992), Jensen (1994), Greiner *et al.* (2000) and Smith and Slenning (2000).

10 DATA MANAGEMENT

Hans Houe, Annette Kjær Ersbøll and Nils Toft

10.1 Introduction

The main purposes of collecting data are establishing surveillance systems and testing hypotheses. In order to be able to perform a valid analysis and find possible significant differences, the study has to be well designed (selection of design, sample size, randomisation, etc.). However, before the analysis can be made, data have to be *collected, checked and organised in a database*. This is called data management. Often, proper data management is neglected with the consequence that data might be erroneous or incomplete. Some companies, especially in the pharmaceutical industry, have a number of so-called data managers. They are specially trained in handling data and their job is to receive, organise and check data to be ready for statistical analysis.

Epidemiological studies often utilise many data that are available from databases of existing recordings. The existing data may then be combined with additional data gathered for specific purposes in the project. Farm records, veterinary clinics or practices, diagnostic laboratories, slaughterhouses and milk recording schemes are examples of sources for existing data. The farmer's organisations usually have large databases that already have combined information on, for example, demographics, disease and production data. The final analyses are therefore dependent on data of different kinds obtained from different sources, may be also data that undergo different transformations and interpretations through different intermediate databases. When the investigator has not performed all the primary observations it is important to be aware of how differences in primary observations and recordings can affect the final analysis. For example, farmers have different thresholds of when a mastitis case should be treated by a veterinarian who is then recording the disease and treatment. The threshold of diagnosing various diseases at meat inspection may vary from person to person, between slaughterhouses and may also change over time. The investigator must always try to adjust for such sources of variability or at least include them in the final discussion of the results.

The aim of this chapter is to stress why and how to perform proper data management. Furthermore, the structure of databases, data quality, data control and data editing will be discussed. It is the aim to give the reader an overview of the pathways of data from the original sampling, observation or measurement, to registration in databases, re-coding of data and finally the analyses of the data. At the end of the chapter, a short overview of some databases in Denmark will be given.

10.2 Primary observation, measurement and data recording

The data needed for epidemiological studies include demographic data on population size, age, breed, etc. together with data on animal performance and risk factors. An outline of these data and their characteristics is given in Chapter 3. As with any historical event, the information, or in this case, the data should be traced back as close as possible to its origin.

Figure 10.1 shows examples of the steps from the event until the information ends up in a database. The origin of data is thus an event followed by observations, decisions and often interpretation of the information. The meat inspector observing and recording a case of atrophic rhinitis in a pig is

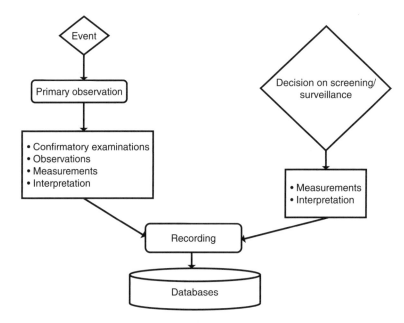

Figure 10.1. *Steps from the event until information is gathered in a database.*

the origin of that information. The case of atrophic rhinitis has of course been present for a longer time, but as recording of clinical signs is usually not routinely performed on individual pigs, the meat inspector's observation makes up the origin of that information. Thus, a clear distinction should be made between the origin of the case or event and the origin of the data. This is, for example, important when evaluating causal relationships.

In many recording systems for animal diseases, the veterinarian making the diagnosis, also enters the information into a database. However, in most cases the farmer or pet owner calling the veterinarian is the original observer. It is the farmer's judgement whether to call the veterinarian or not that determines whether the disease will ever be recorded. If the animal has vague symptoms, the farmer may choose to wait 1–2 days before calling the veterinarian, and therefore there is often a time lag between primary observation and time of confirmatory examination and hence recording. The veterinarian's recording may be a direct observation such as diarrhoea. However, the recording can also be based on an interpretation by the veterinarian. Thus, the presence of diarrhoea in a skinny third-lactating cow with normal appetite may be interpreted as paratuberculosis, which is then recorded. Alternatively, the veterinarian may wait for a laboratory test before recording the exact aetiological diagnosis. See also Chapter 3 for further details on disease classification into the three levels: (1) specific causes; (2) lesions or deranged function; and (3) presenting problem.

In the Danish surveillance scheme for infectious bovine rhinotracheitis (IBR), blood samples from every sixth slaughtered animal are examined for IBR antibodies. The origin of the data is here given by the selection process of animals and the following test results in the laboratory. Thus, many 'original' or raw data are influenced by decisions by humans, e.g. when to take blood samples, when to measure food intake, etc.

For any database the definition of the source is crucial for the later interpretation and handling of possible bias (see Chapter 11). Thus, the threshold among farmers for defining a disease condition may show a higher variation than the diagnostic criteria among veterinarians. Thus, when using database recordings, the history behind the many different variables in the database used must be known as this has implications for judging the data quality and for the interpretations done.

10.3 Sources of data

Several institutions and organisations make more or less systematic recording of data. Each institution or organisation has its specific purposes for collecting data and therefore the sampling criteria vary substantially. The investigator must consider these different criteria before using such databases and not uncritically use the observations for other purposes than they were made for. In the following, different sources and their purposes of sampling data are mentioned. More detailed information on specific databases is given at the end of this chapter (Section 10.8).

10.3.1 *Governmental veterinary institutions and organisations*

In most countries, different governmental institutions have a defined role in surveillance and control of diseases. Therefore, many databases are embedded in legislation especially concerning infectious diseases and in recent years also use of medication and antibiotic resistance. Usually, the governmental diagnostic laboratories manage these data.

10.3.2 *Veterinary practices*

The practicing veterinarian is the main source for data on clinical diagnoses. Many practitioners can enter a disease code directly on their invoices for direct transmission to databases. The number of disease codes is usually limited and some code definitions may be vague (e.g. diarrhoea, thick leg).

10.3.3 *Slaughterhouses – meat inspection*

The main purpose of meat inspection is the protection of consumers from diseased animals and meat with low quality. However, it also gives a lot of valuable information on disease status of the animals that can be used by the farmer. The meat inspection in slaughtered pigs and cattle gives opportunities for detailed investigation of the carcass and hence a lot of valuable information on pathological conditions. As clinically diseased animals go to emergency slaughter, the animals at the routine slaughter line mostly represent animals without clinical symptoms or at least without obvious severe signs. Therefore, the meat inspection and recording of data is especially important for quantification of subclinical conditions or less severe diseases.

10.3.4 *Agricultural organisations and farm records*

In most developed countries the agricultural organisations have organised the collection of several data from their members. In the cattle industry this includes milk recording (yield, cell count). The farmers are given special sheets on which they can record daily events in the herd. This information is then gathered with information from veterinary practices, slaughterhouses, etc. (see examples later on description of specific databases (Section 10.8)).

10.4 Database structure

Until now the word database(s) has been used several times without a proper definition of what we mean by the term *database*. This is because databases have been such an integrated part of daily life as an epidemiologist that the word is considered as common as, e.g. computer. By the word database we refer to a *collection of data*, thus it is a very flexible word that can be used to address anything from a pile of invoices regarding purchase of cat food in a cattery to the organisation of data in the Danish Cattle Database (DCD).

For an introduction to the different types of database concepts such as relational databases, hierarchical databases, object oriented databases, etc. we refer to, e.g. Korth and Silberschatz (1991). Here, we will briefly outline some elements that might be worth considering when designing your own databases.

A central concept of a database structure is the *record* (a record is also called an observation). A record is a collection of registrations of variables of interest. A collection of records might be called a *table*. In order to retrieve the individual records from the table a uniquely defined *key* must be present. The key can be a variable such as the Central Herd Registration (CHR) number, but may also be defined by more variables, such as FarmId + SowId in an anonymised study among several sow farms. Figure 10.2(a) and (b) show examples of a good database structure with a well-defined key and a bad structure where identical tables are used to distinguish between farms. The latter still allows for identification of individual records, but information retrieval quickly becomes rather tedious. Note, that even though the design in Figure 10.2(b) is far from

(a) The key is {FarmId, SowId, parity}

FarmID	SowId	Parity	LitterSize
1	1	1	9
1	1	2	12
2	1	1	9

(b) The key is {SowId, parity}

Farm 1

SowId	Parity	LitterSize
1	1	9
1	2	12

Farm 2

SowId	Parity	LitterSize
1	1	9

Figure 10.2. *Examples of (a) a good database structure and (b) a bad database structure.*

good, it still allows for identification of individual records through variables. The lazy person might be inclined to drop the SowId since identification can be carried out through the position in the table, i.e. by counting the number of parity 1 entries to assign a SowId associated with a given record. However, if the identification is achieved through the position of data, then simple procedures such as merging data sets might produce disastrous results.

While one table might form a database it is the possibility to associate data in different tables when data are on different levels (e.g. recordings of animals and herd information) that is the strength of using a database tool such as Access, Oracle, MySQL or one of the other numerous applications available. By forming tables of records and associating these through relations it is possible to avoid problems of redundancy and inconsistency as well as the possible additional storage capacity introduced by systematic missing values (some systems will reserve the space for a variable in all records, despite the possible missing values).

EXAMPLE 10.1. To illustrate the problem of redundancy we assume that we are conducting a study of management practice on dairy farms and the effect on milk production. For the management issues we have chosen to conduct a questionnaire on a sample of farms. For each farm we are then given access to the production records in the DCD. Eventually, we are faced with information consisting of one questionnaire for each farm and a series of records of milk production for each cow on each of the farms. If we were to combine this in a single table, we would have to repeat all the information contained in variables from the questionnaire for each and every record of milk production. The problem is the hierarchic structure of data (see more details on data levels in Chapter 3). A correct solution will of course be to store information from the questionnaire survey in one table with the CHR number as key. Production records are then stored in a different table with Central Cattle Registration (CKR) numbers as key. Finally, we keep track of which cows are located on which farms by forming a relation between the two tables, where CKR numbers are associated to CHR numbers.

EXAMPLE 10.2. To further promote the use of relational databases in information handling, consider the case of data consisting of registrations in a sow herd. Let us further assume that we only register culling, mating and farrowing (and associated traits). To keep this in a single table, we would have something like the table in Figure 10.3(a). It may be a matter of preference whether to leave the missing values empty or repeat, e.g. the culling date in all records for the sow. If the same information is included in more than one record, one should be very careful not to double count events when performing the data analysis. Note that in production records it is often the case that one or more records are incomplete, i.e. no mating method or culling reason is stated. An alternative to this representation would be in three separate tables, one for each event, i.e. mating, culling and farrowing (Figure 10.3b). In the above table the key is actually formed by the entire record. By dividing into three tables it would be possible to form more reasonable keys: for the Farrowing table the key would be SowId + parity, for the Culling table the key would be SowId and in the Mating table the key would be SowId + Parity + MatingDate. Note how the approach with three tables automatically becomes easier to extend in case we are to start registering other events as well, e.g. veterinary services.

To summarise our recommendations regarding database structure we advise you to adhere to the three principles:

1. Define a key, which makes data retrieval simple, i.e. identify the units of the study (records) with codes.
2. Avoid repeating information, e.g. if there is a hierarchy in the data, keep that in the organisation of data.
3. Avoid systematic empty fields, i.e. do not force variables into the same table if they are not naturally combined as in the case of the three distinct events in the sow herd.

If data are organised according to these principles the issues discussed in the next sections of this chapter might become a little bit more straightforward and less tedious.

(a)

SowId	Parity	Farrow date	Litter size	Mating date	Mating method	Culling fate	Culling reason
1	1			01 Mar 01	Boar		
1	1	25 Jun 01	10				
1	2			10 Aug 01	Insem		
1	2			31 Aug 01	Boar		
1	2					10 Oct 01	ReproFail

(b)

SowId	Parity	Farrow date	Litter size
1	1	25 Jun 01	10

SowId	Parity	Mating date	Mating method
1	1	01 Mar 01	Boar
1	2	10 Aug 01	Insem
1	2	31 Aug 01	Boar

SowId	Parity	Culling date	Culling reason
1	2	10 Oct 01	ReproFail

Figure 10.3. *Possible observations in a sow herd stored as (a) a single table and (b) three tables.*

10.5 Data quality

When using data from other sources (i.e. not directly measured and recorded by the investigator), it is important, in addition to the data, to ask for documentation of data (coding and interpretation) and of data quality. Are there specific protocols for sampling and measurement of variables? Who performed the initial sampling, measurement and interpretation of data? What is the sensitivity and specificity of diagnostic tests used for measurements? Are there specific definitions for interpretation of data into a new code for a disease complex?

The content of databases depends on the purposes and is often influenced by history and traditions. Further, the content and use of databases vary between countries. Therefore, there is a need to evaluate the subject matter and the quality of data whenever data from other sources are used. The final data depend on every link in the data stream. Every step in the data processing should be clearly defined. The following outline some critical elements within different types of data.

10.5.1 *Clinical data*

The farmer or pet owner is often the first person to observe clinical signs or certain behaviour. For many diseases the first sign is reduced feed intake and often this may be the only sign that makes a client call the veterinarian. On other occasions the symptoms are so obvious that the farmer simply calls the veterinarian and says that he has a cow with milk fever or mastitis. But as discussed in Section 10.2 concerning the distinction between primary observation and recording, the variation in thresholds for the farmer to call the veterinarian can be an important source for misclassifications when evaluating clinical or disease data. There are also many situations where the farmer makes an observation without calling the veterinarian, for example abortions or stillborn calves. In these situations the data are highly dependent on the likelihood of the farmer recording the observations.

When the veterinarian is called to a diseased animal, he makes a clinical diagnosis of the animal. It varies how specific he will be in recording the diagnosis. For example, a mastitis case can be recorded simply as 'mastitis' or it can be recorded as 'chronic mastitis' or even more specifically as 'chronic unilateral purulent mastitis'. There must be clear protocols for what happens if the veterinarian makes two or more diagnoses on the same animal. Will only the most serious disease be recorded or will all diagnoses be recorded?

In some situations a positive pregnancy diagnosis followed by a negative pregnancy diagnosis may be interpreted and recorded as an abortion. However, care should be taken not to treat this information in the same way as the directly observed abortions because there are different uncertainties attached to these two situations.

10.5.2 *Pathological data*

In general, the criteria for pathological conditions are better defined than for clinical diagnoses. However, the individual meat inspectors may show variations in the limit before recording, for example, a slight chronic pleuritis. Therefore, it must be investigated, when examining these data, if efforts have been made to harmonise or specify criteria for registrations. The threshold for recording may change over time. Thus, an increase in pleuritis cases over a 5 year period can be due to either increased occurrence or increased recording.

10.5.3 *Laboratory data*

Laboratory data consist of detection of bacteria, virus, fungi and parasites or their respective antibodies. Additionally, a huge number of physiological, patho-physiological or exogenous substances can be detected in body fluids, tissues, excretions, etc. These data are directly influenced by the sensitivity and specificity of the laboratory techniques. Human beings may, however, also be involved in the process – for example, by determination of bacterial species by direct observation of colony morphology of bacterial cultures. Here, the laboratory personnel have their own sensitivity and specificity. In contrast, the results of an ELISA reader are not directly dependent on the personnel.

In addition to the validity of the laboratory techniques, the data are influenced by the people deciding which animals should be tested. For example whether sampling is based solely on clinical cases or on a surveillance programme.

10.5.4 *Medicine consumption*

The data on the medicine type are well defined as there is a code for the medical product. The uncertainties can include the diseases they are actually used for. It would influence the data quality if the legislation is not followed and medicine used for other conditions than it was prescribed for.

10.5.5 *Production data*

Many production data are of high quality. For example milk yield, weight at slaughter and number of sold animals are registered with high accuracy.

10.5.6 *Demographic data*

The farmer usually records many daily events and observations in the herd: date of birth, score of the size of calves, date of culling, etc. These data often have high quality as they are often not influenced by subjective judgement (except for sizes of animals). There may be a pitfall in the quality of recording. If recordings are not performed every day, the exact date of event may have been forgotten.

10.5.7 *Risk factors*

As well as for all the data on disease and production, the quality of data on potential risk factors should also be assessed. An extensive list of risk factors (or determinants in general) is given in Chapter 3. In general, data on host determinants such as age, sex and breed have good quality as they are easily measured (concerning age, see also the previous subsection on demographic data). Agent determinants on the other hand are difficult to quantify and are therefore often not included. In the future, it will probably be possible to include more genetic information of both the host and the agent in databases. Data on production system and climate usually have good quality. However, it should always be noted whether the variables are measured using exact measurement tools or subjective measures (e.g. humidity may be measured exact or by a subjective evaluation of whether it is high or normal). Data on animal handling are often very subjective in nature. Many are obtained through a questionnaire and many aspects of the data quality are related to the quality of the questionnaire (see Chapter 12).

10.6 Data control

A number of possible sources of error in data can be identified. During the process of entering data, typing errors might occur. Typing errors are relatively easy to identify and correct. Other types of errors could be due to wrong notation of results on original forms, problems in the herd with handling and collection of samples (e.g. blood samples), wrong ear tags and problems in the laboratory with analysis of samples. These types of errors are more difficult to identify and correct compared to typing errors. Often we only have an indication of errors without knowing whether to and how to correct them.

An adequate data control includes a number of different data checks. Depending on the actual data set, partial or complete data control should be performed in order to reduce errors in data. In the following, suggestions for data control are given.

Initially, data are entered into a database. In order to reduce typing errors, data should be:

- entered twice, or
- proofread (parts of or all data entered).

By entering data twice and making an automatic comparison between the two data sets, it is possible to identify typing errors. Another possibility is to proofread data in the database with the original data forms.

When errors due to typing errors have been identified and corrected, all other types of error sources have to be checked. The types of data control are summarised in Table 10.1.

Table 10.1. *Overview of data control with examples from a study of dairy cows*

Type of data control	Description	Example
Entering data twice	Enter all data twice	Identify typing errors
Proofreading	Proofread data in database with original forms	Identify typing errors
Missing values	Specific items or parts missing?	Missing somatic cell count in milk sample
Extreme values	Evaluate minimum and maximum values for possible outliers for quantitative measurements	Negative milk yield
Frequency distribution	Frequency distribution of qualitative measurements to identify illegal categories	Distribution of breeds in the study
Graphical illustrations	Scatter plots of relations	The relation between fat and protein content in milk
Logical checks	Relation between variables, check impossible combinations	Pregnancy test of male participants
Dates	The relation between dates	Pregnancy test before delivery date

All missing values should be identified in order to evaluate if the values are missing at random or not. This can be done by evaluating if specific animals or parts of the study have missing values. As an example, blood samples from heifers might be missing more often than blood samples from cows, because it is more difficult to handle heifers. In a study of colic horses, laboratory and chemical samples were taken on arrival of the horses. However, many of the horses with no colic problem or horses with severe colic were not sampled, as they were expected to either recover soon or be euthanised. In this case, data are not missing at random. Evaluation of the laboratory samples might therefore be biased as only some of the horses were sampled.

Quantitative variables (continuous, discrete) such as the daily weight gain and the milk yield can be evaluated for extreme values and by evaluation of different plots (see later in this section). The extreme values can be evaluated by calculating the minimum and maximum values and evaluating if these values lie within the expected interval.

Qualitative variables (ordinal, nominal, dichotomous) such as body condition and breed have only specified values. These variables can be checked by use of frequency distributions. It is hereby possible to identify animals with non-plausible values. If only Jersey and Holstein cows are included in the study, errors in inclusion or entering of data can be identified by making a frequency distribution of breed in the study. In a similar way the body condition of the cows can be checked, since there are a limited number of allowed values.

Graphical illustrations can be used for further evaluation of errors in data. The relation between different variables can be illustrated using different plots. If a specific relation is expected, possible extreme values can be identified. An example from human medicine is the relation between weight and height. Generally, a person in the age group 20–50 will have an increasing weight with increasing height. Extreme values can be identified and possible errors may be identified. Other examples are the inverse relation between the content of fat and milk yield as well as the content of protein and milk yield.

Logical control includes evaluations of relations, where some combinations are known to be impossible, such as, a pregnancy test for male participants. Depending on the type of data there might be a small or a large number of possibilities for performing logical control.

Control of dates can be done by relating the different dates, e.g. by use of a graphical illustration or calculating differences in days between specific dates. The date for farrowing should be later than the date for insemination and the number of days between two inseminations should be around 3 weeks. Also the date of blood sampling minus the date of birth must not be a negative number.

It should be stressed that every time data are transferred from one database system to another, data control should be performed in order to detect possible conversion problems (e.g. transfer of data from Excel to SAS). This is done by comparing summary statistics generated by the different softwares.

EXAMPLE 10.3. In a study of the milk yield of Danish dairy cows, 2056 cows were selected from 28 herds. For this example, a cross-sectional study was used. An example of the data set is given for the first 20 animals in Figure 10.4 (the key is chr and ckr). Data originated from the Danish Cattle Database (DCD), and these was no possibility of proofreading, as we did not have the original forms with the recordings. Therefore, we were only able to perform a part of the data control. First, data for cows with missing values for one or more of the recordings were printed. Seven cows had one or more missing values (Figure 10.5). This is a small number of cows with missing values. In the statistical analysis, these seven cows are suggested to be excluded.

The next step in the data control is evaluation of the qualitative and quantitative variables. Breed and parity are both qualitative, milk yield, somatic cell count, fat and protein content are all quantitative. Frequency distributions for the qualitative variables were made and the minimum and maximum values for the quantitative variables were calculated (see Figures 10.6 and 10.7 respectively). It is seen that the number of cows per herd included in the study from the 28 herds are in the range 3–202 cows. Further, it is seen that five different breeds are included, although only three cows are of breed 4. The parity ranged from 1 to 9, with 92% of the cows in parity 4 or below. The minimum values for milk yield, somatic cell count and fat and protein content are all 0. This is due to the fact that '0' is entered into the database even though the cow has not been milked. Hence, a zero value is the code for no milk sample and therefore these values should be set to missing or deleted. The maximum values for the four continuous variables should be evaluated in relation to the expected values. It is seen that one cow has a protein content above 6%, which is the expected maximum value. None of the other maximum values are extreme.

Different logical checks have been performed as combinations of missing, zero and non-missing values for the milk yield, fat and protein content. This gave no strange combinations. There were no dates in the data set.

Finally, different graphical illustrations of relations between milk yield, somatic cell count, fat and protein content were made (see Figure 10.8). These illustrations identified one cow with an extreme protein content (protein content at 8.3%, i.e. the same cow identified when looking for maximum values). In order to evaluate this figure, comparison of the protein content with the protein content in the previous or the following months could be performed, if data are available.

10.7 Data editing

A statement like 'It is standard to delete the most extreme animals' is absolutely wrong and not accepted as a scientific method for data handling and editing. All animals in a study and all measures collected should be evaluated and

Obs	chr	ckr	scc	milk	fat	protein	parity	breed
1	100	1	0	0.0	0.00	0.00	6	SDM
2	100	2	0	0.0	0.00	0.00	5	Cross
3	100	3	0	0.0	0.00	0.00	4	SDM
4	100	4	0	0.0	0.00	0.00	4	Cross
5	100	5	0	0.0	0.00	0.00	4	Cross
6	100	6	130	22.6	3.00	2.75	5	SDM
7	100	7	1520	4.6	4.50	4.15	4	SDM
8	100	8	0	0.0	0.00	0.00	4	SDM
9	100	9	350	20.4	2.85	2.90	3	Cross
10	100	10	90	16.8	4.05	3.45	3	SDM
11	100	11	0	0.0	0.00	0.00	4	Cross
12	100	12	320	14.0	4.45	4.00	4	SDM
13	100	13	420	8.6	3.80	3.95	4	SDM
14	100	14	570	6.6	4.25	4.25	4	SDM
15	100	15	0	0.0	0.00	0.00	3	SDM
16	100	16	0	0.0	0.00	0.00	3	SDM
17	100	17	0	0.0	0.00	0.00	3	SDM
18	100	18	0	0.0	0.00	0.00	2	SDM
19	100	19	90	16.8	3.95	3.20	4	SDM
20	100	20	120	23.2	4.30	2.65	4	SDM

Figure 10.4. *Outline of the database for the milk yield in Danish dairy herds. Somatic cell count (SCC) is measured in 1000 counts per millilitre. Milk is measured in kilograms per day. Fat and protein are the fat percentage and protein percentage.*

Obs	chr	ckr	scc	milk	fat	protein	parity	breed
1	100	37	.	.	.	.	1	SDM
2	400	282	0	0.0	0.0	0.00	.	Jersey
3	1000	1002	0	0.0	0.0	0.00	.	SDM
4	1900	1555	.	.	.	.	2	Cross
5	1900	1635	.	.	.	.	1	Cross
6	2500	2022	40	19.6	4.2	3.55	.	RDM
7	2800	2055	0	0.0	0.0	0.00	.	SDM

Figure 10.5. *Missing values for one or more of the recordings in the study of the milk yield in Danish dairy cows. Somatic cell count (SCC) is measured in 1000 counts per millilitre. Milk is measured in kilograms. Fat and protein are the fat percentage and protein percentage.*

handled with care. However, it is very difficult to distinguish between an erroneous measurement and a correct measurement, which for some reason is not close to the measurements for the remaining animals.

In general, only a very limited number of measurements should be edited. Some types of errors are of course acceptable to correct such as typing errors. Other types of errors and possible outliers should not necessarily be corrected. It is suggested that data are only edited or deleted if there is a good explanation for doing so. Otherwise, it should be stated that there is a problem with some of the animals and/or measurements, but it is not known how to solve it. The analyses can then be performed with and without these observations and the influence evaluated.

chr	Frequency	Percent	Cumulative Frequency	Cumulative Percent
100	75	3.65	75	3.65
200	158	7.68	233	11.33
300	39	1.90	272	13.23
400	58	2.82	330	16.05
500	86	4.18	416	20.23
600	98	4.77	514	25.00
700	202	9.82	716	34.82
800	24	1.17	740	35.99
900	111	5.40	851	41.39
1000	154	7.49	1005	48.88
1100	79	3.84	1084	52.72
1200	51	2.48	1135	55.20
1300	70	3.40	1205	58.61
1400	65	3.16	1270	61.77
1500	111	5.40	1381	67.17
1600	18	0.88	1399	68.04
1700	82	3.99	1481	72.03
1800	46	2.24	1527	74.27
1900	120	5.84	1647	80.11
2000	62	3.02	1709	83.12
2100	62	3.02	1771	86.14
2200	43	2.09	1814	88.23
2300	193	9.39	2007	97.62
2400	7	0.34	2014	97.96
2500	10	0.49	2024	98.44
2600	3	0.15	2027	98.59
2700	13	0.63	2040	99.22
2800	16	0.78	2056	100.00

breed	Frequency	Percent	Cumulative Frequency	Cumulative Percent
RDM	262	12.74	262	12.74
SDM	930	45.23	1192	57.98
Jersey	381	18.53	1573	76.51
DRK	3	0.15	1576	76.65
Cross	480	23.35	2056	100.00

parity	Frequency	Percent	Cumulative Frequency	Cumulative Percent
1	697	33.97	697	33.97
2	594	28.95	1291	62.91
3	369	17.98	1660	80.90
4	230	11.21	1890	92.11
5	97	4.73	1987	96.83
6	42	2.05	2029	98.88
7	13	0.63	2042	99.51
8	7	0.34	2049	99.85
9	3	0.15	2052	100.00

Frequency Missing = 4

Figure 10.6. *Data control of qualitative variables.*

Different types of errors and outliers described in the previous section can be grouped as:

1. Untypical biological or other characteristics.
2. Untypical measurements.

Obs	type	max	min
1	fat	10.03	0
2	milk	43.10	0
3	prot	8.35	0
4	scc	8100.00	0

Figure 10.7. *Data control of quantitative variables.*

3. Entry or transcription mistakes.
4. Data corruption during transfer between different software.

Items 1–4 may occur in combination. Items 3 and 4 should be corrected when identified. Data editing should be described in the final report paper.

There is no doubt, that identified typing errors or other reasons for data corruption should be corrected in the final data set. All other types of errors are often difficult to identify, e.g. problems with the ELISA test. If possible, a number of replicates can be used, for example, testing the same sample twice. If a large difference between the two replicates of the same sample is seen, there is a problem. However, if the two replicates are similar, there might still be a problem, now related to the whole plate or the sample. This type of problem is only possible to identify if the plate is replicated or repeated sampling of the animal is used. Due to the expenses, this is often not done. Problems with the plate or the sample can sometimes be identified by making plots of the relations between different measures and thereby identifying possible outliers.

10.8 Examples of databases with information on Danish farm animals

It is difficult to give a simple and systematic overview of all the existing databases and their exact content. They are created on many different levels and with many different purposes. Some databases are official with well-defined content and protocols for sampling. Many other databases are more or less internal in the institutions. In addition, a huge number of databases are created by researches for very specific research purposes. Usually, only few people know the exact content of the databases. The databases develop over time and many get special names as we get more acquainted with them ('Cattle database', 'Vetstat', etc.). Some databases may be subsets or parts of other databases. Here, some examples of databases in Denmark are given. The reader should be aware that the information given here of the content of the databases may change over time.

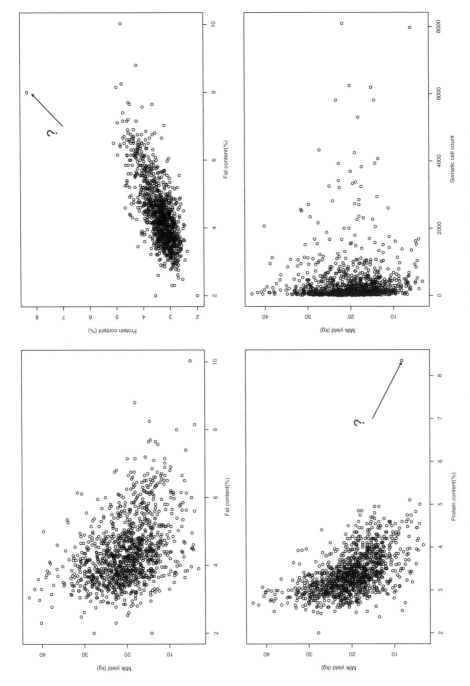

Figure 10.8. *Data control. Graphical illustration of the relations between the quantitative variables. Milk yield in Danish dairy cows.*

10.8.1 Central Farm Animal Register (in Danish: Centrale HusdyrbrugsRegister, CHR-register)

The register is managed by the Ministry of Food, Agriculture and Fisheries in collaboration with the cattle industry. In 1997, the ministry decided that all cattle in Denmark should be registered. The decision of establishing a national database on all cattle was influenced by the outbreak of mad cow disease in England. Thus, the CHR-register is an example of a database rooted in legislation. The CHR-register contains information on all agricultural holdings with farm animals. Every cattle must be registered with information on date of birth, breed, sex and the dam. Further, information on calvings, movements and deaths must be reported. The information in the CHR-register is coordinated with information in the DCD.

10.8.2 Vetstat

Vetstat was established in 1999 with the purpose of studying among other things the correlation between antibiotic consumption and antibiotic resistance. The medicine consumption is recorded in collaboration between The Danish Medicines Agency (in Danish: Lægemiddelstyrelsen), The Danish Agricultural Advisory Service (in Danish: Dansk Landbrugsrådgivning), Mærsk Data and the Danish Zoonosis Centre. Since January 2004, VetStat is maintained at the Section for Animal Health in the Department of Epidemiology and Risk Assessment at Danish Institute for Food and Veterinary Research (DFVF). In Vetstat, all prescription medicine to animals is recorded. Information on farm animals includes species, age, ordination group, drug, authorisation number of veterinarian and the date of expedition. Data on medicine are gathered from pharmacies and veterinarians. Vetstat is managed by the Danish Zoonosis Centre.

10.8.3 DANMAP – Danish Integrated Antimicrobial Resistance Monitoring and Research Program

The objectives of the DANMAP are:

- To monitor the occurrence of antimicrobial resistance among bacteria isolated from food animals, foods and humans.
- To monitor the use of antimicrobial agents for treatment in humans and in animals.
- To demonstrate associations between such use and the occurrence of resistance.

The DANMAP participants are Statens Serum Institut (no English name), The Danish Veterinary and Food Administration, The Danish Medicines Agency, Danish Institute for Food and Veterinary Research and Danish Zoonosis Centre. Each participant has access to their own data and the results are published yearly. DANMAP is managed by the Danish Zoonosis Centre.

Collection of bacterial isolates:

- From food animals, samples consist of random sampling of herds at slaughter and isolates from diagnostic submissions. In addition, *Salmonella* isolates from subclinical infections as well as cases of clinical salmonellosis are included.
- From foods, it is a nation-wide collection of samples from various food categories.
- From humans, results from routine susceptibility testing of *Campylobacter* and *Salmonella* at Statens Serum Institut and routine susceptibility testing of various pathogens in hospitals and general practice are included.

10.8.4   *Danish Cattle Database (in Danish: 'Kvægdatabasen')*

The Danish Cattle Database (DCD) is managed by the Danish Cattle Federation (in Danish: 'Dansk Kvæg') and the database is owned by the farmers. All registered data are gathered in the Danish Cattle Database. Data are handled by Mærsk Data. DCD contains registrations from the farmers, dairies, slaughterhouses, veterinarians and laboratories. The information can be utilised by the farmers, their advisors, agricultural companies and for research and educational purposes (Figure 10.9).

The DCD information is used to calculate breeding values for cows and bulls and is thus important for selection of breeding animals. The DCD is also used to monitor health and production in the herd and many advisors use the information in their routine work. A huge number of predefined printouts can be ordered from the database and used by the farmers, their advisors and others. Also, a special selection of data can be ordered from the database.

10.8.5   *Danish register on bovine virus diarrhoea virus*

The register is managed by the Danish Cattle Federation. Since 1999, the bovine virus diarrhoea virus (BVDV) register has been included in the Central Farm Animal Register. The herds are registered with BVDV infection status, which is based on interpretations of different laboratory examinations. In principle,

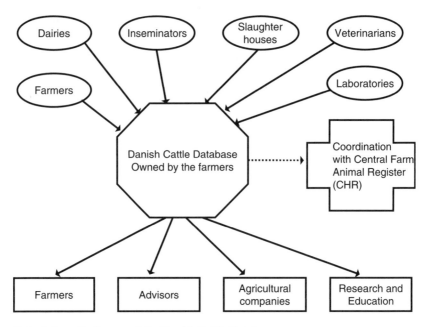

Figure 10.9. *Schematic diagram of the Danish Cattle Database.*

the free status is obtained and maintained by one or more of the following test procedures:

1. Examination of antibodies in bulk milk.
2. Test of three slaughter animals or three animals in the herd for BVDV aniti-bodies in blood.
3. Whole-herd testing for detecting persistently infected (PI) animals, removal of PI animals and follow-up testing.

10.8.6 *The Danish SPF Company Database (specific pathogen-free pigs)*

The Danish SPF Company keeps a database with information on SPF and MS herds. SPF herds are declared free of *Actinobacillus pleuropneumoniae* (AP) (except serotypes 6 and 12), *Mycoplasma hyopneumonia* (MYC), toxin-producing *Pasteurella multocida, Brachyspira hyodysenteriae, Sarcoptes scabiei* and *Haematopinus suis*. SPF herds re-infected with MYC are designated MS herds. All other herds are designated conventional. Approximately, 5% of all herds are SPF herds and 25% are MS herds in Denmark.

10.8.7 The PRRS Database (porcine reproductive and respiratory syndrome) (pigs)

The Danish Bacon and Meat Council (DBMC) keeps a PRRS database, where approximately 50% of all herds participate in a surveillance for PRRS virus. About 80% of all Danish sows and about 50% of all Danish slaughter pigs are in these participating herds.

10.8.8 The database for mandatory meat inspection recordings (pigs)

Data on all mandatory meat inspection recordings are in databases at the DBMC where all registrations on all pigs and sows slaughtered at slaughterhouses managed by the DBMC are recorded together with slaughterhouse identification, day of slaughter, live and slaughtered weight of the pig, meat percentage, sex, etc. There are approximately 50 possible pathological or other types of registrations on every pig, where a pig or sow may have up to four registrations in the database.

10.8.9 The Zoonosis Register (pigs)

A national *Salmonella enterica* surveillance and control programme, for herds delivering more than 200 pigs annually for slaughter, was initiated in 1995 in Denmark. The programme is based on meat-juice samples from carcasses at the abattoirs. The programme categorises the herds into three salmonella levels based on the previous 3 months' seroprevalence: level 1 herds with a low prevalence; level 2 herds with a moderate prevalence and level 3 herds with a high prevalence.

10.8.10 The Efficiency Control (pigs)

Danish pig producers control the performance of sows (weaned piglets per sow, etc.), feed conversion rate, growth of pigs, etc. in their own databases. These data are gathered at the local Agricultural Advisory Services.

10.8.11 The Ante Mortem Database (poultry)

Since 1997, veterinary officers have carried out pre-slaughter examinations at the farm of every broiler chicken and turkey flock slaughtered in Danish abattoirs. Data from these inspections are collected and transferred into a national register (the Ante Mortem Database) containing information such as origin of the flocks (identification, hatchery, age and breed of parent birds), date(s) of delivery, number of individuals and identification of feed mills.

10.8.12 *The Post Mortem Database (poultry)*

Veterinary officers being responsible for post mortem health inspections at Danish abattoirs collect information on every slaughtered poultry flock. This information is compiled in a central register (the Post Mortem Database) containing data such as number of individuals slaughtered, number of individuals condemned and reasons for condemnation.

10.8.13 *The Salmonella Database (poultry)*

Since 1997, data concerning all samples for salmonella in every epidemiological unit (house) of parent birds in the Danish broiler chicken and layer industry, broilers, pullets and layers have been compiled in a central register (the Salmonella Database). The flocks are monitored regularly and extensively by serological and bacteriological methods for all salmonella serotypes.

10.8.14 *The Efficiency Control Database (poultry)*

Every Danish poultry farmer has the opportunity to have production data for every flock registered in a central register in the Danish Poultry Council (the Efficiency Control Database). The database contains information on daily weight gain, egg production, mortality and feed and water consumption.

10.8.15 *Project databases*

Several specific project databases based on the existing databases have been made. For example, the Danish BVD register has been used together with information from the Geographical Information System to investigate risk factors for infection. Figure 10.10 shows a flow diagram of the data that are relevant for a project on BVD. The figure illustrates that there often are several steps before the data are ready for analysis.

10.9 Further reading

For an introduction to the different types of database concepts such as relational databases, hierarchical databases, object oriented databases, etc. we refer to, e.g. Korth and Silberschatz (1991).

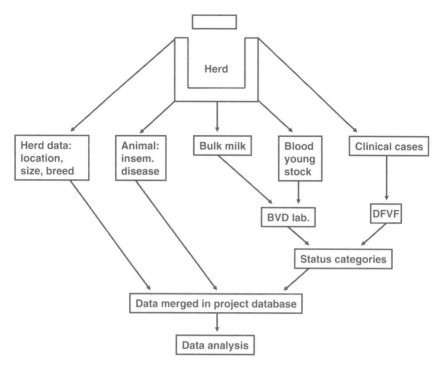

Figure 10.10. *Example of the flow of different data in a project on bovine virus diarrhoea virus (BVDV).*

10.10 Acknowledgements

We thank the employees of DFVF for providing information on their databases. We thank Mimi Folden Flensburg and Annette Cleveland-Nielsen for helping with the description of specific databases.

11 BIAS AND INTERACTION

Jeanett Bruun, Mimi Folden Flensburg
and Annette Kjær Ersbøll

11.1 Introduction

In this chapter, we describe how bias can invalidate the results obtained in a study and also how interaction can change the interpretation of the results. Bias is defined as a systematic error and may occur in, for example, the design, selection of animals, performance of the study and analysis of the results. Whenever a study is performed the issue of bias needs to be considered. Consideration of likely sources of bias is necessary even before the study begins. If bias is present, the obtained results may be invalid and lead to wrong conclusions. The sources of bias are many and varied, but special attention should be paid to:

1. selection bias;
2. information bias (including misclassification);
3. confounding bias.

Bias with specific relevance to questionnaires will be covered in greater detail in Chapter 12.

Two factors may not act independently in their contribution to the outcome (e.g. disease or production). Confounding bias is present when the effect of the confounder completely changes or explains the initial effect seen of the risk factor. The confounder has an effect on both the disease (or production) and the risk factor. Bias can be said to be an effect of the way the study is planned and performed, i.e. data derived. Interaction is not a bias, but is closely linked to confounding bias as both are related to a change in the relationship between a risk factor and the outcome (this will become more evident in Chapter 13). Interaction is a biological phenomenon and describes the modification of the relation between outcome and risk factor(s) by another (risk) factor. When the effect of one factor depends on the level of another factor then interaction is present. This means that the association under study is different depending on the level of the other factor.

Bias needs to be considered during the design phase of any study. Some types of bias can be controlled for in the analysis phase others cannot. Confounding bias and some types of information bias can be controlled during the analysis phase provided we have the necessary information. Therefore, it is important that potential sources of bias have been considered early in the study. Causal diagrams is an excellent tool to identify potential factors that may influence the outcome, but also to identify possible relationships between the different risk factors considered.

11.2   Bias

11.2.1   *Selection bias*

In order to reduce labour and costs, most epidemiological studies do not investigate all individual animals of a population, but rely on data from a sample of individuals from the study population. Bias may be introduced if the sample is not representative of the study population and also if the study population is not representative of the target population (see Chapter 2). This type of bias cannot be controlled for in the analysis phase. It is, for example, important that certain geographical areas are not overly or sparsely represented, and that data do not originate from almost exclusively the same veterinarians or farmers. In order to estimate the prevalence of diseases, data could fairly easily be obtained from diagnostic laboratories. However, such data are not representative of the target population, as material is submitted to diagnostic laboratories because disease problems occur. Therefore, a study population obtained this way would mainly describe herds or animals with the disease and, hence, overestimating the prevalence.

Attention should also be paid to seasonal changes that may influence disease prevalence greatly. Results obtained from salmonella prevalence studies conducted in January will inevitably show results that will differ from salmonella prevalence studies conducted in August and September (Figure 11.1).

Case–control studies aim to test whether there is a significant difference between cases and controls in regard to exposure to a suspected risk factor. When cases and controls are selected it is essential to ensure that both groups had an equal likelihood of exposure to the risk factors. If not, bias will be introduced and the validity of the results of the study compromised.

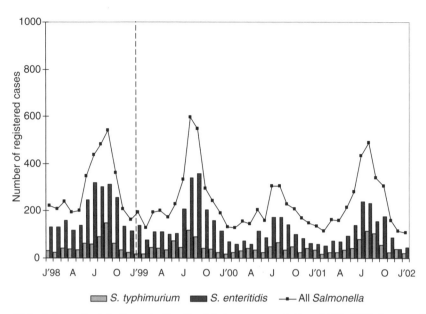

Figure 11.1. *Salmonella infections in the Danish human population, 1998–2001 (source: Danish Zoonosis Center).*

EXAMPLE 11.1. A study on risk factors for diabetes in dogs was performed in a small animal hospital in Sealand of Denmark. Dogs admitted to the hospital with diabetes were selected as cases. The controls were selected from among dogs admitted for routine vaccination. In this example, case dogs might come from the whole area of Sealand because the hospital has special expertise in managing patients with diabetes, whereas controls are more likely to come from the city around the hospital. Therefore, risk factors such as exercise, feeding strategy and age might be affected by the difference in geography. Dogs from the countryside are less likely to be overweight, often enjoy more exercise, but may not be as old. These factors could be risk factors, and therefore cases and controls do not have equal likelihood of exposure.

11.2.2 *Information bias*

Information bias can occur due to a number of reasons: inaccurate diagnostic procedures, questions in a questionnaire and coding thereof, or measurement error when using instruments for measurement of, e.g. weight. Information bias can be broken down into misclassification bias, which includes errors measured on the categorical scale, and measurement error, which are measures on the continuous scale. Misclassification can occur when cases are not recognized as such and may be selected as controls, and vice versa. It is crucial that the criteria for being classified as cases and controls are well defined and described. Perfect diagnostic tests with 100% sensitivities and 100% specificities rarely exist, and thus diagnostic testing almost always results in some degree of misclassification in regard to disease status. There will be both false-positives and false-negatives depending on the decided cut-off between diseased and non-diseased animals. Methods exist to identify the cut-off where both are as low as possible (optimise sensitivity and specificity) or depending on the impact of either false-positives or false-negatives one can be decreased, but at the cost of an increase in the other (see Chapter 9). Therefore, it is evident that the use of diagnostic tests requires careful thinking not only about the background for doing the test, but also about the influence that an increase in the number of tests will have on the resulting sensitivity and specificity of the combination of tests. Misclassification bias due to diagnostic testing can be corrected during the analysis phase provided information regarding sensitivity and specificity has been collected.

Questions in a questionnaire may not measure what they were meant to do, or coding of all the possible measures of, e.g. barn type may not be feasible and therefore may lead to misclassification bias (Chapter 12).

EXAMPLE 11.2. Veterinarians performing pre-slaughter inspection of Danish broilers were asked to give their opinion on the bedding in the house, as they had to mark the following possibilities on an information sheet: "Is the bedding dry □ normal □ or moist □ (please X the relevant)." This question gives room for variable interpretation. Firstly, the quality of the bedding may vary considerably within the same house and secondly, there is no objective quantitative standard to refer to. The perception of dry, normal or moist is highly individual and subjective.

EXAMPLE 11.3. In a survey aiming at estimation of the prevalence of Newcastle disease in a developing country, farmers were asked to answer the following question: "Are you familiar with the symptoms of Newcastle disease?" Some may answer yes because they have experience with the disease. Others may answer yes because they have heard or read about it. Others may answer yes simply because they do not want to be regarded as ignorant.

EXAMPLE 11.4. In a Danish survey concerning a contagious poultry disease, broiler chicken farmers were asked the following question: "Do you make sure, that visitors on your farm behave in a hygienic way?" Surely, it will take a strong personality to answer "No"! Usually, farmers are very aware of "good management practice" and are not inclined to give out information that may disappoint expectations.

When conducting studies involving comparison of data on disease outbreaks in different countries, it is important to bear in mind that the official definitions of certain diseases may in fact vary considerably between countries and possibly lead to misclassifications.

EXAMPLE 11.5. For many years, Office International des Epizooties (OIE) and the European Union (EU) did not share the same definition for Newcastle Disease (ND). The EU definition was: "An infection of poultry caused by an avian strain of the paramyxovirus 1 with an Intra Cerebral Pathogenicity Index (ICPI) in day-old chicks greater than 0.7." The OIE defined ND more vaguely as "a disease of birds caused by strains of paramyxovirus type 1, significantly more virulent than lentogenic strains." The difference in the definitions means that cases of ND occurring in Thailand may not necessarily have been recorded as ND had they occurred in France and vice versa.

Measurement error occurs when an observed value measured by an instrument is different from the 'true' value (Petrie and Watson, 1999). Measurement errors may be corrected if information regarding the error exists.

11.2.3 Confounding bias

Often in epidemiological studies, the objective is to support or reject hypotheses of association between two or more variables. However, attention should be paid to possible variables, which may influence the relationship studied. If a third variable can change the observed relationship between a risk factor and a disease then *confounding* is present.

A confounding variable (confounder) is a factor that fully or partially accounts for the observed effect of the exposure (risk factor) on the disease status. There is a *confusion* of risk factor and confounder. The confounder may either cause an apparent relationship to appear or hide a true relationship. The degree of confounding may vary, but often confounding will lead to underestimation or overestimation of the factor whose effect is being studied.

In studies for risk factors, a confounder is: related to the disease and related to the risk factor (exposure) whose effect is being studied (Figure 11.2, Examples 11.6 and 11.7). A necessary link (*intermediate factor*) between the risk factor and the disease is not a confounder (Example 11.8).

Examples of typical confounders include age, sex and breed, but many more may occur in a study, and several could be present at the same time. Any variable that satisfies the conditions in Figure 11.2 should be considered as a confounder.

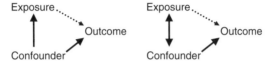

Figure 11.2. *The relationship between confounder, exposure (risk factor) and outcome (disease). The dashed line indicates the possible relation in the study between the exposure and disease. The solid lines indicate the necessary relations for confounding between the confounder, exposure and outcome.*

EXAMPLE 11.6.   In a sample of dogs an apparent relationship between number of litters and mammal tumors may be observed. However, older dogs have a greater risk of having developed tumors over the years. Also, they have had time to deliver more litters. Age is a third factor (a possible confounder), which might explain the observed relationship between number of litters and mammal tumors.

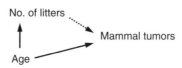

EXAMPLE 11.7.   In a study concerning respiratory disease in pigs, mechanical ventilation was found to be a risk factor. However, the size of the herd was also believed to influence the occurrence of the disease and was therefore included in the investigation. When herd size was included, the effect of mechanical ventilation disappeared. The reason was that large herds almost always had mechanical ventilation, but also carried the highest risk of having respiratory disease. Whereas, smaller herds often had passive ventilation and also a lower risk of having respiratory disease.

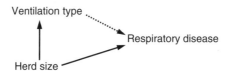

EXAMPLE 11.8.   Bovine somatotropin hormone (BST) can increase the milk yield of dairy cows. However, there has been concern that it also increased the incidence of mastitis. In an analysis of the association between BST and mastitis, the milk yield had been controlled for as a confounder. However, this is wrong because BST causes more mastitis through the increased milk yield. Therefore, milk yield is not a confounder that changes the relationship between BST and mastitis, but an intermediate factor (a direct effect of BST on milk yield).

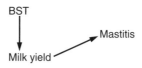

There is no mathematical or statistical test to find whether a factor is an intermediate factor or not. It is the biological knowledge about the problem that should identify when a factor is intermediate. Therefore, it is crucial to carefully consider the direction of the arrows in the causal diagram (Dohoo *et al.*, 2003).

Confounding can be controlled by exclusion, matching or analytical control depending on the purpose of the study. *Exclusion* means only including one level of the confounding variable. However, extrapolation of the results can then only be performed at this particular level of the confounder.

Confounding may also be controlled by matching during the design of the study, either by *frequency matching* or by *individual matching*. In frequency matching, the groups to be sampled must have the same proportion of the possible confounding variable. If, for example, one group contains four times as many males as females, then the other group should also be selected to contain four times as many males as females. In individual matching, each case is matched with a control with respect to the possible confounding variable. It may be cumbersome to match for many possible confounders, but when matching is performed it is usual to match for the main possible ones such as age, breed and sex. A note of caution though is that if there is any potential for a matching variable to be associated with the studied outcome, then this factor should not be used for matching.

EXAMPLE 11.9. During 1998, an outbreak of Salmonella Manhattan (SM) in humans occurred in Denmark. The cause of this outbreak was investigated by the Danish Zoonosis Centre at the Danish Veterinary Institute. There were 16 people with verified SM (cases). Since the number of cases was relatively small, matching on the potential confounders, age, sex and geography was performed in order to be able to focus the analysis on potential causes of the outbreak. On the basis of this matching, 45 people were chosen as controls. The investigation showed that smoked ham was the most probable cause of SM. This was later confirmed by recovering SM from samples collected at the production site.

Finally, confounding can be controlled by including information about the potential confounders in the analysis (see Chapter 13).

11.3 Interaction

In some situations two factors may not act independently in their contribution to disease. The presence of two different factors can influence the occurrence of disease more (or less) than we would expect from the effect that each of the two factors have on their own. This phenomenon is known as *interaction*. When interaction is present the effect of one factor on disease has to be interpreted on each level of the other factor (Figure 11.3).

Some researchers distinguish between different types of interaction: statistical interaction, biological interaction and public health interaction (one does not exclude the other). However, there is no generally accepted standard for this distinction and therefore we will not make it here. When interaction is

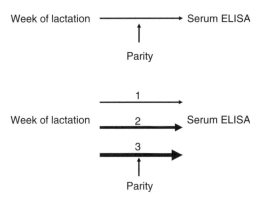

Figure 11.3. *The relationship between two factors and disease when interaction is present. In the situation in the top part there is no interaction, the association between week of lactation and the ELISA response is independent of parity. In the situation in the bottom part the increasing line thickness indicates stronger association between week of lactation and ELISA response with increasing parity.*

present and the joint effect of two factors is more than we would expect, then there is synergism between the two factors, and contrary to this when the joint effect is less than we would expect, the two factors act *antagonistically*. Again, some texts reserve the terms *synergism* and *antagonism* for biologic interaction. In this text we will not make this distinction but merely use the term synergism when there is an increased joint effect and antagonism when the joint effect is decreased (Rothman *et al.*, 1980; Ely, 1992; Rothman and Greenland, 1998). In some texts, *effect modification* is used as a synonym for interaction; however, other authors reserve this term for the effect of interaction in the population (Miettinen, 1974).

EXAMPLE 11.10. A cross-sectional study was conducted where blood samples were collected once in each of 66 herds during August 1999 and February 2000 to investigate whether the ELISA response to *Mycobacterium avium* subsp. *paratuberculosis* changes with parity (factor one) and lactation stage of the cow (factor two) (Figure 11.3). Serum samples were collected from 3796 cows in the 66 herds. The study was divided into two parts, one where cows were classified as positive or negative using a low cut-off value and one where the classification was based on a high cut-off value (in the following noted as low and high, respectively). Results of the study with low cut-off were that both parity and stage of lactation had an influence on the odds of being antibody-positive in a serum ELISA. However, the relationship was not straightforward, since there was an interaction between the two variables. This means that the effect of stage of lactation on the odds for a positive ELISA depends on the parity of the cow and vice versa. This is illustrated in Figure 11.4. Odds for a positive serum ELISA increases through lactation stages 3–12, 13–28 and 29–44 for first and second parity cows, but for third parity and above there is no increase during the same stages of lactation. The interpretation is that effect of stage of lactation depends on parity.

The odds for being ELISA positive does not increase between the two first lactation stages for parity 1 cows, but it does for parity 2 and above 2 (effect of stage of lactation depends on parity).

The interpretation of the effect of parity on the finding of a positive ELISA cannot be reported without also reporting the stage of lactation at blood sampling and vice versa. This finding is very important for practising veterinarians who would like to take blood samples from cows to find out if they are ELISA positive for *Mycobacterium avium* subsp. *paratuberculosis* using the mentioned cut-off. If the cow is a first or second parity cow, late lactation seems to be the best time for sampling to detect antibodies. However, if the cow is a third parity cow or higher, then time of sampling is not important from 3 weeks into the lactation.

In the same study the cut-off for a positive ELISA was changed (the cut-off was set at a higher value) and again the effect of parity and stage of lactation was investigated. It can be seen from Figure 11.5 that no interaction was present. There is no significant difference between the groups either within parity or within lactation.

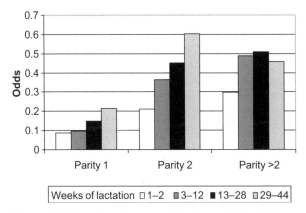

Figure 11.4. *Odds for being ELISA positive for cows at the low cut-off point for cows at different stages of lactation in different parities in 3796 cows from 66 Danish dairy herds.*

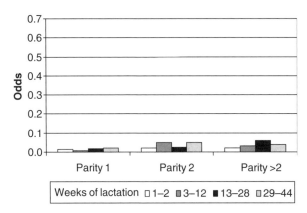

Figure 11.5. *Odds for being ELISA positive for cows at the high cut-off point for cows at different stages of lactation in different parities in 3796 cows from 66 Danish dairy herds.*

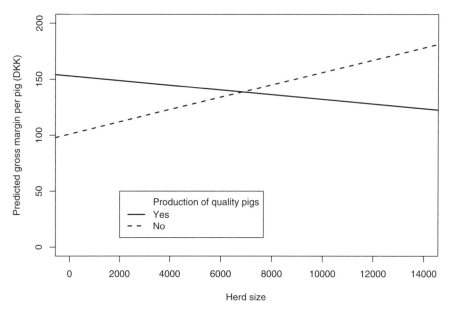

Figure 11.6. *The relationship between predicted gross margin and herd size for pig producers with and without production of quality pigs in a cross-sectional study conducted in Denmark in 2000.*

Disease is used here as an example, but interaction also applies when we are studying other problems such as increase or decrease in, e.g. production variables (weight gain, milk yield, etc.). When we are analysing epidemiological data, it is very important to take interaction into account, since it changes the interpretation of the factors involved. When interaction is present, the effect of one factor has a different interpretation depending on whether the other factor is present or not.

EXAMPLE 11.11. A cross-sectional study was conducted to investigate factors affecting the gross margins per pig (earnings) of pig producers in Denmark. A random sample of pig producers was collected stratified on farmers age, farm area (ha), geographic area and economic size. The significant factors included in the final analysis were whether or not the farm had slatted floors, fully sectioned units, production of quality pigs (organic, Antonius or other welfare requirements) and the herd size. However, the relationship between gross margin per pig, production of quality pigs and herd size was not a simple one. There was an interaction between production of quality pigs and herd size. The effect of increasing the herd size on the gross margin per pig was dependent on whether the production was of quality pigs or not. For pig producers without production of quality pigs, there was a linear relationship between the average gross margin per pig and the herd size with intercept 101.00 DKK and an increase of 5.50 DKK per increase in a herd size of 1000 pigs (see Figure 11.6). For pig producers with production of quality pigs, there was a linear relationship between the average gross margin per pig and the herd size with intercept 153.00 DKK and a decrease by 2.10 DKK for every increase in a herd size of 1000 pigs (Figure 11.6). However, this decrease in gross margin per pig was not significant.

---

12 QUESTIONNAIRES

*Annette Cleveland Nielsen, Jens Frederik Agger
and Annette Kjær Ersbøll*

12.1 Introduction

Questionnaire data are commonly used in veterinary epidemiology to obtain descriptive features of a population and in search for risk factors for health or disease and they are an integral part of epidemiological studies and investigations of disease outbreaks. Some data may not be easily obtained (or not possible to obtain at all) in other ways than asking questions to relevant persons. For example, seeking information about management from farmers, veterinarians and other consultants working in the animal production and health sector. The alternative to questionnaires may be long lasting and expensive prospective observational studies, particularly when we need information about management and working routines and their relations to health.

A questionnaire is a form with written questions. Questionnaires are designed in order to obtain information with a specific purpose, as, for example, evaluation of risk factors for chronic pleuritis in slaughter pig herds.

It should be kept in mind that questionnaire data can be very misleading due to information and selection bias, if not constructed and carried out properly. If the data from the questionnaire are not valid or reliable, the results of the studies will not be reliable. The objective of this chapter is to give guidelines for construction of questionnaires, in order to ensure that we really measure what we want to measure, i.e. secure the validity.

12.2 Types of questionnaires and communication forms

12.2.1 *Questionnaire types*

Generally, there are two types of questionnaires, the quantitative standardized type and the exploratory qualitative free style (Oppenheim, 1992).

Quantitative questionnaires can be used to gather data for hypothesis testing, while qualitative questionnaires are often used to acquire sufficient background knowledge for developing questionnaire investigations.

The *standardized questionnaire* is quantitative in nature and is the one traditionally used in veterinary epidemiology. The purpose of the standardized questionnaire is data collection of facts for subsequent statistical and epidemiological analysis. An example is a standardised questionnaire designed to identify and evaluate risk factors for chronic pleuritis in Danish slaughter pig herds (Cleveland-Nielsen *et al.*, 2002). Here, the risk factors are divided into four risk factor groups: management and production facilities, herd stem data (as, for example, SPF health status), neighbourhood factors (as, for example, distance to other herds) and finally herd-owner characteristics (such as age and participation in study groups on pig production, Figure 12.3). In this context, the word standardized means that the same questions and possibilities of answers are put to all respondents and in the same manner even though there may be more interviewers asking the questions. The questions are designed in order to answer the hypotheses established at the start of the study. This type of questionnaire requires an insight on the topic in question and its possible relation to risk factors.

Exploratory, or qualitative, questionnaires are often used in interviews conducted as conversations. The purpose of this type of questionnaire is often to generate hypotheses by gathering information on attitudes or perceptions (Vaarst *et al.*, 2002) or to pinpoint the essentials on a certain topic. If only very little is known about the topic, the qualitative questionnaire may be a way to ensure that the hypothesis in fact represents a reasonable interpretation and insight in the topic being studied. An example could be a study on why farmers act as they do in relation to occurrence of disease. Such aspects of management are important to understand when veterinary practitioners and agronomists act as consultants and advisors in health or production issues. Only very little is standardised in the qualitative type of questionnaire, but there is often a hidden hypothesis behind the topic one is interested in evaluating. An example of a qualitative questionnaire is given in Figure 12.1.

One method used for exploratory data collection is called grounded theory (Creswell, 1998). It uses a special form of interview technique with semi-structured questionnaires and open questions. It is based on an interplay between data collection and concurrent analysis of the interviews with a range of persons selected in a manner so that they represent the diversity in opinions related to the topic. The sampling and interviewing processes continue until no more new aspects are encountered for developing the theory and hypotheses. Usually, the interviews are tape recorded. Each interview is then typed

Topic: Herd health management

Facts about the herd owner
Background questions. A number of closed questions were asked as an introduction to the conversation. (Names of owner and wife, their education, and type of farm.)

Which social background does the farmer, his family and employed people have?
Please tell a little about the history of the farm.
Why did you and your wife choose to have dairy cows?
Can you give examples from start until now on how the development has had an impact on you and your family as dairy producers?
How do you share the work on the farm?
Please try to describe how you view your life here on the farm?

What is 'consulting' for a farmer?
(The interviewers' hypothesis is here that 'Recording of clinical disease just by being recorded and being presented will add to the cognition both for the farmer and for the veterinarian'.)
Is herd health management conducted in a systematic way in your herd?
How?
What does it mean for you personally that you can get advise?
Please give an example where you felt that you needed advise on problems with your cows and calves.

How is your relations to advisors – how do you use the advisory service in your decision process?
(The interviewers' preliminary hypothesis is that 'There are many non-spoken and non-written conditions that impact on the relation in a negative way compared to the goals that the farmer wanted to meet'.)
How has consultancy developed during the years you have owned the farm?
What is your opinion on this development?
What do you expect from herd health management consultancy?
What do you expect from the veterinary practitioner?
Give an example of good health management consultancy from the veterinary practitioner.
How do you feel the consultants meet your expectations?
How do you really want to use your veterinary practitioner?
How do you view your relations to the advisors that visit your herd?

Final questions
How do you think your life will be in 5 years from now?
How would you like your future on the farm?
What do you actually do in order to reach these goals?

Figure 12.1. *Example of a qualitative questionnaire with the purpose of identifying key areas of farmers' perception of farm consultants. (Adopted from the PhD study of Hans Jørgen Andersen, Danish Dairy Board.)*

on paper with a broad margin, and the text is analysed line by line, where the researcher writes down all types of reflections related to the topic. The result of this 'content analysis' of each interview is then 'constantly compared' to previous results. When no more aspects are identified, the interviewing process is stopped. The results from the initial content analysis and comparison to previous interviews (written in open coding) are then organised in groups and relations between groups (axial coding), leading to a theory that may be tested in new quantitative studies. The purpose is to establish a better theoretical background on a certain topic leading to a better foundation for designing and developing questions and questionnaires for new and more precise data collection for descriptive and analytical epidemiological studies.

The rest of this chapter will only deal with standardized questionnaires.

12.2.2 Communication forms

Interview as a research method is a conversation with some level of structure on a specific target. However, interviews are just one of several methods to obtain answers to the questions. We differentiate between the communication forms (telephone, mail, web based, face to face) and the type of questionnaire (qualitative and quantitative). An overview of the two types of questionnaires and different communication forms is given in Figure 12.2.

There are advantages and disadvantages of all four communication forms, as stated in Table 12.1. A mailed self-administered questionnaire often gives an initial response rate below 40%, whereas interviews often have a 70–80% response rate (Oppenheim, 1992). Two telephone interviews by Alban and Agger (1996) and Cleveland-Nielsen *et al.* (2002) obtained response rates of 90 and 76%, respectively. However, Asch *et al.* (1997) reported a mean response rate of approximately 60% in a study of 236 mailed surveys. Other drawbacks of mailed questionnaires are their unsuitability for respondents of poor literacy, no possibilities to avoid incomplete and/or incorrect responses or questions or avoid the passing on of questionnaires to others. The main advantage of mailed questionnaires is low costs and avoidance of interviewer bias. An advantage of telephone or face-to-face interviews is that the purpose of the study can be explained and misunderstandings of questions can be corrected, both of which can result in a larger motivation for participating and less

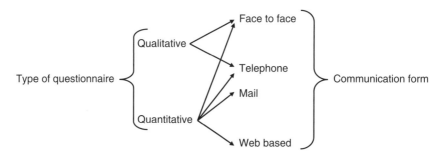

Figure 12.2. *The two types of questionnaires and four different communication forms.*

Table 12.1. *Advantages and disadvantages of different communication forms*

Type of questionnaire	Advantages	Disadvantages
Mailed questionnaire	Low cost Self-administered No interviewer bias	Low response rate Unsuitable to respondents of poor literacy Risk of many incomplete and/or incorrect answers Can be passed on to others Prone to self-selection bias
Web-based questionnaire	Low cost No interviewer bias Fast communicated Self-administered Minimal researcher administration	Requires that the respondents have a computer Low response rate Unsuitable to respondents of poor literacy Risk of many incomplete and/or incorrect answers Prone to self-selection bias
Face-to-face interview	High response rate Purpose can be explained Non-directive guidance can be given	Expensive Time consuming Prone to interviewer bias Risk of pre-judged categorisation of respondent by interviewer
Telephone interview	Low cost Fast to conduct High response rate Purpose can be explained Non-directive guidance can be given	Prone to interviewer bias Risk of pre-judged categorisation of respondent by interviewer

information bias. These topics enhance the validity of the study, if the guidance offered from the interviewer is non-directive. Interviewer bias is a drawback to both face-to-face and telephone interviews. The bias occurs when interviewers do not put the questions in the same manner or do not perceive the answers in the same manner. A special case related to the face-to-face interview is the nonverbal communication between interviewer and respondent and risk of pre-judged categorisation of a respondent by an interviewer (Waltner-Toews, 1983). Telephone interviews are less expensive and faster to conduct than face-to-face interviews. Web-based questionnaires are a fairly new form where the questionnaire is sent by e-mail or is available from a webpage. Hence, they are only suitable if the respondents have access to a computer. The respondents do all the work on their own, both reading and answering the question. This type of questionnaire is fast to conduct and only requires minimal administration by the researcher. Web-based questionnaires have the same drawbacks as mailed questionnaires. Moreover, this type of questionnaire is, together with mailed questionnaires, prone to self-selection bias. Self-selection bias occurs due to the respondents selecting themselves to participate (e.g. only the most interested farmers), opposed to interviews where the farmers are selected for participation and initially reluctant farmers can be motivated to participate.

Web-based and mailed questionnaires should give a positive impression, so the respondent feels it looks interesting and is worth looking into in detail. The layout is important, e.g. use colours and boxes to mark the answer.

12.3   Types of questions and scales of measurement

There are three main kinds of questions: open ended, semi-open ended and closed. An overview of the three types of questions and scales is given in Table 12.2. The open ended questions allow the respondent to answer freely in his/her own words and are valuable for a quantitative outcome (a discrete or a continuous scale) or with prose. The semi-open ended questions have already formulated answers, but have a possibility to include additional information. The closed questions have already formulated answers that should be mutually exclusive and cover all possibilities. All types of questions can use numerical or verbal answering possibilities. Closed and semi-open ended questions can have dichotomous (two possibilities) or polytomous (more than two) answering possibilities and they can be ordinal (order of categories) or nominal (no order). Moreover, closed questions can be designed using ratings or intensity scales with either verbal or numerical scaling (numerical rating scale (NRS), verbal rating scale (VRS) and visual analog scale (VAS)).

A VRS is used for nominal and ordinal variables with, e.g. five different answers. The answer possibilities are given in prose (e.g. question 5 in

Table 12.2. *Types of questions and scales*

	Scales					
	Qualitative outcome			*Quantitative outcome*		*In prose**
	Dichotomous	*Polytomous*		*Discrete*	*Continuous*	
		Nominal	*Ordinal*			
Types of questions						
Closed	X	X	X			
Semi-open	X	X	X			
Open				X	X	X

*When the interviews have been performed, the answers can sometimes be grouped using one of the other scales.

Figure 12.3). An NRS is used for ordinal variables. The answers are given as a number on a scale, e.g. gait score 0–5, where 0 means normal walking and 5 means unable to walk. A VAS is used to quantify a measure, e.g. pain. The scale is, a 10 cm line with no pain in 0.0 cm and severe pain at 10.0 cm. At evaluation an 'X' is put on the line to indicate the severity of the pain. The outcome is the distance from 0.0 cm to the 'X'.

It is recommended to use words, phrases and styles familiar to most people within the relevant population of responders. It is also recommended to use simple and precise words; short, specific and non-vague phrases without ambiguous details. Aim for short questions (as a rule of thumb less than 15–20 words per question) although not so short that it reduces the precision. Further, use only one-dimensional questions, i.e. ask only about one thing in each question and avoid leading questions, e.g. 'You clean the cow barn every day, don't you?' Do not make presumptions, be realistic and use common sense. Consider to include more questions on the same aspect for validation of answers within the questionnaire (see Figure 12.3).

Examples of well-designed questions are given in Figure 12.3: question numbers 2, 4 and 9 are open ended questions, where 2 uses verbal answering in prose and 4 numerical on a continuous scale, whereas number 9 have a discrete answering possibility. Number 6 is an example of a semi-open ended question with verbal, polytomous, nominal answering possibility. Numbers 1, 3, 5, 7 and 8 are closed questions. The examples in Figure 12.3 are well-designed questions, as they are simple, short and use a straightforward language with terms familiar to the respondents. Moreover, there are not more than five answering possibilities to any question and all replies are mutually exclusive.

Examples of poor and misleading questions are given in Figure 12.4(a) and improvements to these poor and misleading questions are shown in

No	Question	Reply					Notes for interviewer	Variable	Code					Coding
		20–30	31–40	41–50	51–60	>60			1	2	3	4	5	
1	How old are you?	20–30	31–40	41–50	51–60	>60		Age						
2	How do you manage the problem of underweight piglets, when the batch is moved to the grower units?						Write down answer	Underpig						
3	Do you move underweight piglets backwards to the next litter?	Yes	No					Pigback	1	2				
4	How large a percentage of barley is in the home-mixed feed?	Percent						Pctbarley	Number					
5	Do tail-biting occur in this unit?	Yes, often	Yes, sometimes	Yes, but seldom	No, never			Tailbite	1	2	3	4		
6	Who euthanise ill pigs?	Me	Staff	Daka	Vet	Others		Euthanper	1	2	3	4	5	
7	What is the SPF-health status of the herd?	SPF	MS	Skd	Skm	Conv		SPF	1	2	3	4	5	
8	How many days do you treat pigs with arthritis?	1 day	2 days	3 days	>3 days			Arthritis	1	2	3	4		
9	How many yearsows do you have?	Number						Yearsows	Number					

Type of question and scale: 1 = closed, ordinal; 2 = open, in prose; 3 = closed, dichotomous; 4 = open, continuous; 5 = closed, ordinal; 6 = semi-open, nominal; 7 = closed, nominal; 8 = closed, ordinal; 9 = open, discrete.

Figure 12.3. *Examples of well-designed questions. The questions are from a large-scale study of risk factors for health status of Danish slaughter pig herds (Cleveland-Nielsen et al., 2002).*

(a)

No.	Question	Reply			Variable	Code			Coding
1	You clean the cow barn every day, don't you?	Yes	No		Clean	1	2		
2	Does it happen often that your cows get stone bruises in the claws because the path from the farm to the field is in bad condition?	Never	Sometimes	Often	Bruises	1	2	3	
3	How many man hours are used for feeding and milking the cows in the morning?	Number			Man-hours	Number			

(b)

No.	Question	Reply				Variable	Code				Coding
1	How often during one week do you remove dung from the floors in the cow barn?	Number				Clean	Number				
2A	Is the path from the farm to the field where the cows grass . . .	with a dry surface without stones?	with a dry surface with stones?	with a muddy surface with stones?	with a muddy surface without stones?	Path	1	2	3	4	
2B	How many cows have had bruises in the claws in the past month?	Number				Bruises	Number				
2C	What is the number of cow years in your herd during the past year?	Number				Year-Cow	Number				
3A	How many man hours are used for feeding the cows in the morning?	Number				MH-feed	Number				
3B	How many man hours are used for milking the cows in the morning?	Number				MH-milk	Number				

Figure 12.4. (a) Examples of poor and misleading questions. (b) Examples of improving the questions from part a).

Figure 12.4(b). The purpose of question number 1 was to get information on removal of dung on the floor of the cow barn. However, we cannot be sure that the farmer perceives the question in this manner, nor that he knows that we are specifically interested in the removal of dung on the floor. So we have to be more specific. Therefore, the question has been rephrased in order to ensure that he knows that we are interested in the removal of dung on the floor and the frequency within a week. Now all respondents reply on the same specific question within the same time span. Number 2 has to be divided into several questions in Figure 12.4(b), where we first establish the condition of the path and, second the number of bruises. Number 3 also has to be divided into two questions related to feeding and milking, respectively, to be able to have specific answers on use of man-hours for the two tasks.

The advantages of closed questions are that they are easy to interpret, code, process and analyse and make group comparisons easy, in contrast to open ended questions (Oppenheim, 1992; Vaillancourt et al., 1991). This makes closed questions less prone to information and misclassification bias. Moreover, closed questions are less time consuming, enabling more questions to be asked within the same time span. The disadvantages of closed questions are that there might be loss of information and they can be tedious to answer. The advantages of open ended questions, on the other hand, are that they are easier to formulate and give freedom and spontaneity of the answers and an opportunity to give a thorough answer. Dichotomous or polytomous answer possibilities in closed questions are eliciting the most reliable answers and re-categorizing polytomous questions into dichotomies, and do not jeopardise the repeatability of the questions. For closed questions no more than five choices should be available in interviews and no more than 10 in mailed questionnaires (Vaillancourt et al., 1991). Polytomous closed questions obtained trough interviews can elicit ordinal information bias (Oppenheim, 1992), where respondents are more likely to choose the last or first of multiple categories. If closed questions are designed as ratings or intensity scales, another ordinal bias can occur, as respondents are more prone to choose middle values. An example could be sizes of calves with three answering possibilities: small, medium and large, where respondents most often answered medium size. To avoid ordinal information bias, categories of the closed questions can be interchanged among respondents.

12.4 Constructing the questionnaire

The questionnaire and questions are designed in order to obtain all relevant information in a way that reduces systematic errors (the so-called bias, see Section 12.6). The language needs to be positive, so that the responders do not feel guilty, embarrassed or personally offended, if questions touch on personal topics, e.g. the way the animal owner handles his animals. Proof-read the questionnaire to ensure correct spelling and grammar.

12.4.1 Pre-coding of answers in structured questionnaires

Pre-coding within a questionnaire may be a great help to the investigator for the construction of the data set, although the possibilities for pre-coding depends on the type of question. Pre-coding can be organised as 1, 2, 3, 4, 5, 6, etc., according to the answer. However, if more than one answer to the same open ended question is acceptable, there are at least two possible ways of coding. One is the numbering system 1, 2, 4, 8, 16, etc. With this method it is possible to record several answers within a single code by adding the numbers, e.g. answers 1, 4 and 8 are recorded as the sum 13. This number is a unique code that can only be obtained in this specific combination of answers. This coding does not take up much space in the questionnaire, and the code can be dissolved in its components in later analyses. The alternative is to do separate coding as dichotomous variables. The advantage is that it is quite easy to proceed with data analysis, and the disadvantage is that it takes up much space in the questionnaire.

12.4.2 Pre-testing

It is always wise to test the questionnaire before the 'real' data collection begins. Pre-testing can initially be done on experts on the subject concerned and afterwards on the intended target group. The purpose is to check for mistakes, whether the respondents understand the questions, to check the logic order of the questions, and also to coordinate when several interviewers participate in the data collection. For example, in a survey with three interviewers this can be done by having each interviewer calling 10 respondents, and then discuss the experiences later. The questionnaire is modified according to the pre-testing, and more than one pre-test may be necessary. The units (farmers, dog owners, etc.) that have been used for the pre-test may still be used in the real investigation, although some researchers omit the use of the pre-tested units in the later analyses. The length of the interview or time needed to answer a mailed questionnaire should be evaluated in the pre-test. An interview (telephone or face to face) should not take more than 30–40 min and a mailed questionnaire not more than 1 h in order for the respondents to be motivated to complete the questionnaire.

12.5 Obtaining the information

Generally, a questionnaire should be as short and specific as possible depending on the topic, and not take too long a time to complete, depending on the method of administration. It is important to remember that the respondent and the interviewer get tired after more than 30–60 min of questioning.

It is always wise to inform respondents before the interview so that they feel secure about the situation and the purpose of the investigation. Thus, it is quite common that the investigator or affiliated supporters sends a letter of introduction (see example in Figure 12.5) encouraging the selected person to participate. It is important to state the confidentiality of participation and of answers. It is important the interviewer acts as a person who can be trusted. Make sure you obey national laws, e.g. the possibility to file personal

---

Letter head for the organisation

13. August 1993

To the herd owner.

MASTITIS CONTROL

Questionnaire regarding infection with Streptococcus agalactiae.

The Danish Dairy Board is responsible for mastitis control in Denmark.

Beyond problems with high somatic cell count, some herds have cases of mastitis caused by Group B Streptococcae. On an annual basis 150–200 herds are infected by this bacteria. The Dairy Board has together with J.F. Agger, Department of Animal Science and Animal Health, The Royal Veterinary and Agricultural University planned an investigation with the purpose to find explanations on why some herds get infected and other herds never contract the infection.

The investigation will take place in all herds newly infected with Str. Agalactiae in 1992, and in a similar number of herds without the infection.

During the next 14 days a student from The Royal Veterinary and Agricultural University will call you by telephone and ask you to answer some questions.

In order to obtain results that are relevant for Danish dairy farmers, The Dairy Board encourage you to answer all the questions in agreement with the current conditions in your herd.

It is emphasised that your participation in the study will be onfidential, and your name and herd id number will not be given in the planned report.

The result of the study will be presented in the Dairy Board newsletter.

The Dairy Board asks you to receive the telephone interviewer in a friendly manner and The Dairy Board wants to thank you for your participation in the investigation.

Sincerely

Figure 12.5. *Example of a letter to the herd owner as an introduction to an interview.*

information that can be considered under the law of register data. Obtain farmers' written permission to extract data from databases if they should be linked to the questionnaire data at a later stage.

It is important to stress that the questionnaire should always be available upon request when using questionnaire data in publications.

12.6 Bias related to questionnaires

Bias is also covered in Chapter 11, but some aspects have specific reference to questionnaires and will be covered here. Bias is a systematic error in contrast to random error in, e.g. sampling of data (see Chapters 3 and 11). Bias jeopardize the validity of results and one is not able to correct for systematic error at the analysing stage (except for confounding, if data on the confounding variable have been collected, see Chapter 11). This section will describe the special kind of bias that questionnaire data are prone to.

The most crucial aspects for questionnaire data are: representativity of the initial sample of respondents enabling inference to the target population and an adequately high response rate, ensuring representativity of the respondents, both of which are associated with selection bias. Moreover, validity of the data is crucial. These issues are related to information bias.

12.6.1 *Selection bias*

Selection bias occurs if the selection odds for the diseased or the exposed groups is different from the selection odds for the non-diseased or unexposed groups (Kleinbaum *et al.*, 1982). Selection bias from questionnaire data is related to a non-random sample and/or a low response rate. In order to avoid selection bias the initial sample of respondents should be a random sample ensuring representativity, thereby enabling inferences of the results from the sample to the target population. A non-random sample as, for instance, a convenience sample, may lead to selection bias. An example of a convenience sample could be only to sample those herds delivering pigs to a special slaughterhouse.

If the response rate is low there are greater possibilities of bias being introduced as both non-respondents and respondents may have special characteristics that make the resulting sample non-representative. This bias is also called volunteer bias. However, even surveys with a high response rate may not provide a representative sample of the population. Still, response rates are a conventional proxy for assessment of bias, which often is difficult to identify (Asch *et al.*, 1997). Definition of the response rate is not straightforward, as correction of either the numerator or the denominator is possible. According to Asch *et al.* (1997), the crudest measure of response rate is dividing the number of questionnaires received by the numbers sent. However, there might be several reasons for correction of the response rate, as, for instance, undeliverable to address, dead respondents, failure to meet inclusion criteria or other things making a respondent non-eligible (Asch *et al.*, 1997). In order to obtain a high response rate a letter with information, giving a good explanation of the study and its purpose should be send to the respondents a couple of weeks before the mailed questionnaire is sent or the interview is going to be conducted (see example in Figure 12.5). The letter of information should also state why the respondent has been chosen and the importance of the respondent's participation. For many respondents it is important that data are treated confidentially and that they do remain anonymous. An offering of a reward for participation might increase the response rate, but it might also introduce selection bias from self-selection. A return envelope should always accompany mailed questionnaires and for interviews the respondents should be able to choose for him or her the most convenient time for the interview in order to obtain a higher response rate. Moreover, it is important to keep a log book in order to send reminders or call non-respondents several times. Reminders, either by mail or by telephone, were shown to increase the response rate with a mean of 13% when Asch *et al.* (1997) evaluated 321 mailed questionnaires, whereas anonymity or rewards did not increase the response rate. The response rate should always be stated in publications enabling readers to judge the possible extent of selection bias. In order to evaluate selection bias due to non-respondents, self-selection of respondents or low representativity of the respondents to the population, values on selected variables for all three groups can be compared, as done in a study by Cleveland-Nielsen *et al.* (2002), see Table 12.3. By inspection of Table 12.3, it can be stated that

Table 12.3. *Comparisons between quartiles for the 265 respondent herds, the 111 non-respondent herds and the target population – 10,628 Danish slaughter pig herds in year 2000*

Variable	Respondent			Non-respondent			Population		
% Chronic pleuritis	Q_1	Median	Q_3	Q_1	Median	Q_3	Q_1	Median	Q_3
Overall	8.5	22.4	41.7	8.6	23.1	39.0	8.1	19.5	31.6
Health status									
SPF herds[a]	4.3	6.1	9.7	5.2	6.5	8.5	4.6	7.0	11.3
MS herds	6.5	12.0	23.4	6.4	12.5	25.9	7.4	11.6	21.5
Conventional herds	10.2	28.5	45.5	10.2	27.0	40.6	9.6	22.2	30.9
Annual deliverance	1304	2566	4214	1000	2316	4056	652	2012	3788

[a]Only five SPF herds in the non-respondent group.

there are no large differences between values for the variables for the three groups, so there does not seem to be any selection bias, non-respondent bias or self-selection bias of the respondent group in the study. Other tests for non-respondent bias are: a repeated survey, which can be conducted on a sample of initial non-responders comparing these results with those from the original respondent group, or comparing information from respondents with known information about the underlying population (Asch *et al.*, 1997).

12.6.2 *Information bias*

Information bias gives a distortion in the effect of risk factors due to measurement error or misclassification of subjects on one or more variables (Kleinbaum *et al.*, 1982). Information bias can occur from: the questionnaire itself, interviewer bias, respondent bias or misclassification bias (misclassification bias is here defined as a special case of information bias and will be dealt with separately below). An example of bias caused by the questionnaire itself can be a question not understandable to the respondents or which the respondents are likely to misunderstand and thereby not answer correctly upon. Interviewer bias can occur if interviewers are asking leading questions to the respondents as: 'Don't you . . .?' Information bias from the respondents are often recall bias and they often appear if one asks a question, on a topic that happened long time ago or on a topic that the respondent only seldom experiences.

Information bias due to the questionnaire itself is best avoided by pre-testing the questionnaire on either experts on the study subject or both experts and a sub-sample of respondents. The pre-testing should ensure that the questions are understandable and all necessary questions are asked, and unnecessary questions omitted. All questions should have a clear purpose and be clear, unambiguous, non-directive and short. Questions should not exceed 15–20 words and one should use language and terms familiar to the respondents (Vaillancourt *et al.*, 1991). Double barrelled (two questions within one) and double negative questions should be avoided (Oppenheim, 1992). If the purpose of the questionnaire is clear, then accurate questions can be asked and reliable data can be collected. There should be an internal logic of questions within logic sequences, for instance, by topic or time order or a funnel approach (gradually narrowing the scope) should be achieved in order to focus the respondents' thinking and enhancing recall (Oppenheim, 1992; Waltner-Toews, 1983). Interviewer bias, due to inconsequent phrasing of questions, differences in perception of answers or directive guidance is best reduced by training of interviewers. The training should ensure that all know the purpose of not only the study, but also of all questions in the questionnaire and the importance of the same phrasing of questions and non-directive guidance. Information bias due to the respondent consists of recall bias and prestige bias. Prestige bias occurs when the respondents give what they believe to be the best answer or what they think the researcher thinks they should be doing (Waltner-Toews, 1983). Recall bias occurs when the respondent does not remember the topic that he is asked. Both types of bias can be reduced by asking logic questions within logic sequences in the questionnaire and by the attitude and presentation by the interviewer, thereby focusing the respondents thinking and recall (Waltner-Toews, 1983). Moreover, it is important only to ask questions that are not too far away in time in order to minimise recall bias.

Misclassification bias is here defined as a special case of information bias that occurs when the investigator codes or enters data in the wrong way, thereby leading to an error in the classification of responses. When coding open ended questions into categories it requires a coding frame for each question developed from a representative sample of responses. The categorization should pay purpose of answering the hypothesis behind the question and not just do justice to the responses. Moreover, there should be a reasonable number of respondents in every category. In order to avoid misclassification bias in closed questions, a consistent coding of categories should be used, i.e. always 1 for yes and 2 for no. There should be a special code for missing information. The program for entering data could be programmed only to be able to accept possible defined values for coding. Correct entering of data should be checked by proofreading the raw data and the data entered. This should be done by both the persons entering the data and by another person. Moreover, the entered data should be checked for outliers and impossible values (see also Chapter 10 on data management).

12.7 Validity of questionnaire data

Validity concerns the problem to measure what we want to measure. The validity of the questions and thereby ultimately our study is best evaluated by observing the true status of the question by visits to the farm or visits to a sub-sample of the farms. Another possibility is to compare the questionnaire data to other sources of information on the same variable, as, for instance, databases including information on health status, herd size, etc., verifying the data (Oppenheim, 1992). One can also ask cross-check questions, asking the same information in a different manner or cross-check questions demanding logical consistency (Waltner-Toews, 1983; Oppenheim, 1992; Cleveland-Nielsen *et al.*, 2002). In Figure 12.6, examples of cross-check questions on all-in all-out production of slaughter pigs are given. The first question in

No.	Question	Reply		Notes for interviewer	Variable	Code		Coding
1	Do you practise batch production with all-in all-out?	Yes	No		AIAO	1	2	
2	Do you move underweight pigs backwards to the next litter?	Yes	No		Back	1	2	
3	Over how long time are new pigs installed in the unit?	Number			Piginst	Number		

Figure 12.6. *Examples of cross-check questions to improve validity of the answers on all-in all-out production. The questions are from a large-scale study of risk factors for health status of Danish slaughter pig herds (Cleveland-Nielsen et al., 2002).*

Figure 12.6 establishes whether the farmer thinks he has all-in all-out production of slaughter pigs. The next two questions check this by asking how he manages underweight pigs and over how long time the units are filled with pigs. Obviously, it cannot be all-in all-out production if underweight pigs are moved backwards and the units are filled continuously.

The repeatability of the data (i.e. will the information given be consistent) is best evaluated by the repeatability of the information. A simple test–retest design can be conducted, where the same respondents or a random sub-sample of respondents are given the same questionnaire again within a reasonable time period (Schukken *et al.*, 1989; Hansen, 2002). The magnitude of the different error types, as coding and typing errors, measurement error or farmer/interviewer error can be evaluated overall or within topics (Schukken *et al.*, 1989). Repeatability of categorical data can be estimated by kappa (κ). Repeatability of continuous data can be evaluated by using Bland Altman plots and by calculating the correlation coefficients (see Chapter 13) (Sallander *et al.*, 2001).

12.8 Perspectives and applicability of questionnaires in the dialogue between farmers and advisors

Veterinary advise to farmers related to herd health management requires knowledge about the biological problems (disease occurrence), the production conditions and the environment, and how these have developed during the past period of, e.g. 6–12 months. Some of the information can only be available from a discussion between the farmer and the advisor. Therefore, it might be a good idea to develop questionnaires that can form a basis for a discussion between the farmer and the veterinarian. The topic should be quite specific; for example, focusing on mastitis, housing conditions and working routines. The questionnaires need to be a combination of quantitative and qualitative questions, in order to get a common understanding of the reasons for the situation. Somehow, this is 'just' a further development of the anamnestic procedure, which veterinarians always deal with before treatment of disease.

12.9   Acknowledgement

We thank Hans Jørgen Andersen, Danish Dairy Board, for providing an example of a qualitative questionnaire.

13 DATA ANALYSIS

Annette Kjær Ersbøll, Jeanett Bruun and Nils Toft

13.1 Introduction

The aim of this chapter is to give a general introduction to data analysis used in veterinary epidemiology. The chapter is initiated by a general discussion on hypothesis testing and selecting the correct statistical test. Before collection of data, the hypothesis, significance level, etc. should be considered. Analyses of continuous and dichotomous outcomes are given as these are the most common. Analysis of a continuous outcome is demonstrated using *t*-test, analysis of variance (ANOVA) and linear regression. Analysis of a dichotomous outcome is described by the χ^2-test, McNemar test, logistic regression and logistic analysis. Agreement between measures is described using kappa (κ) for a qualitative outcome and Bland–Altman plot for a continuous outcome. Only the most important formulas are given in this chapter. References are given for a detailed description, proofs, etc. Appendix E gives the SAS-code (Statistical Analysis System, version 8.2 SAS Institute) and output for selected examples given in this chapter. Appendix F gives the R-code and output for selected examples given in this chapter.

13.2 Introduction to hypothesis testing

In this chapter, *hypothesis* refers to the statistical hypothesis as described in Chapter 2. The basic idea about hypothesis testing is that we make inference about the population using a sample drawn from the population. Random selection (Chapter 8) of the sample is important in order to avoid bias (Chapter 11). However, due to uncertainty, the sample estimates are not exactly the same as the true (but usually unknown) population parameters. We therefore use a probability (p-value) to indicate the chance of getting the result if the hypothesis is true. This is the basic principle in hypothesis testing. Hypothesis testing is initiated by formulating the hypothesis. The statistical hypothesis is a mathematical formulation of the effects on the outcome to test. As an example, consider the effect of breeds on milk yield. The hypothesis could be: The milk yield is the same for all breeds. This is called the null hypothesis, H_0. The null hypothesis is usually stating no effect. Whenever testing a null hypothesis, H_0, there is an alternative hypothesis, H_1.

EXAMPLE 13.1. In order to evaluate the relation between breed, parity and milk yield, data from one herd were selected from a large study of milk yield, cell count, etc. in Danish dairy cows. In total, 111 cows were present in the selected herd. Consider the effect of breed on milk yield. The hypothesis could be: 'The milk yield is the same for all breeds'. This is the null hypothesis, H_0, stating no effect of breed on milk yield. The alternative hypothesis, H_1, is: 'There is a difference in milk yield between at least two of the breeds'.

In order to evaluate the H_0 hypothesis, the value of a test statistic is calculated and compared to a specific distribution. The statistical tests are described in detail in the following sections. For each test statistic there is a critical value of the test statistic and an associated p-value. The p-value is a probability describing the chance of getting the observed value of the test if the null hypothesis is true. The critical value is a cut-off value based on a specified significance level (e.g. 5%) and the statistical test used. The critical value can be used for making a decision of acceptance or rejection of the null hypothesis. If the test statistic is above the critical value, we will reject the null hypothesis and accept the alternative hypothesis. However, if the test statistic is less than or equal to the critical value we accept the null hypothesis. Rejection of the null hypothesis (and thereby acceptance of the alternative hypothesis) means that we conclude that the result of the test is significant. Acceptance of the null hypothesis means that we cannot reject the null hypothesis and we therefore conclude that the result is non-significant. Acceptance or rejection of the hypothesis in relation to the p-value is illustrated in Table 13.1. The p-value depends on the statistical test used and the test statistic value (sample size and standard deviation). Each statistical test has a specific distribution (often normal, t, F, χ^2). The p-value is the area under the distribution curve of the tail of the distribution calculated from the test statistic value (see Figure 13.1).

The decision of acceptance or rejection of the null hypothesis might be wrong. If we reject the null hypothesis and conclude a significant effect, when there is no true difference, we are making a type I error. Alternatively, if we accept the null hypothesis and conclude a non-significant effect, when there is in reality a difference, we are making a type II error (Table 13.2).

Table 13.1. *Acceptance or rejection of the* H_0 *hypothesis. The relations between p-value, critical values* (C_1 *and* C_2) *and the significance level* (α) *are given for the two cases, significance and non-significance. The significance level is traditionally set to* $\alpha = 0.05$

p-*Value*	Test statistic value (tsv)			Hypotheses	
	One-sided		Two-sided	H_0	H_1
	Right	*Left*			
p-value $\geq \alpha$	tsv $< C_1$	tsv $> -C_1$	$-C_2 < $ tsv $< C_2$	Cannot reject	–
p-value $< \alpha$	tsv $\geq C_1$	tsv $\leq -C_1$	$C_2 \leq$ tsv or tsv $\leq -C_2$	Reject	Accept

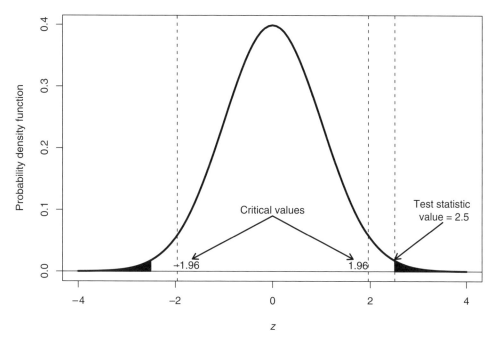

Figure 13.1. *A distribution for testing against a two-sided alternative hypothesis indicating the test statistic value for a specific study (2.5), the critical value (± 1.96) and the p-value (0.012, the sum of the dark areas.)*

Table 13.2. *The type I and type II errors in hypothesis testing*

		True condition	
		H_0 *true*	H_1 *true*
H_0 hypothesis	Accepted (not rejected)	Correct decision $1 - \alpha$: Confidence	Type II error: β
	Rejected	Type I error: α α: Significance level	Correct decision $1 - \beta$: Power

The type I error is denoted by α and is called the significance level, often set to 0.05 (5%). The type II error is usually denoted β and $1 - \beta$ is called the power of the test (β is often set to 20%). By selecting a 5% significance level and 80% power we accept to make a wrong conclusion or a type I and a type II error in 5 and 20% of the cases, respectively (Chapter 8). In 5% of the cases we conclude that there is a significant difference (reject H_0) although there is no true difference. In 20% of the cases we conclude that there is no difference (do not reject H_0) even though there is a true difference. The choice of $\alpha = 0.05$ and $\beta = 0.20$ is conservative. However, we can increase the power (e.g. $\beta = 0.05$), but this implies a dramatic increase in sample size.

13.3 Selection of statistical test

When the hypothesis has been stated, a statistical test has to be selected. The choice has to be based on (1) the type of outcome and (2) the type and number of independent (explanatory) variables to be analysed. For continuous outcomes the analyses could be a t-test, analysis of variance and linear regression. The t-test is used when only one explanatory variable with two levels is to be evaluated, e.g. comparison of two different diets based on daily weight gain. If the explanatory variable has more than two levels and/or there are more than one explanatory variable to be tested, analysis of variance is an appropriate method to use. When the hypothesis concerns evaluation of the association between two continuous variables, linear regression and correlation should be used. For dichotomous outcomes the analyses could be the χ^2-test, McNemar test, logistic regression and logistic analysis. In general, the χ^2-test can be used for evaluation of the association between two qualitative variables. If the association between more than two variables is to be evaluated, logistic regression and logistic analysis could be performed. The association between a dichotomous outcome and a continuous explanatory variable can be analysed using logistic regression. For evaluation of the association between a dichotomous outcome and qualitative explanatory variables, logistic analysis should be used. The choice of statistical test for evaluation of the hypothesis is very important. The significance of the effects, the results and the conclusion are based on the method used. Therefore, it is very important to identify the type and scale of the outcome to be tested (Chapter 3) in order to choose the correct analysis. An overview of different statistical methods depending on the type of outcome and the type and number of explanatory variables is given in Table 13.3.

Table 13.3. Overview of different statistical tests depending on the type of the outcome and the type and number of explanatory variables

Outcome (dependent variable)	Explanatory variable (independent variable)			
	Quantitative	Qualitative		
		Two groups paired	Two groups unpaired	One or more variables each with two or more levels
Quantitative				
Continuous	Linear regression Correlation	Paired t-test	t-test	Analysis of variance (ANOVA)
Discrete*	e.g. Poisson regression	e.g. Poisson analysis	e.g. Poisson analysis	e.g. Poisson analysis
Time-to-event*	Survival analysis	Survival analysis	Survival analysis	Survival analysis
Qualitative				
Ordinal*	Ordinal logistic regression	Ordinal logistic analysis	Ordinal logistic analysis χ^2-test, Fisher exact test	Ordinal logistic analysis
Nominal*	Nominal logistic regression	Nominal logistic analysis	Nominal logistic analysis χ^2-test, Fisher exact test	Nominal logistic analysis
Dichotomous	Logistic regression	McNemar	Logistic analysis χ^2-test, Fisher exact test	Logistic analysis

*These topics are considered beyond the scope of this book and will not be addressed further.

13.4 Analysis of a continuous outcome

13.4.1 *Comparison of a mean with a given value*

In order to compare a mean value with a given value, a *t*-test can be used. The hypothesis is that the mean value is not significantly different from the given value. As an example, consider the hypothesis 'The mean weight at weaning in piglets is equal to 7 kg'. The hypotheses, test statistic value and distribution of the test are

$$H_0: \quad \mu = \mu_0, \qquad H_1: \quad \mu \neq \mu_0$$

$$t = \frac{\bar{y} - \mu_0}{s/\sqrt{n}}$$

$$t \sim t(n-1)$$

where μ_0 is the given value
  μ is the population mean
  t is the test statistic value
  $\bar{y}$ is the estimated mean value
  s is the estimate of the standard deviation
  n is sample size (number of animals)
  $t(n-1)$ is the distribution of the test statistic value (t distribution with $(n-1)$ degrees of freedom)

When the null hypothesis is rejected, we have shown that the mean value is significantly different from the given value μ_0.

EXAMPLE 13.2. In a study of the weaning weight in piglets, data for 379 piglets in one herd were extracted from a database for a 6 month period. The mean weight at weaning was $\bar{y} = 7.27$ kg with a standard deviation at $s = 1.38$ kg. The hypotheses are

$$H_0: \quad \mu = 7.0\,\text{kg}, \qquad H_1: \quad \mu \neq 7.0\,\text{kg}$$

The test statistic value is

$$t = \frac{7.27 - 7.0}{1.38/\sqrt{379-1}} = 3.75$$

The distribution of the test statistic value is

$$t(379 - 1) = t(378)$$

The critical value using a 5% significance level and a two-sided alternative hypothesis is 1.97. As the test statistic value is greater than the critical value, we reject the null hypothesis and conclude that the weaning weight in the herd is significantly different from 7.0 kg.

13.4.2 *Comparison of means for two independent groups: t-test*

In order to evaluate a difference in the milk yield between the two breeds Danish Holstein Friesians (DHF) and crossbreeds (CB), a *t*-test can be performed. The hypothesis is 'There is no difference in milk yield between Danish Holstein Friesians and crossbreeds'. A *t*-test can be used to test the difference in means between two groups. In the present example, we would like to test the difference in mean milk yield between DHF and CB. The outcome should be quantitative on a continuous scale. The hypotheses, test statistic value and distribution of the test statistic are, respectively,

$$H_0: \quad \mu_1 = \mu_2, \qquad H_1: \quad \mu_1 \neq \mu_2$$

$$t = \frac{\bar{y}_1 - \bar{y}_2}{\sqrt{s_P^2 \left(\frac{1}{n_1} + \frac{1}{n_2}\right)}}$$

$$t \sim t(n_1 + n_2 - 2)$$

where μ_1 and μ_2 are the population means for the two groups
       t is the test statistic value
       $\bar{y}_1$ and $\bar{y}_2$ are the mean values for the two groups
       n_1 and n_2 are the numbers of animals in the two groups
       $t(n_1 + n_2 - 2)$ is the distribution of the test statistic value
         (*t*-distribution with $(n_1 + n_2 - 2)$ degrees of freedom)
       s_P^2 is the estimate of the pooled variance for the two groups

The pooled variance is calculated as

$$s_P^2 = \frac{(n_1 - 1)s_1^2 + (n_2 - 1)s_2^2}{n_1 + n_2 - 2}$$

where s_1^2 and s_2^2 are the variances for the two groups. It is assumed that the two population variances are equal. The assumption regarding equal population variances can be tested. If rejected, an alternative *t*-test can be used with unequal variances (Sokal and Rohlf, 1981). The hypotheses are

$$H_0: \quad \mu_1 = \mu_2, \qquad H_1: \quad \mu_1 \neq \mu_2$$

with a two-sided alternative hypothesis. This means that if we reject the null hypothesis and accept the alternative hypothesis, we show that the mean values for the two groups are significantly different, but we do not in principle have prior knowledge about whether μ_1 is greater than or less than μ_2. Both possibilities can occur in a two-sided test. However, if we have a case, where only a one-sided result is of interest, a one-sided test can be used. This is the case when testing e.g. new vaccines. The new vaccine is only of interest, if it

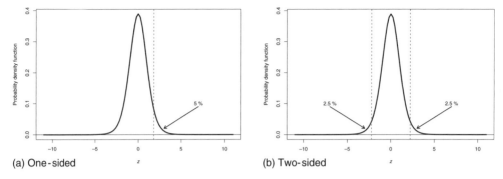

Figure 13.2. *The t-distribution for a one-sided and a two-sided test (df = 10).*

reduces the risk of disease, increases the weight gain, etc. Let μ_p be the weight gain for pigs not vaccinated (placebo) and μ_v the weight gain for vaccinated pigs in the population, respectively. The one-sided hypotheses are then

$$H_0: \quad \mu_v \leq \mu_p, \qquad H_1: \quad \mu_v > \mu_p$$

In most cases, we will use a two-sided alternative hypothesis, as we do not know which level will be the larger. The consequence of using a one-sided versus a two-sided alternative hypothesis is related to the conclusion and how easy it is to obtain significance. Using a two-sided alternative hypothesis, the significance, α (e.g. 5%) is divided between the two tails. Using a one-sided alternative hypothesis, the significance is not divided but is put in one of the tails, depending on the direction of H_1. It is easier to obtain significance by using a one-sided alternative hypothesis, as the absolute critical value is smaller in a one-sided alternative hypothesis compared to the critical value in a two-sided alternative hypothesis. This is illustrated in Figure 13.2.

The assumptions for using a t-test are:

- Data have a normal distribution.
- The observations have the same variance.
- The observations should be independent.

These assumptions should be evaluated whenever the test is performed.

EXAMPLE 13.3. In a study of the relation between milk yield and breed, 111 cows from one herd were included. In the example we will focus on one risk factor: breed (DHF and CB). Descriptive analysis (n, mean, standard deviation, standard error, median, Q1 and Q3) of milk yield is given in Table 13.4. The influence of breed (DHF and CB) on milk yield, has been tested using a t-test. The hypotheses are

$$H_0: \quad \mu_{\text{DHF}} = \mu_{\text{CB}}, \qquad H_1: \quad \mu_{\text{DHF}} \neq \mu_{\text{CB}}$$

The test statistic value is

$$t = \frac{\bar{y}_{DHF} - \bar{y}_{CB}}{\sqrt{s_P^2 \left(\frac{1}{n_{DHF}} + \frac{1}{n_{CB}} \right)}}$$

where

$$s_P^2 = \frac{(31-1)7.77^2 + (80-1)5.41^2}{31 + 80 - 2} = 37.82 = 6.15^2$$

and thereby $s_P = 6.15$. The test statistic value is then

$$t = \frac{22.02 - 21.03}{6.15\sqrt{\left(\frac{1}{31} + \frac{1}{80} \right)}} = 0.76$$

The distribution of the test statistic value is

$$t(31 + 80 - 2) = t(109).$$

The critical value using a significance level at 5% and a two-sided test is 1.98 (the test critical value $t(109)_{0.975}$ is close to 1.96 corresponding to the critical value $N(0,1)_{0.975} = 1.96$ as the number of degrees of freedom is large (df $= 109$)). The test statistic value is less than the critical value and we therefore cannot reject the null hypothesis and conclude that there is no significant difference in the milk yield between the two breeds DHF and CB. The test statistic distribution is illustrated in Figure 13.3 with the test statistic value and the critical values.

The t-test used in the present section to test the difference between two groups of animals (e.g. originating from two different breeds) is an unpaired t-test. It means that we have two different groups of animals, one for each breed. The design will usually be a parallel group design.

Table 13.4. *Descriptive analysis of milk yield (kg) in Danish dairy cows (SD = standard deviation, se = standard error of the mean)*

Variable	Level*				Milk yield			
		n	Mean	SD	se	Median	Q_1	Q_3
Overall		111	21.30	6.14	0.58	21.9	17.7	25.4
Breed	DHF	31	22.02	7.77	1.40	21.9	18.0	26.4
	CB	80	21.03	5.41	0.60	22.0	17.5	24.9
Parity	1	33	18.56	4.95	0.86	18.0	15.6	22.2
	2	36	21.98	5.56	0.93	22.6	18.9	26.4
	3	20	21.88	6.18	1.38	24.4	21.1	25.8
	≥ 4	22	23.79	7.38	1.57	23.1	18.9	29.3

*DHF, Danish Holstein Friesian; CB, crossbreed.

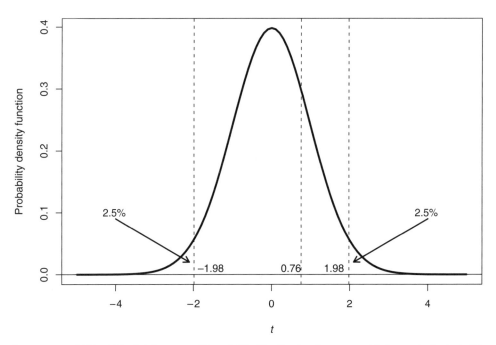

Figure 13.3. *Milk yield of dairy cows. The $t(109)$-distribution for a two-sided unpaired t-test. The critical value and the test statistic value are shown.*

13.4.3 Comparison of means for two dependent groups: paired t-test

Sometimes we have two measurements for the same animal or herd, e.g. evaluation of two diets, where both diets have been tested in the same animal. The design used can be a cross-over design (the animals receive both treatments in a random sequence) or a design with one group of animals with two measures for the same animal. The t-test to perform is different from the previous one as the measurements are not independent: we have two measurements for each animal. Thus, we have paired observations and the test to use is a paired t-test. We calculate the difference between the two observations for each animal and evaluate if the mean difference is significantly different from 0. The hypotheses, the test statistic value and the distribution of the test statistic value are

$$H_0: \quad \mu_d = 0, \qquad H_1: \quad \mu_d \neq 0$$

$$t = \frac{\bar{d} - 0}{s_d / \sqrt{n_d}}$$

$$t \sim t(n_d - 1)$$

where μ_d is the population mean difference
t is the test statistic value
$d = y_1 - y_2$
y_1 and y_2 are the outcomes for the two treatments
$\bar{d}$ is the mean value of the differences between the two treatments
n_d is the number of paired observations
$t(n_d - 1)$ is the distribution of the test statistic value (t-distribution with ($n_d - 1$) degrees of freedom)
s_d is the estimated standard deviation of the difference between the two treatments

---

EXAMPLE 13.4. In order to evaluate a difference in milk yield in dairy cows between January (month 1) and February (month 2), a paired t-test is performed. The mean value of differences in milk yield is 1.52 kg with a standard deviation at 10.3 kg for 104 cows. The test statistic value is

$$ t = \frac{1.52}{10.3/\sqrt{104}} = 1.50 $$

and the distribution of the test statistic value is $t(103)$.

The mean value of the differences is not significantly different from 0 as the test statistic value ($t = 1.50$) is less than the critical value ($t(103)_{0.975} = 1.98$). The $t(103)$-distribution is shown in Figure 13.4 with the test statistic value and the critical value. Therefore, we cannot reject the H_0 hypothesis and must conclude that milk yield in the 2 months is not significantly different.

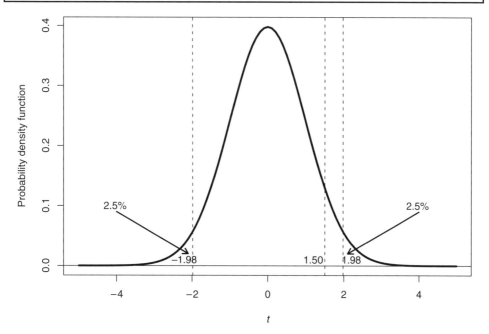

Figure 13.4. *Difference in milk yield of dairy cows in 2 months. $t(103)$-distribution for a two-sided paired t-test. The critical value and the test statistic value are shown. The H_0 is not rejected.*

13.4.4 Comparison of means for more than two groups: analysis of variance

When we have more than two groups to compare, the t-test should not be used any more. However, analysis of variance (ANOVA) is a generalisation of the t-test allowing more than one explanatory variable each with two or more levels. The general idea in the analysis of variance is to split the total variation in the outcome into components corresponding to the explanatory variables. This can be illustrated using an analysis of variance table (Table 13.5) dividing the variation into the different sources that might explain the variation in the outcome.

The variation, which has not been accounted for by the sources of variation, will be denoted the residual variation. Each of the explanatory variables in the analysis will be tested by comparing the variation between the groups of the explanatory variable with the variation between observations within groups (also called the residual variation). If the residual variation is large, it is more difficult to show a significant effect, compared to a situation where the residual variation is small. The general model for a one-way analysis of variance (one explanatory variable) is

$$y_{ij} = a + B_i + \epsilon_{ij}$$

where y_{ij} is the outcome for animal j at level i of the explanatory variable, a is the intercept, B_i is the effect of the explanatory (qualitative) variable with levels, $i = 1, 2, 3, \ldots, k$ and ϵ_{ij} is the random error for animal j at level i of the explanatory variable.

The null hypothesis testing no difference between groups, e.g. four levels of the explanatory variable is

$$H_0: \mu_1 = \mu_2 = \mu_3 = \mu_4, \quad H_1: \exists (m, n) \in [1, 2, 3, 4]^2: \mu_m \neq \mu_n$$

The H_0 hypothesis states that the mean values for all four levels are equal. The alternative hypothesis H_1 states that at least two of the mean values are different.

Table 13.5. *Analysis of variance, splitting the total variation into different sources. df is the number of degrees of freedom, N is the number of animals in the study, MS is the mean square and F is the test statistic value*

Sources of variation	df	MS	F test value	p-value
Explanatory variable with k levels	$k - 1$	MS_B	$F = MS_B / MS_{error}$	
Residual	$N - k$	MS_{error}		
Total	$N - 1$			

The analysis determines whether the discrepancies between the group means are greater than could be expected from the variation between observations within the groups. The F-test statistics is calculated as the variation between groups divided by the variation within groups (here, group mean refers to the mean value of the outcome for a given level of the explanatory variable). The variations between and within groups are called the between and within groups mean squares. The F-test statistics is calculated as

$$F = \frac{MS_B}{MS_{error}}$$

where $\quad MS_B = \frac{SS_B}{df_B} = \frac{\sum_{i=1}^{k} n_i(\bar{y}_i - \bar{y})^2}{k-1}$

$MS_{error} = \frac{SS_{error}}{df_{error}} = \frac{\sum_{i=1}^{k} \sum_{j=1}^{n_i} (y_{ij} - \bar{y})^2}{N-k}$

N is the total number of observations

k is the number of levels of the explanatory variable

SS_B and SS_{error} are the sum of squares between groups and the error sum of square

MS_B and MS_{error} are the mean square between groups and the mean square error

df_B and df_{error} are the degrees of freedom between groups and for the error

y_{ij} is the jth observation in the ith group

$\bar{y}$ is the mean value of all observations

$\bar{y}_i$ is the mean value of the observations in group i

The F-test statistics is tested in an F-distribution with the degrees of freedom $F(k-1, N-k)$. Whenever an explanatory variable has a significant effect on the outcome, pairwise comparison can be performed between levels (categories) of the explanatory variable using a t-test (Section 13.4.2).

EXAMPLE 13.5. In a study of risk factors we are often dealing with more than one risk factor. In the study of the relation between milk yield (Example 13.3), breed and parity, we have seen that there is no significant difference in milk yield between the two breeds. Parity has four levels (parity 1, 2, 3 and ≥ 4). In order to evaluate the influence of parity on the milk yield we have to perform an analysis of variance as the t-test is only able to perform comparison between two mean values. Further, analyses performed using t-test test the risk factors one by one. However, there might be a relation between breed and parity and this might have an influence on milk yield. Therefore, we would like the analysis to include all risk factors in the same analysis. This can be done using an analysis of variance. In the example with milk yield, inclusion of the two risk factors results in a two-way analysis of variance. The hypotheses corresponding to parity are:

H_0: $\quad \mu_{P=1} = \mu_{P=2} = \mu_{P=3} = \mu_{P \geq 4}$

H_1: $\quad \exists(k, l) \in \{P = 1; P = 2; P = 3; P \geq 4\}^2$: $\quad \mu_k \neq \mu_l$

and corresponding to breed:

$$H_0: \quad \mu_{DHF} = \mu_{CB}, \qquad H_1: \quad \mu_{DHF} \neq \mu_{CB}$$

The F-distribution for testing differences between parities is $F(3,106)$ as illustrated in Figure 13.5. The result of the analysis is seen in Table 13.6, where the total variation in milk yield is split into two components (breed and parity), the remaining variation not ascribed by the model is in the residual. A significant difference in the milk yield is seen between parities, and a significant difference in the milk yield between the two breeds is seen. The estimate is read as follows: crossbreed at parity ≥ 4 have a milk yield of 27.83 kg (intercept). For another group, e.g. breed = DHF and parity = 2, the milk yield is $27.83 - 4.23 - 5.74 = 17.86$. When the difference in milk yield between the breeds was analysed using the t-test (Example 13.3) the difference between breeds was not significant. However, when the variation due to differences in parities was taken into account, a significant difference between breeds was seen.

13.4.5 *Correlation*

Correlation or, more correctly, the correlation coefficient, ρ, expresses the degree of linear (*straight line*) association between two continuous variables. There are two methods for calculating the degree of association, depending on the types of variables. The correlation between two continuous variables is given by Pearson's correlation coefficient. The correlation between two qualitative variables can be calculated using Spearman's correlation

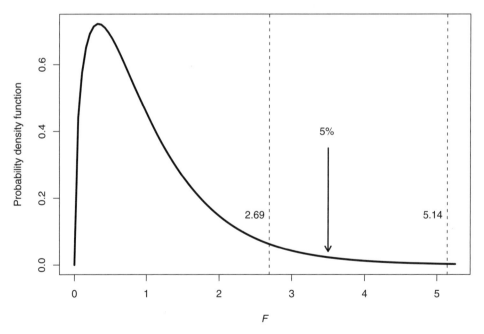

Figure 13.5. *Milk yield (kg) in Danish dairy cows. The $F(3,106)$-distribution with the critical value (2.69) and test statistic value ($F = 5.14$) is shown.*

Table 13.6. *Two-way analysis of variance of milk yield in Danish dairy cows. Breed and parity were included in the model. The least square means estimate (LSmeans), standard error (se), degrees of freedom (df), F-test statistic value and p-value are given*

Variable	Level	LSmeans*	se	df	F-test value	p-value
Breed				1	4.07	0.046
	DHF	18.81	1.47			
	CB	23.05	0.94			
Parity				3	5.14	0.002
	1	16.57^c	1.41			
	2	19.98^b	1.39			
	3	21.46^b	1.32			
	≥ 4	25.72^a	1.57			
Residual				106		

*Levels of parity with different letters as superscript are significantly different at a 5% significance level.

coefficient, which is a non-parametric measure based on ranks. Spearman's correlation coefficient is also used if the continuous variables are highly skewed. Alternatively, Pearson's correlation coefficient can be used if the skewed continuous data are transformed in order to reduce skewness. Both correlation coefficients take values on the interval $[-1;1]$. A correlation close to 0 implies that there is no relation between the two variables. A correlation close to 1 implies a strong positive relation between the two variables, whereas a correlation close to -1 implies a strong negative relation between the two variables. A correlation coefficient equal to -1 or $+1$ means a perfect linear association between the two variables (one variable can be computed from the other without error). The correlation coefficient is a measure of the degree of relation between the two variables without considering which variable is the outcome and which is the explanatory variable. The correlation therefore describes the degree of relation without consideration of causality (Figure 3.1). Pearson's correlation coefficient is estimated as

$$r = \frac{SS_{xy}}{\sqrt{SS_{xx}SS_{yy}}} = \frac{\sum(x_i - \bar{x})(y_i - \bar{y})}{\sqrt{\sum(x_i - \bar{x})^2 \sum(y_i - \bar{y})^2}}$$

where

$$SS_{xy} = \sum(x_i - \bar{x})(y_i - \bar{y}) = \sum x_i y_i - \frac{\left(\sum x_i\right)\left(\sum y_i\right)}{n}$$

$$SS_{xx} = \sum(x_i - \bar{x})^2 = \sum x_i^2 - \frac{\left(\sum x_i\right)^2}{n}$$

$$SS_{yy} = \sum(y_i - \bar{y})^2 = \sum y_i^2 - \frac{\left(\sum y_i\right)^2}{n}$$

ρ is the population correlation coefficient whereas r is the estimated correlation coefficient based on the sample. It is possible to perform a test of a hypothesis regarding the correlation coefficient, e.g. H_0: The correlation coefficient is equal to 0,

$$H_0: \quad \rho = 0$$

meaning no association between the two variables for both Pearson's and Spearman's correlation coefficients. However, the significance of a given value of r depends on sample size. As an example, the Pearson's correlation coefficient estimated at $r = 0.3$ (or $r = -0.3$) is not significant for a small sample size ($n < 44$), but is significant for a large sample size ($n \geq 44$). It is therefore suggested to evaluate the correlation coefficient r (as for other estimates) without too much emphasis on the significance level and rather judge the size of a biologically interesting correlation coefficient (e.g. $r = 0.75$ or $r = -0.75$). For further reading see, e.g. Altman (1995).

EXAMPLE 13.6. The association between temperature, capillary refill time, heart rate, standard base excess (SBE) and packed cell volume (PCV) is illustrated in Figure 13.6 for 472 horses. The horses were referred to the hospital at The Royal Veterinary and Agricultural University with clinical signs of colic (Thøfner et al., 2000). Pearson's and Spearman's correlation coefficients are given in Table 13.7. It is seen that in the present case Spearman's and Pearson's correlation coefficients are very similar. The variables used are all continuous (except capillary refill time (CRT)) and not very skewed, explaining the similarity between Spearman's and Pearson's correlation coefficients.

13.4.6 Linear regression

The aim of performing a linear regression is to evaluate and describe a linear relationship between two (or more) continuous variables and evaluate the effect of one (or more) explanatory variable(s) on the outcome. This is in contrast to the correlation coefficient, where we measure the degree of linear correlation between two continuous variables, without specifying which variable is the outcome and which is the explanatory variable. The linear relation between two continuous variables is illustrated in Figure 13.7.

In simple linear regression the relation between the outcome (y_i) and the continuous explanatory variable (x_i) can be expressed by

$$y_i = \alpha + \beta x_i + \epsilon_i \tag{13.1}$$

where y_i is the outcome (continuous), x_i is the explanatory variable (continuous), α is the intercept on the y-axis for $x = 0$, β is the slope of the line and ϵ_i is the random error.

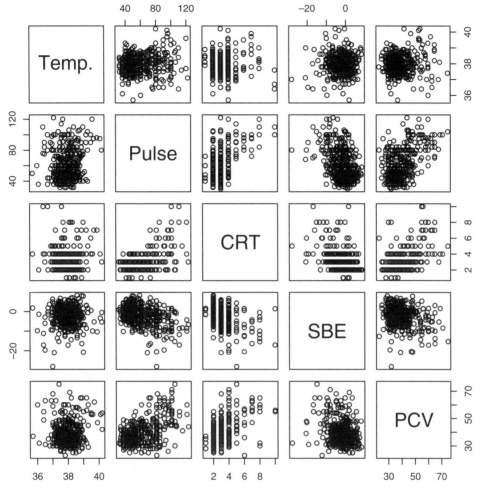

Figure 13.6. *Illustration of the association between temperature, CRT (capillary refill time), pulse, SBE (standard base excess) and PCV (packed cell volume) for 472 horses referred to The Royal Veterinary and Agricultural University with clinical signs of colic (Thøfner et al., 2000).*

The relation between x and y describes the causality, as x has a possible effect on y while the opposite is mathematically not true. In linear regression there is a measurement error on y, but x is assumed measured without error. Linear regression can be used to evaluate the relation between the two variables and calculate how much of the total variation in y the explanatory variable x can explain. Further, the model describing the relation can be used for prediction, say for a given value of x, the expected value of y can be predicted. The two parameters α and β can be estimated by the least squares method. By this method the parameters are given values so that the vertical distances between the observations and the estimated line (residuals) are minimised

Table 13.7. *Pearson's and Spearman's (in italics) correlation coeffi-cients for 472 horses referred to The Royal Veterinary and Agricultural University with clinical signs of colic (Thøfner et al., 2000)*

Pearson's Spearman's	Temperature	Capillary refill time	Pulse	SBE
CRT	0.04			
	0.02			
Pulse	0.17	0.59		
	0.17	*0.52*		
SBE	0.02	−0.42	−0.40	
	0.03	*−0.37*	*−0.36*	
PCV	0.07	0.53	0.56	−0.27
	0.04	*0.45*	*0.46*	*−0.22*

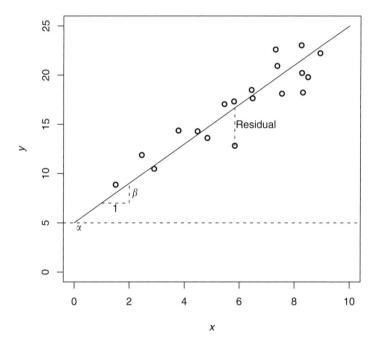

Figure 13.7. *Linear regression. The linear relation between the explanatory variable x and the outcome y. The parameters α and β are intercept and slope, respectively. The observations (dots) and the estimated line are shown.*

(Figure 13.7). The parameters α and β are estimated with some uncertainty given by the standard error of the parameter estimates a and b (se_a and se_b, respectively). The standard errors of a and b can be used for testing hypotheses regarding the estimates and for calculation of confidence intervals.

The estimated slope b and intercept a are given by

$$b = \frac{SS_{xy}}{SS_{xx}} = \frac{\sum (x_i - \bar{x})(y_i - \bar{y})}{\sum (x_i - \bar{x})^2}$$

and

$$a = \bar{y} - b\bar{x}$$

The estimated standard error of the intercept (se$_a$) and slope (se$_b$) are given by

$$se_a = s_{res} \sqrt{\frac{1}{n} + \frac{\bar{x}^2}{SS_{xx}}}$$

and

$$se_b = \frac{s_{res}}{\sqrt{SS_{xx}}}$$

where

$$s_{res}^2 = \frac{SS_{yy} - bSS_{xy}}{n - 2}$$

and

$$SS_{xx} = \sum (x_i - \bar{x})^2$$

$$SS_{yy} = \sum (y_i - \bar{y})^2$$

The relation between x and y is evaluated by testing the null hypothesis: The slope is equal to 0. The hypothesis, test statistic value and distribution of the test statistic value are

$$H_0: \quad \beta = 0$$

$$t = \frac{b - 0}{se_b}$$

$$t \sim t(n - 2)$$

where β is the population slope
   t is the test statistic value
   b is the estimated slope
   $t(n - 2)$ is the distribution of the test statistic value (t-distribution
      with $n - 2$ degrees of freedom)
   n is the number of observations
   se$_b$ is the standard error of the slope, b

If the null hypothesis is accepted, we conclude that there is no relation between x and y as the slope is not significantly different from 0. An alternative null hypothesis regarding the slope could be H_0: The slope is equal to β_0 (e.g. $\beta_0 = 1$). The hypothesis, test statistic value and distribution of the test statistic value are

$$H_0: \quad \beta = \beta_0$$

$$t = \frac{b - \beta_0}{se_b}$$

$$t \sim t(n - 2)$$

A 95% confidence interval (CI) for the estimated slope is given by

$$95\% \text{ CI}_b: \quad b \pm t(n - 2)_{0.975} se_b$$

In order to evaluate the causality between x and y, the amount of variation in y, explained by x, can be calculated. This measure is called the coefficient of determination, is denoted R^2 and takes values on the interval [0,1] or 0–100%. When we are close to 100%, the model is close to fitting perfectly. However, often R^2 is less than 50%, due to animal variation and a number of unexplained variables. In simple linear regression (here, meaning one explanatory variable) as given in Model 13.1, there is a unique relation between the coefficient of determination, R^2, and the correlation coefficient, r, given by

$$R^2 = r^2 \text{ (for Model 13.1)}$$

If the correlation coefficient between two variables is $r = 0.5$, the coefficient of determination is $R^2 = 0.25$. The explanatory variable x then explains 25% of the total variation in y. For a small correlation coefficient, e.g. $r = 0.3$, $R^2 = 0.09$, indicating a poor predictive ability of the model where x only explains 9% of the total variation in y. In order to obtain a reasonable coefficient of determination, e.g. $R^2 = 0.80$, the correlation coefficient between the two variables should be a least $r = 0.89$.

Until now, we have been dealing with simple linear regression, meaning that we have only included a single explanatory variable (x) in the model. However, we are often confronted with a more complicated causality, where not only one, but a number of variables are expected to have an influence on the outcome y. This is called multiple linear regression, in which more than one explanatory variable is included in the model. The simple linear regression

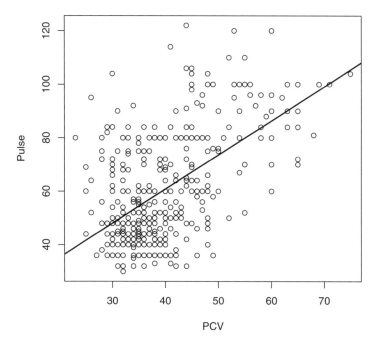

Figure 13.8. *Linear regression between the outcome variable (pulse) and the explanatory variable (PCV).*

model (Equation 13.1) is extended to

$$y_{ij} = \alpha + \beta_1 x_{1j} + \beta_2 x_{2j} + \cdots + \beta_k x_{kj} + \epsilon_{ij} = \alpha + \sum_{i=1}^{k} \beta_i x_{ij} + \epsilon_{ij} \qquad (13.2)$$

where y is the outcome, $x_{1j}, x_{2j}, \ldots, x_{kj}$ are the explanatory variables, α is the intercept on the y-axis for $x_{1j} = 0, x_{2j} = 0, \ldots, x_{kj} = 0$, $\beta_1, \beta_2, \ldots, \beta_k$ are the slopes corresponding to the explanatory variables $x_{1j}, x_{2j}, \ldots, x_{kj}$, respectively, and ϵ_{ij} is the random error.

EXAMPLE 13.7. In a study of colic horses referred to the hospital at The Royal Veterinary and Agricultural University, Copenhagen, Denmark (see also Example 13.6), the relation between pulse, capillary refill time (CRT), temperature, standard base excess (SBE) and packed cell volume (PCV) was evaluated (Thøfner *et al.*, 2000). In total, 472 horses were included in the study. The correlation coefficients (Pearson's and Spearman's) between the variables are given in Table 13.7. In Figure 13.6 scatter plots of the relation between each pair of variables two by two are given. The relation between pulse (outcome) and PCV (explanatory) has been further evaluated by linear regression. The observations and the estimated regression line are seen in Figure 13.8. The estimated parameters are given in Table 13.8. The relation is seen to be significant and is given by the model

$$y = 9.781 + 1.275x$$

where y is the pulse and x is the explanatory variable PCV. The correlation coefficient is 0.56 and the coefficient of determination is therefore 0.31. Hence, PCV can explain 31% of the variation in pulse.

Table 13.8. *Linear regression analysis of the relation between pulse (outcome) and PCV (explanatory) in colic horses*

Parameter	Estimate	Standard error	Test statistic value	p-value
Intercept	9.781	3.778	2.59	0.010
Slope	1.275	0.094	13.63	<0.001
$R^2 = 0.31$				

13.5 Analysis of a dichotomous outcome

Proportions originate from qualitative variables such as the proportion of animals with salmonella. On the animal level, we are dealing with a qualitative variable on a dichotomous scale: occurrence of salmonella or not. In the previous sections we have been dealing with hypotheses regarding a continuous outcome. In this and the following sections, we are focusing on testing hypotheses, when the outcome is qualitative.

13.5.1 *Comparison of a proportion with a given value*

A proportion (as a percentage of animals with endometritis) can be tested for difference from a given value. The hypotheses, test statistic value and distribution of the test are

$$H_0: \quad \pi = \pi_0, \qquad H_1: \quad \pi \neq \pi_0$$

$$z = \frac{|p - \pi_0| - \frac{1}{2n}}{\sqrt{\frac{\pi_0(1-\pi_0)}{n}}}$$

$$z \sim N(0, 1)$$

where π is the population proportion
π_0 is the given value
z is the test statistic value
p is the observed proportion
n is sample size (number of animals)
$N(0, 1)$ is the approximate normal distribution of the
test statistic value (normal distribution)

We subtract $\frac{1}{2n}$ in order to improve the normal distribution approximation to the binomial distribution. The approximation using the normal distribution should only be used when n is large, that is when $np > 5$ and $np(1 - p) > 5$.

When the null hypothesis is rejected, we have shown that the observed proportion is significantly different from the given value π_0.

EXAMPLE 13.8. A farmer would like to know if the proportion of cows with endometritis is greater than 10%. He has 700 cows and 110 of these have endometritis, giving an observed probability for endometritis, $p = 0.157$. The hypotheses are

$$H_0: \quad \pi \leq 0.1, \qquad H_1: \quad \pi > 0.1$$

This is a one-sided test as we are only interested in a proportion greater than 10%.
The test statistic value is

$$z = \frac{|0.157 - 0.1| - \frac{1}{2 \times 700}}{\sqrt{\frac{0.1(1-0.1)}{700}}} = 4.96$$

The distribution of the test statistic value is approximate $N(0, 1)$. The critical value using a 5% significance level and a one-sided test is $N(0, 1)_{0.95} = 1.64$. As the test statistic value is greater than the critical value, we reject the null hypothesis and conclude that the proportion of cows with endometritis in the herd is significantly greater than 10%.

13.5.2 *Comparison of proportions for independent groups: Fisher exact test and χ^2-test*

An example of a hypothesis is: There is no relation (or association) between occurrence of endometritis and breeds. The outcome could be endometritis (yes or no) and the explanatory variable could be breed. The hypothesis can be tested using Fisher exact test. Fisher exact test is complicated to calculate by hand calculator. Therefore, the χ^2-test can be used as an alternative. The χ^2-test is an approximation of the correct test (Fisher exact test). Today, statistical software is often used for statistical analyses and Fisher exact test can therefore be used without problems. Fisher exact test and the χ^2-test are both used for testing an association between two qualitative variables.

Data can be illustrated by a 2×2 table if both the outcome and the explanatory variable have two levels (Table 13.9). Generally, it is an $r \times c$ table (r rows and c columns).

Table 13.9. *A 2×2 table used for testing hypotheses regarding a dichotomous outcome*

		Outcome		Total
		Level 1	Level 2	
Explanatory variable	Level 1	a	b	$a + b$
	Level 2	c	d	$c + d$
	Total	$a + c$	$b + d$	n

The hypotheses (no association between outcome and explanatory variable) and the test statistic value for the χ^2-test for a 2×2 table are given by

$$H_0: \quad \pi_1 = \pi_2, \qquad H_1: \quad \pi_1 \neq \pi_2$$

$$\chi^2 = \frac{(|ad - bc| - n/2)^2 n}{(a+b)(c+d)(a+c)(b+d)} \qquad (13.3)$$

where π_1 and π_2 are the probabilities for disease in the population (one of the levels of the outcome) for each of the two levels of the explanatory variable. The distribution for this test statistic is $\chi^2(1)$, i.e. a χ^2-distribution with one degree of freedom. In order to improve the approximative χ^2-test compared to Fisher exact test an adjustment is made subtracting $n/2$. This adjustment is called Yates correction. The approximative χ^2-test can be used instead of Fisher exact test when the expected values in all cells are greater than or equal to 5. The expected values, $E(a), E(b), E(c), E(d)$ for a 2×2 table are calculated as

$$E(a) = \frac{(a+c)(a+b)}{N}, \qquad E(b) = \frac{(b+d)(a+b)}{N},$$

$$E(c) = \frac{(a+c)(c+d)}{N}, \qquad E(d) = \frac{(b+d)(c+d)}{N}$$

EXAMPLE 13.9. An example could be the evaluation of the association between occurrence of endometritis and breed. In total 700 dairy cows were included in a cohort study, 500 Danish Holstein Friesian and 200 Jersey cows. Of these 700 cows, 110 experienced endometritis in the study. The 2×2 table is given in Table 13.10. The hypotheses are:

$$H_0: \quad \pi_1 = \pi_2, \qquad H_1: \quad \pi_1 \neq \pi_2$$

with estimated probabilities for endometritis $p_1 = \Pr\{\text{endometritis} \mid \text{Holstein}\} = 0.20$ and $p_2 = \Pr\{\text{endometritis} \mid \text{Jersey}\} = 0.05$.
The test statistic value with Yates correction is

$$\chi^2 = \frac{(|100 \times 190 - 400 \times 10| - 700/2)^2 \times 700}{500 \times 200 \times 110 \times 590} = 23.1$$

The critical value for acceptance or rejection of the hypothesis is

$$\chi^2(1)_{0.95} = 3.84$$

It is seen that the test statistic value is much greater than the critical value. We can therefore reject H_0 and conclude that there is a significant association between occurrence of endometritis and breed. The $\chi^2(1)$-distribution is shown in Figure 13.9. The relative risk (RR) for endometritis for Holstein cows compared to Jersey cows is

$$RR = \frac{100/500}{10/200} = 4.0$$

Table 13.10. *Endometritis in Danish dairy herds in relation to breeds*

		Endometritis		Total
		Yes	No	
Breed	Holstein	100	400	500
	Jersey	10	190	200
	Total	110	590	700

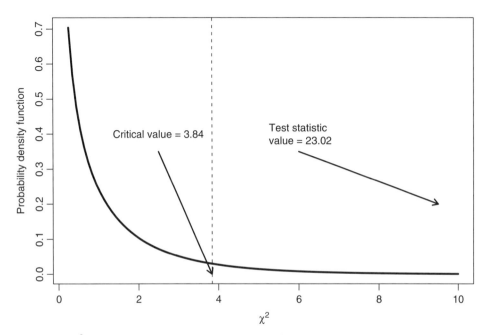

Figure 13.9. $\chi^2(1)$-*distribution. The relation between endometritis and breed in Danish dairy herds. The critical value and the test statistic value are shown.*

The test statistic value for the χ^2-test for an $r \times c$ table is given by

$$\chi^2 = \sum_{i=1}^{r} \sum_{j=1}^{c} \frac{(O_{ij} - E_{ij})^2}{E_{ij}}$$

where O_{ij} and E_{ij} are the observed and expected number of the ith row and jth column in the $r \times c$ table. The expected value of the cell ij is calculated as

$$E_{ij} = \frac{n_i n_j}{N}$$

where n_i and n_j are the number of observed animals in the ith row and jth column and N is the total number of animals.

The distribution for this test statistic is

$$\chi^2((r-1)(c-1))$$

Evaluation of association between two variables such as outcome (e.g. infected: yes/no) and an exposure factor is based on unpaired data. Each animal is either infected or not, and each animal is either exposed or not. In the next section, analysis of paired qualitative data is described.

13.5.3 Comparison of paired proportions: McNemar test

In a study of *Campylobacter* spp. in turkey samples, we are interested in a comparison between two methods (automated enzyme immunoassay (EiaFoss) and conventional bacteriogical culture) for diagnosing *Campylobacter* spp. For each sample, we have a result (a positive or negative) for each of the two methods. This type of data is called paired observations. Comparison of the two methods for diagnosing *Campylobacter* spp. can be performed using McNemar test. The null hypothesis states that there is no difference in the probability of being tested positive using the two methods and is given by

$$H_0: \quad \lambda_1 = \lambda_2, \qquad H_1: \quad \lambda_1 \neq \lambda_2$$

where λ_1 and λ_2 are the population probabilities, $p_1 = (e+f)/m$ and $p_2 = (e+g)/m$ are the estimated probabilities of being tested positive using method 1 (p_1) and method 2 (p_2). Data from this type of study can generally be presented in a 2×2 table given in Table 13.11.

The test statistic value is

$$\chi^2 = \frac{(|f-g|-1)^2}{f+g}$$

and the distribution of the test statistic value is $\chi^2(1)$.

Table 13.11. *McNemar test evaluating equal probabilities for being positive using the two diagnostic methods*

		Method 2		Total
		Positive	Negative	
Method 1	Positive	e	f	$e+f$
	Negative	g	h	$g+h$
	Total	$e+g$	$f+h$	m

Table 13.12. *McNemar test evaluating equal probabilities for being positive using the two methods for detection of Campylobacter spp. in turkey faecal samples (Borck et al., 2002)*

		EiaFoss		Total
		Positive	Negative	
Conventional culture	Positive	32	21	53
	Negative	4	4	8
	Total	36	25	61

EXAMPLE 13.10. The frequency distribution of the results for comparison of the two diagnostic methods for detection of *Campylobacter* spp. in turkey samples is given in Table 13.12. The hypotheses are

$$H_0: \quad \lambda_1 = \lambda_2, \qquad H_1: \quad \lambda_1 \neq \lambda_2$$

where the estimates are $p_1 = \text{Pr\{positive | conventionalculture\}} = 0.869$ and $p_2 = \text{Pr\{positive | EiaFoss\}} = 0.590$.

The test statistic value is

$$\chi^2 = \frac{(|21 - 4| - 1)^2}{21 + 4} = 10.24$$

and the critical value is

$$\chi^2(1)_{0.95} = 3.84$$

As the test statistic value (10.24) is greater than the critical value (3.84), we reject the H_0 hypothesis and conclude that the probability of being tested *Campylobacter* positive is significantly different for the two methods.

13.5.4 Logistic regression

In linear regression (see Section 13.4.6) the relation between two continuous variables is described. However, we are often dealing with studies in which the outcome is dichotomous (e.g. presence or absence of infection) and not continuous. The relation between the dichotomous outcome and a continuous explanatory variable can be evaluated using logistic regression. In Figure 13.10(a) the relation between the probability of being infected and a continuous explanatory variable is illustrated. It is seen that when using logistic regression the relation has an S-shaped curve. In order to estimate the relation between the outcome and the explanatory variable, a logit-transformation is needed. The logit-transformation is given by

$$\text{logit}(p(x)) = \ln\left(\frac{p(x)}{1 - p(x)}\right)$$

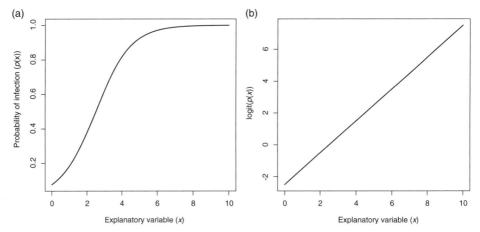

Figure 13.10. *Logistic regression: (a) The relation between a continuous explanatory variable (x) and the probability of being infected (p(x)) given a value of x and (b) the relation between a continuous explanatory variable, x and logit(p(x)).*

where x is the continuous explanatory variable, $p(x)$ is the probability for being, e.g. infected given a value of the explanatory variable, x, $1 - p(x)$ is the probability for not being infected given a value of the explanatory variable, x, and $\ln(\ )$ is the natural logarithm.

The relation between the dichotomous outcome and the explanatory variable (x) is given by

$$\text{logit}(p(x)) = \alpha + \beta x$$

where x is the continuous explanatory variable, $p(x)$ is the probability for being infected given a value of the explanatory variable, x, α is the intercept and β is the slope.

The estimated relation between $\text{logit}(p(x))$ and x is linear and is illustrated in Figure 13.10(b).

The parameters α and β in the logistic regression are estimated (a and b) using maximum likelihood estimation. This is done using statistical software, such as Statistical Analysis System (version 8.2, SAS Institute).

As in standard linear regression it is possible to test hypotheses about the parameters α and β. In order to evaluate an association between the outcome and the explanatory variable, the slope can be tested for difference from 0. The hypotheses are

$$H_0: \quad \beta = 0, \qquad H_1: \quad \beta \neq 0$$

$$z = \frac{b}{se_b}$$

$$z \sim N(0, 1)$$

Table 13.13. *Descriptive analysis of the milk yield for dairy cows at high and low somatic cell count levels (SCC, cut-off value = 125,000 per millilitre)*

			Milk yield				
		n	Mean	se	Median	Q_1	Q_3
SCC level	High	600	19.2	0.28	18.8	14.4	23.3
	Low	540	20.7	0.25	20.4	16.6	24.2

where β is the population slope, b is the estimated slope, z is the test statistic value, $N(0, 1)$ is the test statistic distribution (approximative normal distribution) and se_b is the standard error of the slope.

The hypothesis is accepted at the 5% significance level if the test statistic value, z, lies within the interval -1.96 to 1.96 (see Figure 13.1).

Logistic regression can be used to evaluate the association between a dichotomous outcome and a continuous explanatory variable. Further, it can be used to establish a prediction model. Once the parameters are estimated (a and b), the logistic regression model can be used to estimate the probability of infection, given a specific value of the explanatory variable, x. This is done using

$$\text{logit}(p(x)) = \ln\left(\frac{p(x)}{1 - p(x)}\right) \quad \Leftrightarrow \quad p(x) = \frac{1}{1 + \exp(-(a + bx))}$$

Odds ratio (OR) (see Chapter 7) can be calculated using the estimated slope as

$$\text{OR} = \frac{\text{odds}(x')}{\text{odds}(x'')} = \frac{\frac{p(x')}{1-p(x')}}{\frac{p(x'')}{1-p(x'')}} = \exp(b(x' - x''))$$

where x' and x'' are two specific values of the explanatory variable, x. This is the OR for infection for a given difference in the explanatory variable x of size $x' - x''$. The 95% CI for OR for a change in x from x' to x'' is given by

$$\exp(b(x' - x'') \pm 1.96|x' - x''|se_b)$$

EXAMPLE 13.11. The relation between a high somatic cell count (SCC) and milk yield in dairy cows is evaluated. The original continuous variable SCC has been dichotomised to a high or a low level of SCC. The cut-off value for a SCC is here selected at 125,000 per millilitre. In total, 1140 cows were included in the study. The mean milk yield was 19.9 kg. The mean milk yield for cows with low SCC was 20.7 kg and 19.2 kg for cows with high SCC. The descriptive analysis is given in Table 13.13. The association between high SCC and milk yield (x) has been evaluated using logistic regression (Table 13.14). The model with estimated parameters is

$$\text{logit}(p(x)) = 0.819 - 0.036x$$

---

where $p(x)$ is the probability of high SCC for a given value of the milk yield (x). The association between high SCC and milk yield is evaluated. The hypotheses are

$$H_0: \quad \beta = 0, \qquad H_1: \quad \beta \neq 0$$

and the test statistic value is

$$z = \frac{b}{se_b} = -0.036/0.0093 = -3.87$$

The critical values are -1.96 and 1.96, with acceptance of the hypothesis, if the test statistic value lies within the interval. The test statistic value is less than -1.96 and we therefore reject the null hypothesis and conclude that there is a significant association between a high SCC and the milk yield. It is seen, that the slope is negative, meaning that the probability for a high SCC decreases with an increasing milk yield. The relation between high SCC and milk yield is seen in Figure 13.11 and Table 13.14. OR and 95% CI for high SCC for a change in milk yield of 5 kg (e.g. from 20 to 25 kg) are

$$OR = \exp(-0.036(25 - 20)) = 0.84$$

and

$$95\% \text{ CI:} \quad \exp(-0.036(25 - 20) \pm 1.96 \mid 25 - 20 \mid 0.0093) = [0.76; 0.91]$$

Other variables might have an influence on SCC. One of these extra explanatory variables could be breed. Four breeds were included in the study (RDM, SDM, Jersey and Cross Breeds). Breed is a nominal variable. In order to evaluate the relation between a high SCC and breed, we have to modify the analysis, as there is no longer a linear relation between logit(p) and breed. The analysis can be done using logistic analysis, including breed as a categorial variable in the model.

13.5.5 Logistic analysis

If the explanatory variable is continuous, logistic regression is performed (Section 13.5.4), assuming a linear relation between logit($p(x)$) and x. However, when the explanatory variable is qualitative, e.g. nominal, logistic analysis can be performed. Most textbooks use the term 'logistic regression' for both analyses (with a quantitative and a qualitative explanatory variable, respectively). However, in the present textbook the term 'logistic analysis' has been used for

Table 13.14. *Logistic regression of the relation between high somatic cell count (SCC) in Danish dairy cows and milk yield (se: standard error of estimate)*

Variable	Estimate	se	p-value	OR[†]	95% CI
Intercept	0.819	0.1954	<0.001	–	–
Milk	−0.036	0.0093	<0.001	0.97*	0.95–0.98

[†]OR is for a change in milk yield of 1 kg.

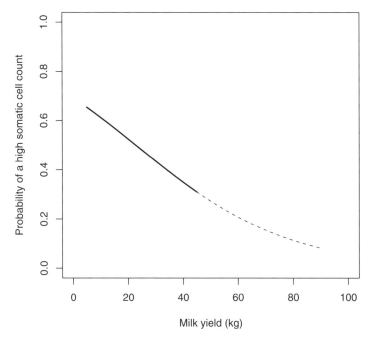

Figure 13.11. *Logistic regression. The relation between high somatic cell count and milk yield in dairy cows. The solid line represents the interval where data support the analysis, and the extrapolated dashed line has been added to illustrate that the relationship between probability of high somatic cell count and milk yield is non-linear.*

the analysis of a dichotomous outcome and a qualitative explanatory variable in order to explicitly indicate the difference between the two methods (such as linear regression and analysis of variance for a continuous outcome).

The model is given by

$$\text{logit}(p_i) = \alpha + B_i$$

where α is the intercept and B_i is the effect of the qualitative explanatory variable, $i = 1, 2, \ldots, I$.

If there are both qualitative and quantitative variables the model is given by

$$\text{logit}(p_{ij}) = \alpha + B_i + \gamma x_{ij}$$

where α is the intercept, B_i is the effect of the qualitative explanatory variable, $i = 1, 2, \ldots, I$, x_{ij} is the continuous variable, $j = 1, 2, \ldots, J$, and γ is the slope for the continuous variable.

EXAMPLE 13.12. The relation between a high somatic cell count (SCC) and milk yield in dairy cows was evaluated in Example 13.11. The influence of breed on high SCC will be evaluated in the following. The descriptive analysis is given in Table 13.15. The association between high SCC and breed was significant ($p = 0.002$) (Table 13.16).

A combined logistic analysis, evaluating the effect of both breed and milk yield on high SCC, was also performed. The resulting model is

$$\text{logit}(p_{ij}) = \alpha + B_i + \gamma x_{ij}$$

where α is the intercept, B_i is the effect of breed, $i = 1, 2, 3, 4$, x_{ij} is the milk yield and γ is the slope for the milk yield.

The resulting model is illustrated in Figure 13.12 and Table 13.17. Both explanatory variables were significant.

13.6 Model control

Statistical analyses are based on different assumptions. These assumptions should be fulfilled in order to obtain valid results of the analyses. In the following, evaluation of fulfilment of the assumption, the so-called model control, will be described for performing an analysis of a continuous and a dichotomous outcome.

Table 13.15. *Descriptive analysis using frequency distribution of breeds in the study of high* somatic cell count (SCC) in Danish dairy cows*

N (%)		SCC		Total
		High	Low	
Breed	RDM	92 (57.1)	69 (42.9)	161
	SDM	296 (57.1)	222 (42.9)	518
	Jersey	85 (43.4)	111 (56.6)	196
	Crossbreed	127 (47.9)	138 (52.1)	265

Table 13.16. *Logistic analysis of the relation between high somatic cell count (SCC) in Danish dairy cows and breeds*

Variable	Level	Estimate*	se	p-value	OR	95% CI
Intercept		−0.083	0.123			
Breed				0.002		
	RDM	0.371[ab]	0.201		1.45	0.98 – 2.15
	SDM	0.371[a]	0.152		1.45	1.08 – 1.95
	Jersey	−0.184[c]	0.190		0.83	0.57 – 1.21
	Crossbreed	0[bc]	0		1	–

*Estimates with different letters as superscript are significantly different at a 5% significance level.

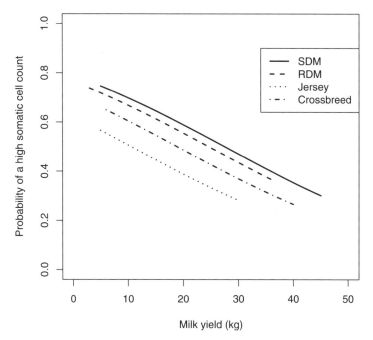

Figure 13.12. *Combined logistic analysis. The relation between high somatic cell count, milk yield and breeds in dairy cows.*

Table 13.17. *Combined logistic analysis of the relation between high somatic cell count (SCC) in Danish dairy cows, breeds and milk yield*

Variable	Level	Estimate*	se	p-value	OR	95% CI
Intercept		0.905	0.240	<0.001		
Milk		−0.048	0.010	<0.001	0.79[†]	
Breed				<0.001		0.71–0.87
	RDM	0.275[ab]	0.204		1.32	0.88–1.96
	SDM	0.414[a]	0.154		1.51	1.12–2.04
	Jersey	−0.399[c]	0.196		0.67	0.46–0.99
	Crossbreed	0[b]	0		1	–

*Estimates with different letters as superscript are significant at the 5% significance level.
[†]For a change in milk yield of 5 kg.

13.6.1 Model control of analyses of a continuous outcome

In the previous sections, the *t*-test, linear regression and analysis of variance have been described. The assumptions for these analyses are

• Data are normally distributed.
• All observations have equal variances.
• Observations are independent.

These three assumptions can be evaluated as a part of the analysis.

In order to evaluate a normal distribution of the observations, a test for a normal distribution of the residuals can be performed. A number of tests are available, among these the Shapiro–Wilks or Kolmogorov–Smirnov tests are suggested. The null hypothesis is that data have a normal distribution. The assumption can be further evaluated using a normal probability plot of the residuals or a comparison of the histogram of the residuals with the expected normal curve.

The assumption of equal variances of all observations is also called homogeneity of variances or homoscedasticity. The equality of variances can visually be evaluated using a residual plot. Alternatively, Bartlett's test for homogeneity of variances can be used (Sokal and Rohlf, 1981). However, Bartlett's test is very sensitive to departures from normality. A significant test may therefore indicate non-normality rather than heteroscedasticity.

The last assumption is that the observations are independent. Dependence between observations can be due to repeated measures in time on the same animals, as the observations made on the same animal often will be more alike compared to observations from different animals. Independence between observations is usually evaluated based on the information of design and data collection procedure. However, a test can be performed using, e.g. a run test (Sokal and Rohlf, 1981). There is no simple adjustment for lack of independence except changing the design of the study and/or data collection procedure.

EXAMPLE 13.13. In Example 13.5 we performed an analysis of variance in order to evaluate the effect of parity group and breed on the milk yield. The assumptions for performing the analysis will be evaluated in the present example. In Figure 13.13 the normal probability plot (Figure 13.13a), a histogram of residuals (Figure 13.13b) and the residual plot (Figure 13.13c) are shown. The normal probability plot indicates departures from normality as observations in both tails depart from the straight line. Comparison of the histogram of residuals with the normal distribution further indicates that observations in the tails might be a problem. Test for normality using Shapiro–Wilks test (p = 0.011) or Kolmogorov–Smirnov's test (p > 0.15) further confirmed problems with the assumption of normality. The observations are independent as we have only a single milk yield from each cow. The assumption regarding equality of variances can be evaluated using the residual plot. It does not indicate problems regarding non-equality of variances.

13.6.2 Model control of analyses of a dichotomous outcome

When dealing with a dichotomous outcome the possibilities for assessing model fit are slightly more complicated compared to the continuous outcome case. Here, we will use the goodness-of-fit test with the estimated dispersion

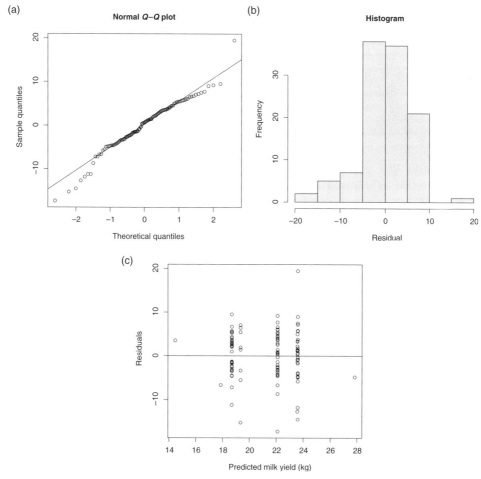

Figure 13.13. *Evaluation of assumptions for the two-way analysis of variance of milk yield in Danish dairy cows: (a) the normal probability plot; (b) histogram of residuals with the expected normal curve superimposed; and (c) residual plot with residuals against predicted values.*

parameter as a measure. Further methods are given by, e.g. Hosmer and Lemeshow (2000). The dispersion parameter is a measure of how well the model fits data. The dispersion parameter should be close to 1. It takes values above (overdispersion) or below 1 (underdispersion).

EXAMPLE 13.14. In Example 13.12 we performed a logistic analysis in order to evaluate the effect of breed and milk yield on the probability of a high somatic cell count (SCC). The dispersion parameter was estimated to 1.36 using the deviance and to 1.003 using Pearson's methods. Both indicate a good fit.

13.7 Model reduction

Many diseases are multifactorial, meaning that a number of causes and factors influence the occurrence, extent and spread of the disease. In order to evaluate the importance of the factors, analyses are often performed including a large number of possible explanatory variables (causes and risk factors). Depending on the type of the outcome, the analyses can be made using multiple linear regression (continuous outcome), multiple logistic regression (dichotomous outcome), analysis of variance (continuous outcome) or logistic analysis (dichotomous outcome). Among the possible risk factors (explanatory variables) included in the model, we are often interested in identification of the (few) variables with a significant influence on the outcome. This identification can be done by model reduction.

There are different strategies for model reduction. The three standard strategies are

- forward selection,
- backward elimination,
- stepwise selection.

When using forward selection, we start with an empty model. Each variable is evaluated for inclusion as the first variable in the model. The most significant variable will initially be included (evaluated individually). The next variable to be included in the model with one variable will be the most significant variable of those left, when one variable has been included. This continues until the variables to be included are not significant.

Backward elimination starts with a full model including all possible variables. In the first step, the most non-significant variable is excluded. In the second step, the most non-significant variable, of those left, is excluded. This continues until all variables in the model are significant.

A stepwise procedure is a combination of forward selection and backward elimination. It starts by an empty model (or a full model) and forward selection. The first variable to include is the most significant variable when evaluated individually. The next variable to include is selected by a forward procedure, as described above. When two variables are included in the model, it is evaluated if the first included variable is significant. If not, it is excluded, otherwise it stays in the model. The procedure continues, including the next variable. If a new variable is included, the other variables in the model are evaluated for significance. If inclusion of one variable changes the significance of one of the other variables in the model, this variable is then evaluated and excluded, if needed. This continues until no more variables can be included or excluded.

It is recommended to evaluate the variables excluded during model reduction in the final model for possible significance. It should be remembered that the variables are excluded from the model at different steps in the reduction procedure. The variables in the model at the time of exclusion of a variable have an influence on the significance of the variable to be excluded. This is due to correlation and confounding between the explanatory variables.

Depending on which analysis is performed, significance might be evaluated by different measures (such as p-value).

13.8 Confounding and interaction

Confounding and interaction were described in Chapter 11. Confounding is a systematic error (bias) whereas interaction is a biological phenomenon. In this section confounding and interaction will be discussed in relation to data analysis.

13.8.1 *Confounding*

Confounding is a systematic error (bias), describing the confusion of effects between two (or more) explanatory variables as introduced in Chapter 11. Confounding can be handled in a number of different ways, by exclusion, matching or analytical control. The last method will be described in the following. The type of analysis depends mainly on the type of outcome studied (e.g. dichotomous or continuous).

Generally, confounding is evaluated by comparing a crude estimate of the association between the outcome and the explanatory variable with an estimate of the association adjusted for the confounding variable. The crude estimate of the association is the relationship between the outcome and the explanatory variable without including the confounding variable. The adjusted estimate of the association is obtained after adjusting for the confounding variable. How large the difference should be is debated but a change between 10 and 30% in the estimates of association can be considered large enough to argue that the variable is confounding the association between the explanatory variable and the outcome. The confounding variable does not need to be a significant risk factor in the specific analysis in order to be a confounder. However, it is important also to evaluate the interpretation of the change in effect. Hence, the parameter estimates from a logistic regression analysis may be changed 30%, but if the odds ratio of a disease only changes from 1.21 to 1.18 then the interpretation of the association under study does not change, and it could be argued that there may be statistical confounding but it is not of biological importance (as is the case in general).

The methods used to obtain the estimate of the association adjusted for the confounding variable depend on the types of variables involved (the outcome, the explanatory and the confounding variables).

For a dichotomous outcome (e.g. disease or not) and a dichotomous explanatory variable (e.g. exposure or not) confounding can be evaluated by comparing the crude ratio with the adjusted ratio (odds ratio or relative risk depending on design and purpose). The confounding variable can be dichotomous, nominal, ordinal, discrete or continuous. The crude ratio is calculated from the relationship between the outcome and explanatory variables without considering the confounding variable. The adjusted ratio is a weighted average of the ratios for each level (stratum) of the confounder. The ratio can be adjusted using different methods. In the following we will show adjustment according to Mantel–Haenszel. The stratification of a 2×2 table is illustrated in Table 13.18 where the relation between the risk factor and the disease is stratified by a possible confounding factor with K levels (K strata). The odds ratio or relative risk for the 2×2 table before stratification is called the *crude* odds ratio or the *crude* relative risk. These are calculated as

$$OR_{crude} = \frac{ad}{bc}$$

$$RR_{crude} = \frac{a(c+d)}{c(a+b)}$$

The Mantel–Haenszel method calculates the *adjusted* odds ratio or *adjusted* relative risk where the relation between risk factor and disease is adjusted for the confounder. The Mantel–Haenszel adjusted odds ratio is calculated as:

$$OR_{adj} = \frac{\sum_{i=1}^{K} \frac{a_i d_i}{n_i}}{\sum_{i=1}^{K} \frac{b_i c_i}{n_i}}$$

which for a two-level confounder is:

$$OR_{adj} = \frac{\frac{a_1 d_1}{n_1} + \frac{a_2 d_2}{n_2}}{\frac{b_1 c_1}{n_1} + \frac{b_2 c_2}{n_2}}$$

The Mantel–Haenszel adjusted relative risk:

$$RR_{adj} = \frac{\sum_{i=1}^{K} \frac{a_i(c_i+d_i)}{n_i}}{\sum_{i=1}^{K} \frac{c_i(a_i+b_i)}{n_i}}$$

Table 13.18. *The crude 2 × 2 table and the resulting 2 × 2 tables when stratifying according to a possible confounder with K levels. In this table $a = \sum a_i$, $b = \sum b_i$, etc*

		Disease		
		Yes	No	
Risk factor	Yes	a	b	$a+b$
	No	c	d	$c+d$
		$a+c$	$b+d$	n

$$OR_{crude} = \frac{ad}{bc}$$

$$RR_{crude} = \frac{a(c+d)}{c(a+b)}$$

		Stratum 1 (confounder level 1)				Stratum 2 (confounder level 2)					Stratum K (confounder level K)		
		Disease				Disease					Disease		
		Yes	No			Yes	No		$\cdots$		Yes	No	
Risk factor	Yes	a_1	b_1	a_1+b_1		a_2	b_2	a_2+b_2	$\cdots$		a_K	b_K	a_K+b_K
	No	c_1	d_1	c_1+d_1		c_2	d_2	c_2+d_2	$\cdots$		c_K	d_K	c_K+d_K
		a_1+c_1	b_1+d_1	n_1		a_2+c_2	b_2+d_2	n_2	$\cdots$		a_K+c_K	b_K+d_K	n_K

$$OR_1 = \frac{a_1 d_1}{b_1 c_1}$$

$$RR_1 = \frac{a_1(c_1+d_1)}{c_1(a_1+b_1)}$$

$$OR_2 = \frac{a_2 d_2}{b_2 c_2}$$

$$RR_2 = \frac{a_2(c_2+d_2)}{c_2(a_2+b_2)}$$

$$\cdots$$

$$OR_K = \frac{a_K d_K}{b_K c_K}$$

$$RR_K = \frac{a_K(c_K+d_K)}{c_K(a_K+b_K)}$$

which for a two-level confounder is:

$$RR_{adj} = \frac{\frac{a_1(c_1+d_1)}{n_1} + \frac{a_2(c_2+d_2)}{n_2}}{\frac{c_1(a_1+b_1)}{n_1} + \frac{c_2(a_2+b_2)}{n_2}}.$$ (13.4)

From these equations we see that the adjusted ratio is a weighted average of the stratum-specific ratios. To assess the degree of confounding one must compare these adjusted ratios with the crude ratios from Table 13.18. Whenever these differ, there is confounding. The problem is to determine when they differ enough for this confounding to be relevant. There is no solution to this problem and our advice is to judge whether including the confounder alters your conclusions about the underlying biological hypothesis.

Statistical test of the association between the risk factor and the outcome, adjusted for the confounder, is given by

$$\chi^2 = \frac{\left(\left|\sum_{i=1}^{K} a_i - \sum_{i=1}^{K} E(a_i)\right| - \frac{1}{2}\right)^2}{\sum_{i=1}^{K} V(a_i)}$$

where

$$E(a_i) = \frac{(a_i + c_i)(a_i + b_i)}{n_i}$$

is the expected number of observations in category a_i, and

$$V(a_i) = \frac{(a_i + c_i)(a_i + b_i)(b_i + d_i)(c_i + d_i)}{n_i^2(n_i - 1)}$$

is the associated variance. The distribution of the test statistic is $\chi^2(1)$. Regardless of the number of strata of the confounder variable, there will always be only one degree of freedom when outcome and risk factor both have two levels.

The adjusted ratio can be calculated for qualitative variables with more than two levels and can be stratified on more than one potential confounding variable. However, as we stratify on more variables, it becomes increasingly difficult to keep track, both of the 2×2 tables and of the calculations. Therefore, with more than one potential confounding variable and/or with variables with more than 2–3 levels, statistical modelling becomes a more reasonable option.

Confounding can be evaluated using statistical modelling in multivariable analyses (multivariable meaning more than one explanatory variable in the analysis) for both a quantitative and a qualitative outcome. The type of analysis used depends on the type of the outcome and the explanatory variables (see Table 13.3).

Described in general model notation the association between the outcome (y_i) and the explanatory variable (x_{1i}) could be expressed in the following way:

- Model without the potential confounding variable (crude estimate)

$$y_i = \alpha' + \beta' x_{1i} + \epsilon_i \tag{13.5}$$

- Model with the potential confounding variable x_{2i} (the association is adjusted for the effect of x_{2i})

$$y_i = \alpha'' + \beta'' x_{1i} + \gamma'' x_{2i} + \epsilon_i \tag{13.6}$$

The response variable y_i can be either continuous or the logit of the probability of disease (dichotomous outcome). For a dichotomous outcome there is no ϵ_i in the formulas. To evaluate confounding we compare the estimate for x_{1i} in Model 13.5 with the estimate for x_{1i} in Model 13.6.

13.8.2   *Interaction*

Interaction is a biological phenomenon, expressing the effect of combinations of two (or more) variables on the outcome. Interaction can be evaluated using the same tables of stratification (Table 13.18) as were used for evaluation of confounding when the outcome is dichotomous (e.g. disease or not) and one of the explanatory variables is dichotomous (e.g. exposure or not). Interaction is evaluated by comparing the stratum-specific ratios. When they are very different (e.g. one ratio twice the size of one of the others) then interaction is present. Interaction in this case means that the ratios are different for each level of the variable we stratify on. Interaction can be tested using statistical models. Where in the model building process possible interaction should be tested is debated. Some argue that the initial multivariable model first should be reduced to only include significant variables and then biologically plausible interactions between variables should be tested (Hosmer and Lemeshow, 2000). Others argue that interactions should be tested before leaving out non-significant variables (controlling for confounding) since leaving out main effects would be unreasonable in the presence of strong interaction (Kleinbaum *et al.*, 1982). Whether to test all two-way interactions (first order), all three-way interactions (second order) or only the biologically plausible is also debated. One could argue that we will never find anything new by just testing interactions governed by the biological knowledge we already have (biologically plausible). However, by testing a lot of interactions the possibility of including significant interactions just by chance increases with the number of statistical tests used (risk of a type I error: with $\alpha = 0.05$ we have a probability of 5% that a test is falsely significant for each interaction tested).

To illustrate the concept of interaction consider the following models:

Two quantitative explanatory variables:

$$y_i = \alpha + \beta x_{1i} + \gamma x_{2i} + \epsilon_i \qquad (13.7)$$

Two qualitative explanatory variables:

$$y_{ij} = \alpha + B_i + C_j + \epsilon_{ij} \qquad (13.8)$$

One quantitative and one qualitative explanatory variable:

$$y_{ij} = \alpha + \beta x_{1i} + C_j + \epsilon_{ij} \qquad (13.9)$$

where y is the outcome
α is the general mean
B_i and C_j are the effect of two qualitative explanatory, variables
$i = 1,\ldots,I$ and $j = 1,\ldots,J$
x_1 and x_2 are two continuous explanatory variables
β and γ are the slopes
ϵ is the random error

Again, the outcome y can be either continuous or the logit to the probability for disease (dichotomous outcome). If there is a surplus or less effect in the case where two explanatory variables are present then we would have to add another term which can explain this surplus or less; this is the interaction term. The interaction term is added to the model by adding a multiplication term of the two factors involved to the model:

Two quantitative explanatory variables:

$$y_i = \alpha + \beta x_{1i} + \gamma x_{2i} + \delta(x_{1i} \times x_{2i}) + \epsilon_i \qquad (13.10)$$

Two qualitative explanatory variables:

$$y_{ij} = \alpha + B_i + C_j + BC_{ij} + \epsilon_{ij} \qquad (13.11)$$

One quantitative and one qualitative explanatory variable:

$$y_{ij} = \alpha + \beta x_{1ij} + C_j + \delta_j x_{1ij} + \epsilon_{ij} \qquad (13.12)$$

where δ and δ_j are regression coefficients, $\delta(x_{1i} \times x_{1j})$, BC_{ij} and $\delta_j x_{1ij}$ are the interaction terms and B_i and C_j are the effect of two qualitative explanatory variables $i = 1,\ldots,I$ and $j = 1,\ldots,J$.

Based on these models we will work through four different situations depending on whether the two explanatory variables are qualitative, quantitative or both.

1. Both explanatory variables B_i and C_j are dichotomous, i.e. $B_i = (0, 1)$ and $C_j = (0, 1)$ (Models 13.8 and 13.11). The effect of interaction between B_i and C_j is shown in Figure 13.14. Interaction will result in different stratum-specific ratios (e.g. $OR_1 \neq OR_2$) (see Table 13.18). Assessing the degree of interaction by this approach is again a matter of judgement: is the interaction of biological importance? If so, then we have an interaction. The alternative is to analyse Model 13.11 using an analysis of variance or logistic analysis depending on the nature of the outcome. Interaction will result in a significant estimate of BC_{ij} in Model 13.11.

2. A generalisation of the previous situation is when the explanatory variables B_i and C_j are qualitative, but not necessarily dichotomous, e.g. $B_i = (0, 1, 2)$ and $C_j = (0, 1, 2, 3)$ as illustrated in Figure 13.15 (Models 13.8 and 13.11). Again, we can assess interaction by analysis of variance or logistic analysis. If BC_{ij} in Model 13.11 is significant then we have an interaction.

3. One qualitative explanatory variable (e.g. $C_j = (0, 1)$) and one continuous variable (x_1) (Models 13.9 and 13.12). Again, interaction is present if δ_j in Model 13.12 is significant in an analysis of covariance (which is an analysis of variance where some explanatory variables are continuous) or a logistic analysis depending on the nature of the outcome. In Figure 13.16 the effect of interaction is illustrated. Interaction between C_j and x_1 results in a change in slope of the continuous variable x_1 as the value of the qualitative variable C_j changes.

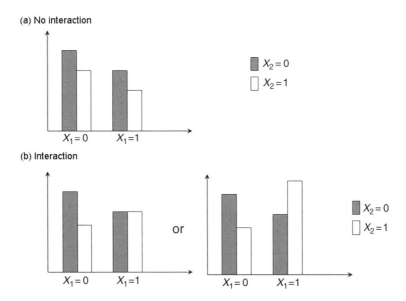

Figure 13.14. *Illustration of the effect of interaction between two dichotomous explanatory variables.*

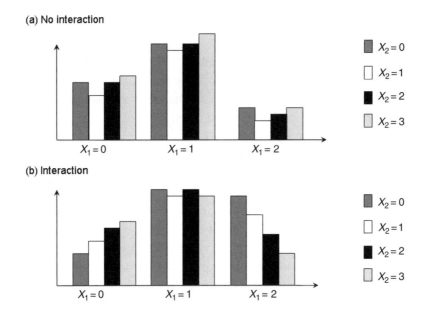

Figure 13.15. *Illustration of the effect of interaction between two qualitative variables.*

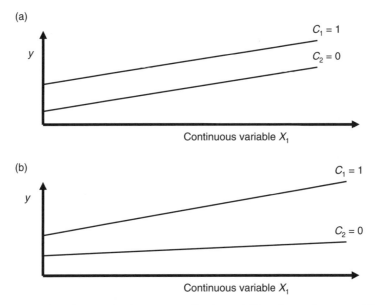

Figure 13.16. *The effect of interaction between a qualitative variable and a continuous variable. (a) When there is no interaction, the slopes of the two curves are equal. (b) Interaction results in different slopes for the lines.*

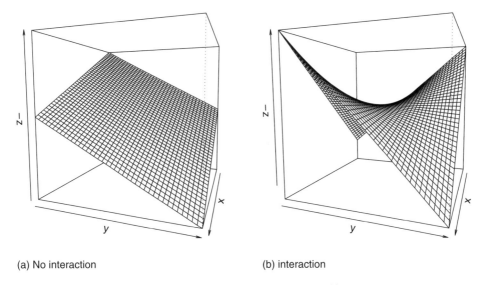

(a) No interaction   (b) interaction

Figure 13.17. *The effect of interaction between two continuous variables.*

4. When both explanatory variables are continuous (Model 13.7), interaction is seen as a significant estimate of δ in Model 13.10. In Figure 13.17 we illustrate the effect of interaction between two continuous variables.

13.8.3 *The relationship between confounding and interaction*

Earlier, we saw that confounding is evaluated by comparing the crude odds ratio with the adjusted odds ratio. However, this adjustment (weighted average) is only reasonable when the stratum-specific odds ratios are similar. Therefore, when strong interaction is present, confounding is not relevant to evaluate since the weighted average does not make sense. Below we give two examples of how to assess whether confounding or interaction is present using the setup of Table 13.18.

> **EXAMPLE 13.15.** A study was carried out in Denmark to study the influence of *Bordetella bronchiseptica* on atrophic rhinitis in pigs. In cooperation with eight veterinary practices, 68 pig herds were included in the study. Each herd was classified as having clinical atrophic rhinitis defined as presence of pigs with short or distorted snout deviating clearly from the breed and any natural variation in snout form. Nasal swaps were taken from ten 4 week old pigs and from ten 8 week old pigs in each herd and tested for toxin producing *Pasteurella multocida* (*P.m. tox+*). The same swaps were also tested for the presence of *Bordetella bronchiseptica* (*B.b.*). Each herd was classified as positive for *P.m. tox+* if the pathogen could be isolated from at least one of the nasal swaps and herds were classified as positive for *B.b.* if the pathogen could be isolated from at least one of the nasal swaps. The results of this study are presented in Table 13.19. We see that there is some difference between the two strata-specific RR's (RR$_1$ = 1.25 and RR$_2$ = 0.94), indicating some interaction between

Pasteurella multicida toxin producing bacteria and *Bordetella bronchiseptica*. The adjusted RR is (Equation 13.4):

$$RR_{adj} = \frac{22(12+3)/37 + 5(5+10)/31}{12(22+0)/37 + 5(5+11)/31} = 1.167$$

The difference between the *crude* RR (1.25) and the adjusted RR (1.17) indicates no or very little confounding between *Pasteurella multicida* toxin producing bacteria and *Bordetella bronchiseptica* in relation to the outcome atrophic rhinitis. The same calculations can be performed using the formulas for odds ratio.

Interaction and confounding were further examined using logistic analysis with atrophic rhinitis as the outcome and *Bordetella bronchiseptica* and presence of toxin producing *Pasteurella multicida* as risk factors. Due to a limited number of observations in some of the combinations (Table 13.19) it was not possible to test an interaction between *Bordetella bronchiseptica* and toxin producing *Pasteurella multicida*. The logistic analysis of the effect of *Bordetella bronchiseptica* and toxin producing *Pasteurella multicida* on atrophic rhinitis showed that presence of toxin producing *Pasteurella multicida* was a significant risk factor (p < 0.001), whereas *Bordetella bronchiseptica* had no significant effect on atrophic rhinitis (p = 0.29). The analysis indicated no confounding between *Bordetella bronchiseptica* and toxin producing *Pasteurella multicida*, as the parameters estimated for each of the risk factors were only slightly changed when the model was modified (from having both variables in the model at the same time to two models including just one of the variables).

EXAMPLE 13.16. The farmer in a Danish sow herd had experienced problems with a high number of stillborn piglets. He wanted to identify the risk factors that were important in relation to the increased number of stillborn piglets. Therefore, production records were collected for the herd during the period January 1 to July 1 2002. The production variables that were recorded were among others: sow identification number, litter number, farrowing date, number of liveborn and number of stillborn piglets. Since some of the sows could have more than one farrowing in this period, data were restricted to include only one randomly selected farrowing for each sow in the herd. Data included 379 sows.

The farmer had observed that the problem seemed to be more prominent in some parities (litter numbers). One or more stillborn piglets was found in 184 of the 379 farrowings and of these 81 were among first-parity sows, whereas 117 of the litters without any stillborn piglet were among first-parity sows. The farmer wanted to know if there was a difference in the number of litters with at least one stillborn piglet between first parity and higher parities.

The study is an observational cross-sectional study, although the study period is long (6 months). Data are given in Table 13.20.

The OR and RR were calculated as:

$$OR_{crude} = \frac{103/78}{81/117} = 1.91$$

$$RR_{crude} = \frac{103/181}{81/198} = 1.39$$

The association between stillborn and parity is tested using a χ^2-test (Equation 13.3). The test statistic value is

$$\chi^2 = \frac{(|103 \times 117 - 78 \times 81| - 379/2)^2 \times 379}{184 \times 195 \times 181 \times 198} = 9.06$$

This test statistic value has a χ^2-distribution with one degree of freedom, $\chi^2(1)_{0.95} = 3.84$. As the test statistic value is greater than 3.84, the hypothesis is rejected and we conclude that there is a significant association between stillborn and parity.

Interaction between farrowing month and parity was evaluated by comparison of the stratum-specific measures of association (Table 13.21). Here, the ORs and RRs are calculated for the relation between parity and stillborn, stratified by farrowing month. The 95% CIs are given in order to evaluate the differences between the ORs or the RRs. The ORs vary from 1.00 to 4.78, i.e. a change of several hundred percent. However, when considering the width of the confidence intervals (e.g. 0.33–41.59), the differences are not that large. It is also seen, that the interval for the ORs (1.00–4.78) is wider than for the RRs (1.00–2.20). If the stratum-specific ORs (or RRs) were compared without considering the uncertainty of the estimates, we would probably conclude that there is an interaction between farrowing month and parity. The interaction was tested for significance using a logistic analysis, including farrowing month, parity and the interaction. The analysis shows that the interaction is not significant, p $= 0.51$.

In order to evaluate possible confounding between farrowing month and parity, the adjusted association measures were calculated.

$$OR_{adj} = 2.12, \quad \text{with 95\% CI:} \quad [1.36; 3.30]$$

and

$$RR_{adj} = 1.45 \quad \text{with 95\% CI:} \quad [1.17; 1.80]$$

The adjusted OR and RR compared to the *crude* OR (1.91) and RR (1.39) do not indicate any confounding.

13.9 Measuring agreement

Most measurements (e.g. diagnostic tests) are not precise. Due to this uncertainty in measurements there are usually a number of tests available. In order to select or replace a method, comparison or agreement between methods is evaluated. The measurements can be either quantitative or qualitative. Depending on the scale of the measurements, different methods can be used for evaluation of agreement. Kappa (κ) is a measure of agreement between two methods (or observers) used when the measure is on a qualitative scale, e.g. presence of *Campylobacter* spp. in turkey samples. When comparing measurements on a quantitative scale, Bland–Altman plot can be used to evaluate agreement.

Agreement between two tests for detection of *Campylobacter* spp. has been evaluated. The two tests were conventional bacteriological culture and automated enzyme immunoassay (EiaFoss). For each turkey sample, detection of

Table 13.19. *The crude 2 × 2 table for* Bordetella bronchiseptica (B.b.) *as a risk factor for atrophic rhinitis and the resulting 2 × 2 tables when stratifying for presence of toxin producing* Pasteurella multocida *(P.m. tox+)*

		Atrophic rhinitis		
		Yes	No	
Bordetella	Yes	27	11	38
bronchiseptica	No	17	13	30
		44	24	68

$$RR_{crude} = \frac{27(17+13)}{17(27+11)} = 1.25$$

		P.m. tox + present (confounder level 1)			P.m. tox + not present (confounder level 2)		
		Atrophic rhinitis			Atrophic rhinitis		
		Yes	No		Yes	No	
Bordetella	Yes	22	0	22	5	11	16
bronchiseptica	No	12	3	15	5	10	15
		34	3	37	10	21	31

$$RR_1 = \frac{22(12+3)}{12(22+0)} = 1.25 \qquad RR_2 = \frac{5(5+10)}{5(5+11)} = 0.94$$

Table 13.20. *Distribution of stillborn and parity in an observational study of risk factors for increased number of stillborn piglets in a Danish pig herd*

		Stillborn		Total
		>0	0	
Parity	>1	103	78	181
	1	81	117	198
	Total	184	195	379

Campylobacter spp. was performed using both tests. Agreement between the tests was evaluated using kappa (κ). This is further discussed in Example 13.17.

Agreement between raters (or observers) classifying animals into one of several groups can also be calculated using the kappa (κ). Differences between raters (e.g. veterinarians) is considered a problem, whenever more than one

Table 13.21. *Stratum-specific ORs and RRs for the association between presence of stillborn piglets and parity stratified by month of farrowing in a cross-sectional study of risk factors for increased number of stillborn piglets in a Danish pig herd*

Measure of association	Farrowing month					
	January	February	March	April	May	June
OR	3.66	1.00	2.06	1.28	2.50	4.78
95% CI (OR)	0.33–41.59	0.21–4.71	0.90–4.74	0.50–3.29	0.96–6.50	1.43–15.97
RR	2.20	1.00	1.54	1.15	1.50	1.80
95% CI (RR)	0.38–1.26	0.54–1.86	0.92–2.57	0.67–1.98	0.97–2.31	1.26–2.57

rater is involved in a study, e.g. in order to measure the disease prevalence. The inter-rater (or between observer) agreement is calculated using kappa. This will be discussed further in Example 13.18.

As a third example, consider two methods for measuring blood pressure in cats, a direct and an indirect method. The direct method (arterial catheter) is very precise, but complicated to use as the cat has to be in anaesthesia. The indirect method (Cardell oscillometric monitor) is very cheap and easy to use without anaesthesia. Therefore, it is of interest to compare the two methods in order to replace the cumbersome and expensive indirect method with the easy and cheap direct method. Agreement between the two methods has been evaluated using a Bland–Altman plot. This will be discussed further in Example 13.19.

13.9.1 *Agreement for qualitative variables: Cohen's kappa (κ)*

Agreement between two methods can be calculated when both methods have been used on the same sample, e.g. the two tests used to diagnose *Campylobacter* spp. (Example 13.17). In the simple case, we have only two levels for the two methods (e.g. positive and negative). However, calculation of kappa is not limited to variables with two levels, but can be generalised for $g \times g$ tables, where $g \geq 2$. Data can be illustrated as in Table 13.22 when the method has two categories or as in Table 13.23, when g categories are used. O_{ij} is the observed number of observations in category ij (that is row $= i$ and column $= j$). r_i and c_j are the number of observations in row i and number of observations in column j, respectively.

The κ is a measure of agreement adjusted by the agreement by chance. The κ is based on proportions rather than numbers. The observed proportion of agreement (p_o) between two methods for an outcome with only two levels

Table 13.22. *Comparison of two methods each with two levels*

Comparison of two methods		Method 1		Total
		Positive	Negative	
Method 2	Positive	O_{11}	O_{12}	r_1
	Negative	O_{21}	O_{22}	r_2
	Total	c_1	c_2	n

Table 13.23. *Comparison of two methods each with g levels*

Comparison of two methods		Method 1				Total
		1	2	$\cdots$	g	
Method 2	1	O_{11}	O_{12}	$\cdots$	O_{1g}	r_1
	2	O_{21}	O_{22}	$\cdots$	O_{2g}	r_2
	$\vdots$	$\cdots$	$\cdots$	$\vdots$	$\cdots$	$\cdots$
	g	O_{g1}	O_{g2}	$\cdots$	O_{gg}	r_g
	Total	c_1	c_2	$\cdots$	c_g	n

(Table 13.22) is given by

$$p_\text{o} = \frac{O_{11} + O_{22}}{n}, \quad \text{for } g = 2$$

or in general for $g \geq 2$ (Table 13.23)

$$p_\text{o} = \frac{\sum_{i=1}^{g} O_{ii}}{n}$$

The κ is a measure of chance-corrected agreement and is calculated as the observed proportion of agreement (p_o) adjusted by expected proportion of agreement by chance (p_e). Furthermore, the κ is standardised by dividing the difference between observed and expected agreement by the maximum proportion of agreement minus the proportion of agreement by chance, i.e. $1 - p_\text{e}$:

$$\kappa = \frac{\text{observed agreement} - \text{expected agreement}}{\text{maximum agreement} - \text{expected agreement}}$$

i.e.

$$\kappa = \frac{p_\text{o} - p_\text{e}}{1 - p_\text{e}}$$

where p_e is the expected proportion of agreement by chance given as

$$p_e = \frac{\sum_{i=1}^g r_i c_i}{n^2}$$

This means that κ expresses the proportion of agreement beyond chance.

EXAMPLE 13.17. In a study of *Campylobacter* spp. in turkey samples, two methods for diagnosing *Campylobacter* spp. (presence or not) were compared (Borck *et al.*, 2002). The methods were conventional bacteriological culture and automated enzyme immunoassay (EiaFoss). In total, 61 turkey samples were used. Each sample was tested using both methods (Table 13.24). The agreement between the two methods was measured using κ. The observed agreement was calculated, using the observed values given in Table 13.24 as

$$p_o = \frac{O_{11} + O_{22}}{n} = \frac{32 + 4}{61} = 0.5902$$

The expected agreement by chance is

$$p_e = \frac{\sum_{i=1}^g r_i c_i}{n^2} = \frac{53 \times 36 + 8 \times 25}{61^2} = 0.5665$$

hence,

$$\kappa = \frac{p_o - p_e}{1 - p_e} = \frac{0.590 - 0.567}{1 - 0.567} = 0.055.$$

κ has a maximum of 1 when agreement is perfect. A zero value indicates no agreement beyond chance and a negative value indicates agreement worse than chance. Different interpretations of κ in the interval [0,1] have been suggested. Landis and Koch (1977) and Fleiss (1981) suggested the interpretation given in Table 13.25.

The usefulness of κ has been debated as there are a number of problems associated with the interpretation (see, e.g. Altman, 1995). κ depends on the prevalence in each category, as seen in Table 13.26. Due to this problem, it is misleading to compare κ values from different studies, where the prevalence in the categories is different. A second problem with interpretation is that κ depends on the number of categories (the value of g). If a $g \times g$ table (where

Table 13.24. *Comparison of EiaFoss and conventional culture for detection of* Campylobacter *spp. in turkey (Example 13.17)*

		EiaFoss		Total
		Positive	Negative	
Conventional culture	Positive	$O_{11} = 32$	$O_{12} = 21$	$r_1 = 53$
	Negative	$O_{21} = 4$	$O_{22} = 4$	$r_2 = 8$
	Total	$c_1 = 36$	$c_2 = 25$	$n = 61$

Table 13.25. *Interpretation of κ in the interval [0,1] suggested by Landis and Koch (1977) and Fleiss (1981)*

Value of κ	Landis and Koch (1977)	Value of κ	Fleiss (1981)
$\kappa \leq 0.2$	Poor		
$0.2 < \kappa \leq 0.4$	Fair	$\kappa \leq 0.40$	Poor
$0.4 < \kappa \leq 0.6$	Moderate	$0.4 < \kappa < 0.75$	Good
$0.6 < \kappa \leq 0.8$	Good	$0.75 \leq \kappa$	Excellent
$0.8 < \kappa$	Very good		

Table 13.26. *Comparison of two methods with the same observed agreement of $p_o = 0.60$, but with different prevalences in the two categories, resulting in different κ values*

		Method 1 +	Method 1 −	Total
$\kappa = 0.20$				
Method 2	+	40	10	50
	−	30	20	50
	Total	70	30	100
$\kappa = -0.01$				
Method 2	+	5	10	15
	−	30	55	85
	Total	35	65	100

$g \geq 2$) is collapsed into a smaller table, e.g. a 2 × 2 table, κ is changed. This is illustrated in Table 13.27, where $\kappa = 0.119$ for the original 3 × 3 table. However, when the table is collapsed to a 2 × 2 table $\kappa = 0.158$ or $\kappa = 0.05$, depending on how the table is collapsed.

A third problem with κ is that it does not take into account the order of categories when the variable is on an ordinal scale. Therefore, a weighted kappa $\kappa(w)$ has been developed in which the degree of disagreement is weighted according to the magnitude of discrepancy. Observations close to the diagonal represent differences of only one category, whereas observations far from the diagonal represent discrepancies of two or more categories. A large discrepancy (e.g. two or three categories) is considered more serious than a smaller one (e.g. one category).

Table 13.27. *Comparison of two methods with three categories or collapsed to two categories, where categories A–B and B–C are collapsed*

		Method 1			Total
		A	B	C	
$\kappa = 0.119$					
Method 2	A	30	20	50	100
	B	20	20	10	50
	C	5	15	30	50
	Total	55	55	90	200

		Method 1		Total
		A + B	C	
$\kappa = 0.158$				
Method 2	A	90	60	150
	B	20	30	50
	Total	110	90	200

		Method 1		Total
		A	B + C	
$\kappa = 0.05$				
Method 2	A	30	70	100
	B + C	25	75	100
	Total	55	145	200

The weighted $\kappa(w)$ is calculated as

$$\kappa(w) = \frac{p_{o(w)} - p_{e(w)}}{1 - p_{e(w)}}$$

where

$$p_{o(w)} = \frac{1}{n}\sum_{i=1}^{g}\sum_{j=1}^{g} w_{ij}O_{ij}$$

$$p_{e(w)} = \frac{1}{n^2}\sum_{i=1}^{g}\sum_{j=1}^{g} w_{ij}r_i c_j$$

and

$$w_{ij} = 1 - \frac{|i-j|}{g-1}$$

Table 13.28. *Agreement between two clinicians evaluating udder asymmetry*

		\multicolumn{5}{c}{Clinician 2}				Total
		0	1	2	3	4	
Clinician 1	0	7	3	2	0	0	12
	1	0	1	0	0	0	1
	2	1	0	0	1	0	2
	3	0	0	1	0	0	1
	4	1	0	0	0	3	4
	Total	9	4	3	1	3	20

The $\kappa(w)$ has been used to measure agreement between two observers evaluating udder health on dairy cows.

EXAMPLE 13.18. In a study of udder health in dairy cows, two clinicians made systematic clinical recordings of the udder on the same 20 cows (data from Houe *et al.*, 2002). The agreement between the two clinicians evaluating udder asymmetry is shown in Table 13.28. Asymmetry was evaluated using an ordinal scale, where 0 means no asymmetry, 1 is slight, 2 is moderate, 3 is pronounced and 4 is severe. As the scale is ordinal, the $\kappa(w)$ have been calculated in order to evaluate agreement between the two clinicians. The κ has been given for comparison, but should not be used due to the ordinal scale of udder asymmetry.

The (unweighted) κ is calculated as

$$\kappa = \frac{p_o - p_e}{1 - p_e}$$

$$= \frac{0.55 - 0.3275}{1 - 0.3275}$$

$$= 0.33$$

where

$$p_o = \frac{7 + 1 + 0 + 0 + 3}{20} = 0.55$$

$$p_e = \frac{12 \times 9 + 1 \times 4 + 2 \times 3 + 1 \times 1 + 4 \times 3}{20^2} = 0.3275$$

The weighted $\kappa(w)$ is calculated as

$$\kappa(w) = \frac{p_o(w) - p_e(w)}{1 - p_e(w)}$$

$$= \frac{0.8125 - 0.59875}{1 - 0.59875}$$

$$= 0.53$$

where

$$p_o(w) = \frac{1}{20}\left(1 \times 7 + \frac{3}{4} \times 3 + \frac{2}{4} \times 2 + \frac{1}{4} \times 0 + 0 \times 0 + \frac{3}{4} \times 0 + 1 \times 1 + \frac{3}{4} \times 0 + \frac{2}{4} \times 0\right.$$

$$+ \frac{1}{4} \times 0 + \frac{2}{4} \times 1 + \frac{3}{4} \times 0 + 1 \times 0 + \frac{3}{4} \times 1 + \frac{2}{4} \times 0 + \frac{1}{4} \times 0 + \frac{2}{4} \times 0 + \frac{3}{4} \times 1$$

$$\left. + 1 \times 0 + \frac{3}{4} \times 0 + 0 \times 1 + \frac{1}{4} \times 0 + \frac{2}{4} \times 0 + \frac{3}{4} \times 0 + 1 \times 3\right)$$

$$= 0.8125$$

and

$$p_e(w) = \frac{1}{20^2}\left(1 \times 9 \times 12 + \frac{3}{4} \times 4 \times 12 + \frac{2}{4} \times 3 \times 12 + \frac{1}{4} \times 1 \times 12 + 0 \times 3 \times 12 + \frac{3}{4} \times 9 \times 1\right.$$

$$+ 1 \times 4 \times 1 + \frac{3}{4} \times 3 \times 1 + \frac{2}{4} \times 1 \times 1 + \frac{1}{4} \times 3 \times 1 + \frac{2}{4} \times 9 \times 2 + \frac{3}{4} \times 4 \times 2$$

$$+ 1 \times 3 \times 2 + \frac{3}{4} \times 1 \times 2 + \frac{2}{4} \times 3 \times 2 + \frac{1}{4} \times 9 \times 1 + \frac{2}{4} \times 4 \times 1 + \frac{3}{4} \times 3 \times 1 + 1 \times 1 \times 1$$

$$\left. + \frac{3}{4} \times 3 \times 1 + 0 \times 9 \times 4 + \frac{1}{4} \times 4 \times 4 + \frac{2}{4} \times 3 \times 4 + \frac{3}{4} \times 1 \times 4 + 1 \times 3 \times 4\right)$$

$$= 0.59875$$

and the weights w_{ij} are

w_{ij}		Clinician 2				
		0	1	2	3	4
Clinician 1	0	1	$\frac{3}{4}$	$\frac{2}{4}$	$\frac{1}{4}$	0
	1	$\frac{3}{4}$	1	$\frac{3}{4}$	$\frac{2}{4}$	$\frac{1}{4}$
	2	$\frac{2}{4}$	$\frac{3}{4}$	1	$\frac{3}{4}$	$\frac{2}{4}$
	3	$\frac{1}{4}$	$\frac{2}{4}$	$\frac{3}{4}$	1	$\frac{3}{4}$
	4	0	$\frac{1}{4}$	$\frac{2}{4}$	$\frac{3}{4}$	1

13.9.2 *Agreement for quantitative variables: Bland–Altman plot*

Agreement between two methods using a quantitative scale can be presented using Bland–Altman plot. This is a graphical presentation of the differences between the two methods against the mean of the two methods. The correlation coefficient between the two methods is sometimes incorrectly used for measurement of agreement. However, the correlation is a measure of linear association, rather than agreement.

Assume measurements Y_{Ai} and Y_{Bi} of two methods A and B for animal i, $i = 1, \ldots, n$ where Y_{Ai} is the outcome measured for animal i with method A and Y_{Bi} is the outcome measured for animal i with method B.

The Bland–Altman plot is constructed by calculating the difference between the two methods for each animal (d_i) as well as the mean of the two methods for each animal (m_i)

$$d_i = Y_{Ai} - Y_{Bi}$$

$$m_i = \frac{Y_{Ai} + Y_{Bi}}{2}$$

The mean difference ($\bar{d}$) between the two methods is an estimate of the bias of one method relative to the other method

$$\text{bias} = \bar{d} = \frac{\sum_{i=1}^{n} d_i}{n}$$

Whenever $\bar{d} \sim 0$ there is on average agreement.

The Bland–Altman plot illustrates for each animal the difference between the two methods versus the mean difference. This can be used to evaluate if the differences are constant for increasing mean differences or the differences are proportional with the mean differences (see Figure 13.18 in Example 13.19).

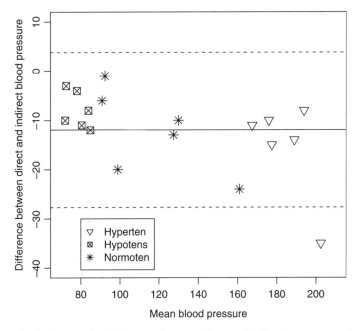

Figure 13.18. *Bland–Altman plot. Differences between direct and indirect measurements of the systolic blood pressure in six cats in three blood pressure intervals: hypotension, normotension and hypertension. The solid line indicates the bias, estimated as −11.9. The dashed lines indicate the limits of agreement [−27.70; 3.81].*

Finally, limits of agreement can be calculated as 95% confidence limits for individual observations as

$$\bar{d} \pm 1.96 s_d$$

where $\bar{d}$ is the mean difference given above and s_d is the standard deviation of the differences given as

$$s_d = \sqrt{\frac{\sum_{i=1}^{n}(d_i - \bar{d})^2}{n-1}}$$

Two methods used for measuring blood pressure in cats are compared in Example 13.19 using the Bland–Altman plot.

EXAMPLE 13.19. Two methods (a direct and an indirect method) for measuring blood pressure in cats have been studied (data from Pedersen, 2002). The direct blood pressure was measured using an arterial catheter in the right femoral artery. The indirect measurement was obtained from the left antebrachium using the Cardell oscillometric monitor. The direct measure is very precise, but complicated to use as the cats have to be anesthetised. Therefore, there has been an interest to replace this direct method with an indirect method. In order to evaluate how well the indirect method is, a study has been performed comparing the two methods. In total six cats were included in the study. The systolic arterial blood pressure was measured during hypotension, normotension and hypertension. The Bland–Altman plot is seen in Figure 13.18. It is seen that the bias between the two methods is 11.9 mmHg, calculated as the mean difference between the two methods. The limits of agreement are

$$-11.9 \text{ mmHg} \pm 1.96 \times 8.04 \text{ mmHg} \quad \text{or} \quad [-27.70; 3.81] \text{ mmHg}.$$

With these limits of agreement we expect that the blood pressures measured for a new cat will differ less than 16 mmHg.

13.10 Overview of statistical analyses

The different statistical analyses and techniques described in this chapter are summarised in Tables 13.29–13.32. Each of the tables contains references to the appropriate section in this chapter as well as the suggested SAS procedure including options (see Appendix E for SAS programs and output for most of the examples in this chapter).

In Table 13.29 an overview of the statistical analyses and SAS procedures for problems with one explanatory and one outcome variable is given.

Table 13.30 gives the statistical analyses and SAS procedures for problems with one outcome variable and two or more explanatory variables.

Analyses of relations without a specific causal relationship are given in Table 13.31.

Finally, Table 13.32 gives an overview of the methods for assessing agreement.

Table 13.29. Overview of statistical analyses and SAS procedures for analysis of causal relations for one explanatory variable (also called risk factor or exposure) divided by type and scale of the outcome and explanatory variables and whether or not there is independence between observations (IO)

Outcome type (scale)	Explanatory variable Type (scale)	No. of levels	IO	Statistical analysis (section in Chapter 13)	SAS (version 8.02) procedure Procedure name	Options/statements
Quantitative (continuous)	Qualitative (dichotomous)	2	Yes	t-test (13.4.2)	PROC TTEST	
	Qualitative (dichotomous)	2	No*	Paired t-test (13.4.3)	PROC TTEST	PAIRED
	Qualitative (dichotomous, nominal or ordinal)	≥2	Yes	Analysis of variance (13.4.4)	PROC MIXED	
	Quantitative	–	Yes	Linear regression (13.4.6)	PROC REG	
Qualitative (dichotomous)	Qualitative (dichotomous)	2	Yes	χ^2-test (13.5.2)	PROC FREQ	
				Fisher exact test (13.5.2)	PROC FREQ	
				Logistic analysis (13.5.5)	PROC GENMOD	
	Quantitative (continuous)	–	Yes	Logistic regression (13.5.4)	PROC GENMOD	
				Fisher exact test (13.5.2)	PROC FREQ	EXACT FISHER
	Qualitative (dichotomous, nominal or ordinal)	≥2	Yes	χ^2-test (13.5.2)	PROC FREQ	
				Logistic analysis (13.5.5)	PROC GENMOD	

*Two observations per animal.

Table 13.30. *Overview of statistical analyses and SAS procedures for analysis of causal relations for more than one explanatory variable (also called risk factor or exposure) divided by types and scales of the outcome and explanatory variables and whether or not there is independence between observations (IO)*

Outcome type (scale)	Explanatory variable		IO*	Statistical analysis (section in Chapter 13)	SAS (version 8.02) procedure	
	Types (scales)	No. of levels			Procedure name	Options/statements
Quantitative (continuous)	Qualitative (dichotomous, nominal or ordinal)	≥2	Yes	Analysis of variance (13.4.4, 13.7, 13.8)	PROC MIXED	
	Qualitative (dichotomous, nominal or ordinal)	≥2	No†	Mixed models (not covered in this book)	PROC MIXED	REPEATED RANDOM
	Qualitative (dichotomous, nominal or ordinal)	≥2	Yes	Analysis of covariance (not covered in this book)	PROC MIXED	
	Quantitative (discrete, continuous)	–				
	Quantitative (discrete, continuous)	–	Yes	Multiple linear regression (13.4.6, 13.7, 13.8)	PROC REG	
	Quantitative (discrete, continuous)	–				
Qualitative (dichotomous)	Qualitative (dichotomous, nominal or ordinal)	≥2	Yes	Logistic analysis (13.5.5, 13.7, 13.8)	PROC GENMOD	
	Qualitative (dichotomous, nominal or ordinal)	≥2				
	Qualitative (dichotomous, nominal or ordinal)	≥2	Yes	Logistic analysis (13.5.5, 13.7, 13.8)	PROC GENMOD	
	Quantitative (discrete, continuous)	–				
	Quantitative (discrete, continuous)	–	Yes	Multiple logistic regression (13.5.4, 13.7, 13.8)	PROC GENMOD	
	Quantitative (discrete, continuous)	–				

*There can be two or more observations for the same animal for all analyses; however, only one case is shown in the table.

†Two or more observations per animal.

Table 13.31. Overview of statistical analyses and SAS procedures for analysis of (non-causal) relations between two variables divided by types and scales of the variables

Variable 1		Variable 2		Independent variables	Statistical analysis (section in Chapter 13)	SAS (version 8.02) procedure	
Type (scale)	No. of levels	Type (scale)	No. of levels			Procedure name	Options/statements
Quantitative (continuous)	–	Quantitative (continuous)	–	Yes	Pearson's correlation coefficient (13.4.5)	PROC CORR	
Quantitative (continuous, discrete)	–	Quantitative (continuous, discrete)	–	Yes	Spearman's correlation coefficient (13.4.5)	PROC CORR	SPEARMAN
Qualitative (dichotomous, ordinal)	>2	Qualitative (dichotomous, ordinal)	>2				
Qualitative (dichotomous, nominal or ordinal)	≥2	Qualitative (dichotomous, nominal or ordinal)	≥2	Yes	χ^2-test (13.5.2) Fisher exact test (13.5.2)	PROC FREQ PROC FREQ	EXACT FISHER
Qualitative (dichotomous)	2	Qualitative (dichotomous)	2	No	McNemar test (13.5.3)	PROC FREQ	EXACT AGREE

Table 13.32. *Overview of statistical analyses and SAS procedures for analysis of agreement between two tests (intra-observer) or between two observers (inter-observer)*

Test 1 or observer A *Type of variable (scale)*	Test 2 or observer B *Type of variable (scale)*	Statistical analysis *(section in Chapter 13)*	SAS (version 8.02) procedure	
			Procedure name	*Options/statements*
Qualitative (dichotomous, nominal or ordinal)	Qualitative	Cohen's kappa (13.9.1) (dichotomous, nominal or ordinal)	PROC FREQ	EXACT AGREE
Qualitative (ordinal)	Qualitative (ordinal)	Weighted kappa (13.9.1)	PROC FREQ	EXACT AGREE
Qualitative (dichotomous)	Qualitative (dichotomous)	McNemar test (13.5.3)	PROC FREQ	EXACT MCNEMAR
Quantitative (continuous)	Quantitative (continuous)	Bland–Altman plot (13.9.2)		

13.11 Further reading

Further reading for statistical analysis in general, see e.g. Altman (1995), Daniel (1995), Samuels and Witmer (1999) and Sokal and Rohlf (1981).

For more information about linear regression, see e.g. Petrie and Watson (1999), Weisberg (1985) and Altman (1995); for logistic regression and analysis, see Hosmer and Lemeshow (2000).

For further reading regarding agreement, see e.g. Bland and Altman (1986) and Fleiss (1981).

APPENDIX A: EXERCISES

Exercises for Chapter 1

Question 1: What does the word epidemiology mean?

Question 2: What is a population?

Question 3: Give a short definition of epidemiology.

Question 4: Consider that all cattle in each herd on the Island of Samsø are blood tested for BVDV. At the same time for each herd it is recorded whether they practice to put animals on pasture. State for the following groups whether it can be considered as a population, an epidemiological unit or an observational unit (there can be none, one or more answers to each statement):

A: The mean body weight of animals in the study
B: The time duration of an epidemiological study
C: All cattle on Samsø
D: One herd on Samsø
E: One individual cow

Question 5: Which of the following studies are dealing with descriptive epidemiology and which are dealing with analytical epidemiology?

A: Frequency of mastitis in Danish dairy herds
B: The role of bedding for occurrence of diarrhoea in piglets
C: Difference in occurrence of milk fever in different parities
D: Mean milk yield in Jersey cows
E: Relation between housing system and somatic cell count

Question 6: Arrange the following steps according to the logical sequence in an epidemiological study:

A: Decide the duration of the study
B: Decide sampling method
C: Collect data and perform other data management
D: Draw conclusions from the study

E: Define the target and the study population
F: State the hypothesis
G: Choose a study design
H: Data analysis
I: Estimate the necessary sample size

Exercises for Chapter 2

Question 1: Why is it important to state the hypothesis before initiation of an epidemiological study (state true or false)?

A: To be able to define the relevant disease and determinants
B: The hypothesis is the basis for deciding which information must be collected

Question 2: Characterise the following statements as whether they are a hypothesis, a purpose or an objective.

A: Improvement of animal welfare
B: High humidity increases the risk of calf pneumonia
C: Establishing the association between housing (loose housing and tie housing) and occurrence of lameness

Question 3: Which of the following statements define the concept of disease?

A: Non-compensated perturbation of one or several functions of an organism
B: Reduced production (e.g. milk yield)
C: The animal drinks extra amount of water
D: Pathological condition occurring in a susceptible population
E: The farmer observes abnormal behaviour of the animal

Question 4: Four hundred dogs are studied for 2 years. There are 100 white, 100 red, 100 brown and 100 black dogs. Thirty brown dogs develop fever. One white dog develops fever. One hundred black dogs develop fever. No red dogs develop fever.

Which hypotheses can be studied from this population and the available information?

A: Development of fever in black and brown dogs
B: The proportion of fever in black dogs is the same as the proportion of fever in blue dogs

C: The proportion of fever in black dogs is the same as the proportion of fever in brown dogs

D: The gene coding for black colour is responsible for fever

E: Coloured dogs have more fever than white dogs

F: The relation between development of fever and colour

Question 5: The Danish Cattle Federation is interested in knowing the prevalence of a new parasite among rodents in Denmark. The parasite can be transmitted to cattle and cause severe infestation in Jersey cows. Faecal samples from 300 rodents and 400 cows are collected randomly from the island Bornholm, where many cows are grazing. Quite often, grazing cows and rodents have snout-to-snout contact. During wintertime, no cows on the island Samsø shows symptoms of the parasite.

1. What is the target population?
2. What is the study population?
3. What is the sample population?

A: Rodents on Bornholm

B: All cows on Bornholm

C: 400 cows on Bornholm

D: 300 rodents on Samsø

E: 300 rodents on Bornholm

F: Rodents on Samsø

G: Cows on Samsø

H: Cows in Denmark

I: Rodents in Denmark

J: All rodents in the world

K: 300 rodents and 400 cows on Bornholm

Exercises for Chapter 3

Question 1: What is a disease determinant?

A: A variable with a constant level

B: Any characteristic that affects disease in a population

C: A farmer that is very determined on effective production

D: A particular feed additive

E: Outcome

Question 2: Determine for each of the following variables if they are an intrinsic or an extrinsic determinant.

A: Age
B: Housing system
C: Climate
D: Breed
E: Gender
F: Nutrition

Question 3: Give a short definition of a risk factor.

Question 4: Which of these statements constitutes the five conditions that usually increase the likelihood of a causal relationship between a factor and the outcome?

A: A large difference between mean and median of the factor
B: The relationship is found in different populations and under different circumstances (consistency and repeatability)
C: Removal of the factor decrease the probability of disease (reversibility)
D: That the factor is a qualitative, rather than quantitative variable
E: Dose–response relationship
F: Biological explanation
G: Strong statistical association
H: Both factor and outcome are present in the population

Question 5: Determine which of the following statements describe infectivity, infectiousness, pathogenicity and virulence, respectively.

A: The possible pathological changes that the agent may induce in a host
B: The ability of an agent to be transmitted from one host to another
C: The ability of an agent to enter and multiply in a host animal
D: The ability of an agent to cause disease in terms of severity

Question 6: Determine which of the following statements describe latent infection, chronic infection, slow infection and reservoir, respectively?

A: The agent is detectable and the host may be shedding the agent continuously
B: Animals or inanimate substances serving as a habitat for the pathogen and upon which the pathogen depends on for survival

C: The agent is hidden in the host and may not be detectable for periods. At other times the agent may be reactivated and thereby be associated with recurrence of disease

D: The number of pathogens (e.g. bacteria) and pathological lesions gradually increase from a subclinical stage to become a lethal disease

Question 7: Establish the possible hypotheses for causality for the following pairs of variables:

A: Milk yield and breed
B: Gender and weight gain
C: Somatic cell count (SCC) and milk yield
D: Weaning diarrhoea in piglets and birth weight
E: Litter size and parity

Question 8: Give the types of variables and scales for the following measures:

A: Gender
B: Body weight
C: Body temperature
D: Body condition score
E: Breed

Question 9: Which of the following descriptive measures are relevant for a quantitative variable or a qualitative variable – or both?

A: Standard deviation
B: Number of observations
C: Mean
D: Frequency distribution

Question 10: Order the following data levels from highest to lowest.

A: Herd
B: Pen
C: Animal
D: District

Question 11: A farmer is measuring the weight of all his slaughter pigs. The scale will usually measure the correct weight, but one day a 5 kg rubber mat has been removed from the weight without adjusting the empty weight to zero. What is the accuracy and precision (characterised as high versus low) on that day?

Exercises for Chapter 4

Question 1: Which types of observational studies are the following examples? State if they are prospective or retrospective.

A: A study of the relation between breed (Danish Holstein Friesian (DHF) and Jersey) and occurrence of mastitis after calving. One hundred DHF cows and 100 Jersey cows were included in the study. All clinical signs of mastitis in the cows were observed during 30 days. None of the cows had mastitis at study onset.

B: A study of the relationship between presence of fleas in the hair coat and the living environment of dogs. Thirty dogs were examined during 1 day. The owners were asked about the living environment of the dogs.

C: The relation between diarrhoea in piglets and the type of feeding. In total 50 farms with piglet diarrhoea and 50 farms without piglet diarrhoea were chosen. The farmers were interviewed regarding feeding of the piglets.

D: The relation between mastitis and housing system was evaluated for dairy cows. Data from the Danish Cattle Database were used. For this study, 50 herds with tie stalls and 50 herds with loose housing were selected. For each herd, 20 cows were randomly selected. All the recordings from the last year were included in the study.

Question 2: Health status in dogs in Copenhagen was examined at the Small Animal Hospital, Copenhagen. In total, 150 dogs were examined once during 2 weeks. Specify:

A: The study design
B: The target population
C: The study population
D: The sample
E: The study unit (unit of observation)

Question 3: The association between living conditions (access to outdoor activity or not) and the occurrence of feline urological syndrome (FUS) in cats is studied. Which study designs have been used?

A: Two groups of cats are included with 10 healthy cats in each group. One group has assess to outdoor activity, the other has not. The cats will be examined several times during the following 3 years for occurrence of FUS.

B: 300 cats were randomly chosen and examined for FUS. The cat owners were interviewed regarding outdoor activity of the cats.

C: 20 healthy cats and 20 cats with FUS were selected. The cat owners were interviewed regarding outdoor activity.

Question 4: For each of the three study designs in Question 3, answer with true or false the following statements:

A: Outdoor activity (exposure) is prior to FUS
B: Incidence risk can be calculated
C: Prevalence can be calculated

Question 5: A flock of 20 000 chickens is examined for diseases three times at the age of 18, 25 and 45 weeks. At each examination 20 chickens were randomly sampled. What type of study is this?

Question 6: The investigator of a flock of 30 000 chickens randomly chooses 50 chickens and marks them with blue colour and a number. He examines the same chickens at the age of 18, 25 and 45 weeks of age. Which type of design is this?

Exercises for Chapter 5

Question 1: Which of the following designs are either observational or experimental?

A: A cross-sectional study
B: A parallel group design
C: A case–control study
D: A cohort study
E: A factorial design
F: A cross-over design

Question 2: Is an experimental study with or without interventions?

Question 3: State true or false for the following statements regarding an experimental study compared with an observational study.

A: The variation between animals in an experimental study is greater than between animals in a similar observational study
B: Results from an experimental study reflects 'real life'
C: All conditions except intervention are equal in an experimental study

Question 4: A veterinarian wants to test the differences in antibody production of a vaccine between male and female dogs. The study population consists of 27 male and 23 female Beagle dogs. Which type of design can be used?

Question 5: The effect of both age (young, old) and gender (male, female) is evaluated in a new vaccination trial. Which type of design can be used?

Question 6: The effect of two types of claw disinfectants (A and B) for dairy cows was evaluated in 100 cows during a period of 3 months. The purpose was to test which disinfectants prevented claw diseases best. During the first 45 days, 50 cows were washed with type A, while the remaining 50 cows were washed with type B. During the next 45 days treatments were switched between the two groups of cows. Which type of study design was used?

Exercises for Chapter 6

Question 1: Decide whether the following statements are true or false:

A: The prevalence is an estimate of the proportion of diseased animals in a defined group (population) of animals at a given point in time
B: Incidence rate is a number between 0 and 1
C: Incidence risk is an estimate of the probability that an animal which is present at the onset of the study develops the disease during a specified time period, given that the animal does not die or leave the study for any other reason
D: Incidence rate is an estimate for the rate of new cases per unit of animal time during a specified period of time
E: Risk estimates can be referred to the individual animal while the rate refers to a group of animals
F: The prevalence is the probability that an individual animal has the disease at a given point in time
G: Incidence risk can be perceived as a probability when referring to the individual animal or as a proportion when referring to the group
H: Incidence and prevalence are not related
I: Incidence is the number of new cases during a specified period of time

Question 2: A farmer wants to describe the occurrence of pigs with diarrhoea in his herd of 5000 pigs. On Friday morning, 4 April 2003, at 7 am, he counts 100 pigs with diarrhoea. Three weeks later, on Friday morning, 25 April, at 7 am, he counts 109 pigs with diarrhoea. There are now 4982 pigs in the herd. Based on this, what measures of disease frequency can be calculated? Do the calculations.

Question 3: A farmer has 100 turkeys. In the morning of 1 May 2003 he counts 20 turkeys with feather pecking. During the following 30 days he identifies 10 new cases of turkeys with feather pecking. No turkeys leave or enter the herd during the 30 days. Based on these observations which measures of disease frequency can be used to describe the occurrence of feather pecking? Do the calculations.

Question 4: The incidence rate of disease is $I_{rate} = 0.2$ cases per animal day (24 h). What is the probability that an animal which is healthy in the morning becomes diseased in the next 24 h?

Question 5: Assume the incidence rate of a disease is constant over a period of 3 months. If $I_{rate} = 0.2$ cases/animal month, what is the incidence rate during the 3-month period?

Question 6: Assume the incidence risk is constant over a period of 3 months. If $I_{risk} = 0.2$ what is the I_{risk} during the 3-month period?

Question 7: Assume that we have estimated the following incidence rates for May, June and July: $I_{rate}(May) = 0.06$ cases/animal month, $I_{rate}(June) = 0.11$ cases/animal month, $I_{rate}(July) = 0.08$ cases/animal month. What is the probability that an animal that is present and healthy on 1 May and stays in the study for the entire period has not been diseased on 1 August?

Question 8: The duration of a case of mastitis in dairy cows is set to 10 days. What is the prevalence of mastitis when $I_{rate} = 0.2$ case/day at risk?

Question 9: An epidemic of foot and mouth disease breaks out in a region of Central Africa, where it has not been seen for 15 years. There is about 10 000 heads of cattle in the region at the onset of the epidemic. When the epidemic is over, 770 heads of cattle have died while showing clinical symptoms of foot and mouth disease. A study of seroprevalence estimates that about 6200 live animals had seroconverted, i.e. had been infected with the virus. Assume that no cattle leave or enter during the outbreak of foot and mouth disease and that deaths due to other causes can be ignored. What is the incidence risk of infection with foot and mouth disease virus? What is the mortality risk? What is the lethality (case fatality) of foot and mouth disease?

Exercises for Chapter 7

Question 1: Which of the following statements are correct?

A: Measures of association quantify the relative relationship between the exposure and the outcome

B: Measures of effect quantify the overall importance of a risk factor to the outcome

C: Relative risk is a measure of effect

D: Relative risk can only be calculated when the sample is representative of the target population

E: Attributable risk is a measure of association

F: Attributable fraction is the difference in risk between the exposed and unexposed group

G: Population attributable fraction is a measure of effect of exposure in the population

H: Population attributable risk is a measure of importance of the risk factor

I: Incidence risk and odds are measures of association

J: Odds ratio can always be used as a measure of association

Question 2: Which measure of association should be calculated in:

A: A case–control study

B: A cohort study

C: A cross-sectional study

Question 3: Which of the following statements about relative risk (RR) are correct?

A: RR is always based on incidence risk

B: RR may be based on incidence risk or prevalence risk

C: RR can be approximated by the odds ratio if the true prevalence is low in both the exposed and unexposed groups

Question 4: The 2 × 2 table below is from a cross-sectional study of eczema in Boxer and Alsatian dogs.

		Eczema	
		Yes	*No*
Dog breed	Boxer	12	8
	Alsatian	3	12

A: Calculate the relevant measures of association
B: Calculate the relevant measures of effect
C: Calculate the relevant measures of importance

Question 5: A case–control study to evaluate the association between a skin reaction for wood tick bites and infections with the bacteria *Borrelia burgdorferi* was carried out with 42 hunting dogs that were bitten by wood ticks. The study gave the following 2 × 2 table:

		Skin reaction	
		Yes	No
Antibodies against	Positive	2	7
Borrelia burgdorferi	Negative	6	27

The odds ratio for this study is OR = 1.29. Answer the following questions regarding the study with true or false:

A: The interpretation of the OR = 1.29 is that odds are 1.29 times higher for having a skin reaction among antibody positive dogs than among dogs without antibodies against *Borrelia burgdorferi*.

B: The estimated attributable fraction AF_{est} = 0.22 is an estimate of the fraction of skin reactions in the group of antibody positive dogs that can be attributed to them being antibody positive.

C: The 95% CI for the OR is: [0.21; 7.80]. This implies that antibodies against *Borrelia burgdorferi* can be considered as a protective factor and a risk factor at the same time.

D: The population attributable fraction (PAF = 4.6%) is a measure of the importance of *Borrelia burgdorferi* as a risk factor.

Question 6: A beef farmer purchases all his animals as 10 day old calves. The calves come from two herds, A and B. No calves have pneumonia at arrival. The two groups of calves are mixed on arrival at the beef farm, and thus live in the same environment. During the first 3 months after arrival the calves from farm A have an incidence risk of pneumonia of 20% and calves from farm B have an incidence risk of pneumonia of 50%. Consider the study as a cohort study.

A: What is the relevant measure of association between farm of origin and the risk of pneumonia? Do the calculation.

B: Calculate the effect of coming from farm B compared to farm A and give your interpretation.

C: Calculate the attributable fraction and give your interpretation.

Exercises for Chapter 8

Question 1: Which of the following statements are true or false in relation to sampling?

A: We want to study the patterns of a population without investigating all animals in the population

B: It is not very important to specify the hypothesis and the outcome before estimating the sample size

C: The more animals we include in the sample, the more certain is the estimate of the population parameter of interest

D: The larger the sample size the higher is the confidence in the result

E: Random sampling is an underlying assumption for all formulae presented in the chapter about sample size

F: The sample is always selected from the target population

Question 2: A farmer needs to know the prevalence of scabies in his herd with 95% confidence. The farmer believes the prevalence is around 15% and wants a maximum allowable error of 5%. Calculate the necessary sample size.

Question 3: The farmer in Question 2 has only 100 cows in his herd. How many animals does he really need to test?

Question 4: Which sampling strategies have been used in the following situations?

A: In order to obtain an estimate of the frequency of pneumonia in slaughter pigs the investigator chose the five swine farms closest to the university

B: A PhD student is examining the development of drug resistance. She randomly selects and cultures samples from 5–10 cows every day for analysis of drug resistance

C: Assume a case–control study on the relationship between colic in horses and age. From a database the investigator randomly selected 40 horses among those with colic and 40 horses among those without colic

D: The necessary sample size for a study on *Campylobacter* infections was estimated as 200 chickens. The researcher decided to select 20 herds, and within each herd she selected 10 chickens

E: For his masters thesis a veterinary student planned to study the occurrence of worm infections in dogs. He identified 10 dog kennels and examined one faecal sample from each dog in all 10 kennels

F: In order to study infection dynamics of *Salmonella* Dublin in dairy herds, eight herds known to be infected were selected

G: A case–control study on risk factors for *Streptococcus agalactiae* mastitis in Danish dairy cows included all 100 test positive herds in 1992 in the case group. A control group of 100 herds was selected among all non-infected herds. From a list with all 9000 negative herds in 1992 arranged in a random order, the researcher randomly selected herd no 43 among the first 90 herds and after this selected every 90th herd for the study

Question 5: A company tests a batch of 250 white mice for the possible presence of a bacteria in the gut. What sample size should be tested in order to be 95% sure that the bacteria is not present. Assume, that if present the prevalence of the bacteria will be 20%?

Question 6: What would happen to the required sample size in Question 5, if:

A: The expected prevalence if disease is present is lowered from 20% to 10%?

B: The company decides that they need to be 99% sure to detect disease, but still believe that the prevalence is 20% if disease is present?

Question 7: Suppose that 50 mice are actually tested in Question 5. What is the maximum prevalence of the bacteria that can be expected if all 50 mice tested negative?

Question 8: Two farmers discuss if there is a significant difference between the average milk yields of their dairy herds. Calculate the necessary sample size in order to determine whether there is a significant difference in milk yield (ECM) assuming a difference of at least 200 kg ECM and a standard deviation in milk yield of 100 kg ECM. Choose a two-sided test with confidence level of 95% and a power of 80%.

Exercises for Chapter 9

Question 1: Which of the following statements about tests are true in a given population/sample?

A: Diagnostic tests, prognostic tests and screening tests are the same

B: Some tests are subjective, others are objective

C: It is not necessary to have cut-off values for tests that have a continuous outcome

D: A gold standard test is usually the test that is found most valid

E: For tests with continuous outcome only one cut-off is valid

Question 2: Which of the following characterise the performance of a test?

A: Sensitivity

B: Apparent prevalence

C: Specificity

D: Positive predictive value

E: Negative predictive value

F: True prevalence

G: Likelihood ratio of a positive test

H: Likelihood ratio of a negative test

I: Positive differential rate

J: ROC curves

Question 3: Estimate Se, Sp, PPV, NPV, LR+ and LR− of the test based on the following table:

	Truly diseased		Total
	Yes	No	
Test			
Positive	60	3	63
Negative	10	97	107
Total	70	100	170

Question 4: Which of the following statements about tests are true?

A: A test always measures the apparent prevalence

B: The predictive value of a positive test is a measure of prevalence

C: Sensitivity is a true estimate of the prevalence

Question 5: Which of the following statements about the predictive values of a test are true?

A: Predictive values are constant for a given test

B: Predictive values depend on the prevalence of the disease in the sample

C: Predictive values depend on sensitivity and specificity

Question 6: A test for an important cattle disease has Se $= 0.81$ and Sp $= 0.98$. The true prevalence TP $= 0.30$.

A: What is the probability that a test positive is truly positive?
B: What is the probability that a test negative is truly negative?
C: What is the likelihood ratio of a negative test?
D: What is the likelihood ratio of a positive test?

Question 7: Calculate the 95% confidence interval for the estimate of Se $= 0.70$, when 100 truly diseased animals are tested.

Question 8: What is the purpose of estimating the differential positive rate?

A: To have an overall measure for the performance of the test.
B: To identify the cut-off values that maximizes the test relative to a given purpose of the test

Question 9: Are these statements about ROC curves true?

A: ROC curves can be used to determine the overall validity of a test
B: ROC curves can be used to determine the prevalence in a population where a diagnostic test with a continuous outcome has been used

Question 10: Two diagnostic tests for the same disease are performed simultaneously. Test 1 has Se $= 0.70$ and Sp $= 0.95$, and Test 2 has Se $= 0.95$ and Sp $= 0.95$.

A: What is the name for the best method of combining the tests to increase the sensitivity? Estimate the combined sensitivity and specificity
B: What is the name for the best method of combining the two tests to increase the specificity? Estimate the combined sensitivity and specificity
C: What assumptions are necessary for the calculations?

Question 11: A dairy herd with 100 cows is tested for a contagious disease. The apparent prevalence and the specificity of the test are AP $= 0.10$ and Sp $= 0.95$. Estimate the herd sensitivity and the herd specificity when 10 randomly selected cows are tested and just one test positive animal constitutes a test positive herd.

Exercises for Chapter 10
Question 1: Data management includes

A: Collection of data
B: Data control

C: Analysis of data

D: Organising data in a database

E: Organising results in tables and figures

Question 2: Organize the following steps about data recording in chronological order.

A: The veterinarian records the diagnosis

B: The veterinarian examines the animal

C: The animal owner calls the veterinarian

D: The veterinarian enters the data into a database

E: The animal owner observes an event – a sick animal

F: The veterinarian makes the diagnosis

Question 3: Consider the following database for a number of mink farms containing information on date of event, live and dead born puppies and disease treatment per mink bitch (diagnosis):

Farm id	Bitch id	Date of event	Event*	Puppies born alive	Puppies stillborn	Diagnosis
2002	35	20/05/2003	1	5	1	
2002	35	21/05/2003	2			11
1999	47	28/05/2003	2			12
1999	54	28/05/2003	1	4	0	

*1 = production record; 2 = disease treatment.

What is the key of the table?

Question 4: Consider that you want to avoid many empty cells in the database in the previous question. How could this be solved by making a new database structure?

Question 5: Which of the following issues are important to address when evaluating the quality of data?

A: Sampling procedures of the analytical units in the database

B: Information about who recorded the data and the purpose of data collection

C: How well defined the measurement is for each variable

D: How well defined the interpretation is for each measurement

Question 6: A database contains recordings on milk production in dairy herds and includes: herd and cow identification number, month, year, parity and diagnosed diseases. Which of the following steps could be part of a data control?

A: Print the database and reenter data in a new database. Compare this to the first
B: Proof-read by comparing the database with the original data forms
C: Make frequency tables of parity to check for legal values
D: Make frequency tables of diseases to check for legal values
E: Make frequency tables of milk yield to check for legal values
F: Check milk yield for extreme values (i.e. evaluate minimum and maximum)
G: Compare the mean milk yield of first and second parity cows
H: Print observations with missing values to check whether missing values occur randomly
I: Delete diseases occurring more than once for each cow

Exercises for Chapter 11

Question 1: State true or false of the following statements about bias and interaction:

A: Bias is a systematic error
B: Bias and interaction might be present at the same time
C: Confounding is a bias
D: When interaction between variables is present, confounding is not relevant to consider
E: Bias and interaction are two words for the same phenomenon

Question 2: Identify the potential bias and/or interaction in the following examples. Give your answer based on the available information.

A: A researcher planned a descriptive study on behaviour in dogs. He called for volunteers in the local newspaper.
B: The age of horses are often determined on the form and wear of the front teeth.
C: Treatment and problems with milk fever in dairy cows were evaluated using a questionnaire and telephone interviews. The farmers were asked about problems the previous year, and which treatments were used.
D: The behaviour of forest ants was found to be related to daylight, i.e. the behaviour was different in daylight compared to darkness. However, the

temperature might have an effect on the behaviour. There was no relation between daylight and behaviour when the temperature was constant.

E: A random sample of cats was selected in Copenhagen in order to perform a descriptive study of the geographical distribution of diseases in cats in Copenhagen.

F: A study showed that the relation between age and aggression in large dog breeds was different from the association between age and aggression in small dog breeds.

Question 3: In a study of risk factors for pneumonia in pigs data were collected during July in 100 pig herds in the Northern part of Denmark. The aim of the study was to evaluate risk factors for pneumonia in pig herds in Denmark. Information about the herds and the farmers was obtained by interview (mechanical ventilation (yes/no), age of the farmer, herd size). Which of the following statements are true?

A: Selection bias may occur because the pig herds in the Northern part of Denmark might not be representative of the pneumonia frequency and causal patterns for Denmark

B: Selection bias might occur due to seasonal variations (sampling in July)

C: Information about risk factors was obtained using interviews. Information bias may occur

D: Confounding bias might occur between age of farmer and ventilation

Question 4: Data on herd size, pneumonia and type of feeding (wet or dry) was collected in Question 3. In order to evaluate the relation between pneumonia, type of feeding and herd size, draw a path diagram illustrating the relation between the variables.

Question 5: In the study in Question 3 the investigators believed there was not the same relation between type of feeding and pneumonia for pigs of LD crossbreed as for pigs of LY crossbreed. Which of the following statements describe the relation?

A: Interaction between type of feeding and breed

B: Confounding between type of feeding and breed

Question 6: Illustrate in a graph the relation between milk production and herd size when there is interaction between herd size and cow breed (Holstein Friesians and Jerseys).

Exercises for Chapter 12

Question 1: Which of the following statements about a questionnaire are true?

A: A questionnaire is a form with questions prepared for obtaining data from a number of respondents

B: A questionnaire is an interview with the respondent

C: A quantitative questionnaire is a form with structured questions requiring short and precise answers

D: A questionnaire is a print of a data set ready for analysis

E: A qualitative questionnaire is a form with semi-structured or unstructured questions

Question 2: Which of the following statements about communication forms are true?

A: A face-to-face communication can be used for both quantitative and qualitative interviews

B: Questionnaires sent by mail usually give very high response rates

C: Web-based questionnaires are prone to more self-selection bias than any of the other types of communication

D: Qualitative interviews are better conducted using face-to-face or telephone communication than using mail or web communication

Question 3: Two veterinary students want to spend 6 months investigating the relationship between calf mortality and milk feeding during the first 2 days after calving. They plan interviews with 100 farmers about their calf management procedures. Give the most logical order of the following elements of the study:

A: Estimation of sample size

B: Grouping of questions into topics in the questionnaire form

C: Coding of possible answers

D: Pre-testing the questionnaire

E: Identify potential bias in the questionnaire

F: Specify the hypothesis

G: Specify the purpose of the study

H: Formulate the questions for the questionnaire

I: Choose the type of study design

J: Identify possible interviewer bias

K: Sending letter of information to the farmer

Question 4: Which types of questions are the following examples?

A: Are you a farmer?
    ☐ Yes   ☐ No
B: How old are you?
    —— (Give your age in years)
C: Housing system?
    ☐ Tie Stall   ☐ Loose Housing
D: How do you prevent milk fever?
    ☐ Do Not
    ☐ Oral calcium
    ☐ Maintain low cation/anion balance in diet
    ☐ Other ——
E: What is the body condition score for this cow?
    ☐ 1: very thin   ☐ 2 ☐ 3 ☐ 4 ☐ 5: very fat

Question 5: Which types of scales are used to record answers in Question 4?

Question 6: A PhD student studies the pain of cows with mastitis, and rates the observations as 1: no pain, 2: weak pain, 3: moderate pain, 4: strong pain and 5: severe pain. Which type of scale is being used?

Question 7: For the following types of questionnaire state whether they are little, moderate or very time consuming to conduct.

A: Questionnaire send by mail
B: Telephone interview
C: Web based
D: Face to face

Question 8: A researcher had conducted 150 interviews and over time got the habit to change a question from: 'Do you like to have a dog?' to 'You like to have a dog, don't you?'. Which of the following statements are true?

A: Selection bias is present
B: Recall bias is present
C: Interviewer bias is present
D: Information bias is present

Question 9: If the interviewer stating the question above (Question 8) does not believe the reply, he may actually on purpose record the answer as 'No, I don't like to have a dog'. Which of the following statements are true?

A: Information bias (misclassification) is present
B: Interviewer bias is present
C: Recall bias is present
D: Selection bias is present

Exercises for Chapter 13

Question 1: Which of the following statements about hypothesis testing is true?

A: Make inferences about the population based on a sample drawn from the population
B: Hypothesis testing is initiated by formulating the hypothesis
C: Estimating the sample size is important after data have been collected
D: Comparison of the test statistic to a specific distribution is necessary
E: Selection of a statistical test is not necessary
F: The critical value is used for making decisions of rejection of the null hypothesis
G: The sample size is important for the rejection of the null hypothesis

Question 2: Are the following a type I error, a type II error or a correct decision?

A: The null hypothesis is true and we reject it
B: The null hypothesis is true and we do not reject it
C: The null hypothesis is false and we reject it
D: The null hypothesis is false and we do not reject it

Question 3: We would like to test the hypothesis: $H_0: \mu_1 = \mu_2$. Which of the following items have an influence on the test?

A: The significance level
B: The power
C: The sample size
D: The standard deviations s_1 and s_2
E: The difference between $\bar{x}_1$ and $\bar{x}_2$

Question 4: A dog breeder has alsatians, dachshunds and terriers. He wants to know if there are any differences between the breeds with respect to growth rates (weight gain per week) during the first 3 months of life. Which of the following statements are true?

A: The null hypothesis is: There are no differences between the weekly weight gain of the three breeds

B: The *t*-test should be used to test the differences in weekly weight gains

C: An analysis of variance should be used to test the differences in weekly weight gains

D: A χ^2-test should be used to test the differences in weekly weight gains

E: A scatter plot should be used to test the differences in weekly weight gains

F: Linear regression should be used to test the differences in weekly weight gains

Question 5: A sheep farmer wants to know if there is an effect of the body weight on milk production. Which of the following statements are true?

A: The null hypothesis is: The body weight has no influence on the milk production

B: The *t*-test should be used to test the hypothesis

C: An analysis of variance should be used to test the hypothesis

D: A χ^2-test should be used to test the hypothesis

E: A scatter plot should be used to test the hypothesis

F: Linear regression should be used to test the hypothesis

Question 6: The correlation in Question 5 was estimated to be $r = 0.4$. Which of the following statements are true?

A: The correlation is positive, meaning that there is increasing milk production with increasing body weight

B: The degree of determination can be calculated as $R^2 = 0.4 \times 0.4 = 0.16$

C: The degree of determination is $R^2 = 0.4$

D: $r = 0.4$ means that that an increase in body weight of 1 kg, increases the milk production by 0.4 kg

Question 7: The analysis in Question 5 yields the following table:

Parameter	Estimate	Standard error	Test statistic value	p-Value
Intercept	−3.00	1.16	2.59	0.010
Slope	0.20	0.015	13.33	<0.001
R^2	0.16			

Which of the following models is true?

A: $y = -3.00 + 0.20 \times x$

B: $y = 0.20 - 3.00 \times x$

C: $x = -3.00 + 0.20 \times y$
D: $x = 0.20 - 3.00 \times y$

where x = body weight, y = milk production.

Question 8: The following is a cross-tabulation of skin reactions in dogs with and without *Borrelia* antigens.

		Borrelia *antigens*	
		Yes	*No*
Skin reaction	Positive	7	6
	Negative	2	27

The study is a cross-sectional study of dogs with ticks. Which of the following statements are true?

A: The null hypothesis is: No relation between skin reaction and *Borrelia* antigens
B: The null hypothesis is: A relation between skin reaction and *Borrelia* antigens
C: The relevant measure of association is OR
D: The relevant measure of association is RR
E: The hypothesis could be tested using a t-test
F: The hypothesis could be tested using a χ^2-test
G: The hypothesis could be tested using Fisher exact test
H: The hypothesis could be tested using an analysis of variance

Question 9: The effect of breed, calving season and housing system on occurrence of endometritis (infected or not) is studied on dairy cows in one herd. The relation can be examined using?

A: A logistic regression
B: A logistic analysis
C: A χ^2-test
D: An analysis of variance
E: Linear regression

Question 10: A study showed the risk was four times higher of abortion in dairy cows if they were infected with bacterium A, compared to not being infected. However, the investigators found that when they stratified for age (high and low), they found $RR_{young} = 9.4$ among the young cows and

$RR_{old} = 1.07$ among the old cows. The investigators also wanted to obtain an 'average' estimate for the association between infection and abortion when adjusting for age. The adjusted $RR_{adj} = 3.56$. Which of the following statements are true?

A: The results indicate strong interaction between age and presence of bacterium A

B: The results indicate strong confounding between age and presence of bacterium A

C: It is not relevant to consider adjustment for confounding, because there is a strong interaction

D: Interaction could be tested in an analysis of variance

E: Interaction could be tested in a logistic analysis

Question 11: Two clinicians compared their diagnostic skills on the same group of dogs (125 dachshunds) in a study of radiographs of slipped columnar discs. Data are given in the table below.

		Clinician 1		Total
		Positive	Negative	
Clinician 2	Positive	25	10	35
	Negative	0	90	90
	Total	25	100	125

Which of the following statements are true?

A: The variables are dichotomous

B: Kappa (κ) is a relevant measure for the agreement between the two clinicians

C: The Bland–Altman plot is relevant to use in order to consider agreement between the two clinicians

D: The difference in proportion of positive dogs between the two clinicians can be tested using McNemar test

E: The difference in proportion of positive dogs between the two clinicians can be tested using a χ^2-test

Answers to Exercises

Chapter 1

Answer 1: The study (logos) of what is upon (epi) the population (demos).

Answer 2: The totality of individuals that share or have certain attributes in common.

Answer 3: The study of occurrence and distribution of diseases (and health) in populations as well as the study of factors that influence disease occurrence.

Answer 4: A: None, **B:** None, **C:** Population (and epidemiological unit if compared to, e.g. rest of Denmark), **D:** Observational unit (i.e. pasture), epidemiological unit and population (depending on the context), **E:** Observational unit.

Answer 5: A: Descriptive, **B:** Analytical, **C:** Analytical, **D:** Descriptive, **E:** Analytical.

Answer 6: F, E, G, A, I, B, C, H, D.

Chapter 2

Answer 1: True: A and B. **False:** None.

Answer 2: A: Purpose, **B:** Hypothesis, **C:** Objective.

Answer 3: A and D.

Answer 4: Hypotheses C, E and F can be studied. A is not a hypothesis. B involves blue dogs, which are not included in the study. D cannot be studied with the available information.

Answer 5: 1: I, **2:** A, **3:** E.

Chapter 3

Answer 1: B.

Answer 2: Intrinsic: A, D and E. **Extrinsic:** B, C and F.

Answer 3: A factor that is associated with an increase in the probability of occurrence of an outcome (sometimes also used for a factor associated with a decreased probability of an outcome, protective factor).

Answer 4: True: B, C, E, F and G. **False:** A, D and H.

Answer 5: A: Pathogenicity, **B:** Infectiousness, **C:** Infectivity, **D:** Virulence.

Answer 6: A: A chronic infection, **B:** A reservoir, **C:** A latent infection, **D:** A slow infection.

Answer 7: A: Breed affects milk yield, **B:** Gender affects weight gain, **C:** SCC affects milk yield or milk yield affects SCC (i.e. the possible causality goes both ways), **D:** Birth weight affects occurrence of weaning diarrhoea, **E:** Parity affects litter size.

Answer 8: A: Qualitative, dichotomous, **B:** Quantitative, continuous, **C:** Quantitative, continuous, **D:** Qualitative, ordinal, **E:** Qualitative, nominal.

Answer 9: A: Quantitative, **B:** Both, **C:** Quantitative, **D:** Qualitative.

Answer 10: District (D) > Herd (A) > Pen (B) > Animal (C).

Answer 11: The precision is high, but the accuracy is low.

Chapter 4

Answer 1: A: Prospective cohort study, **B:** Cross-sectional study, **C:** Case–control study, **D:** Retrospective cohort study.

Answer 2: A: Cross-sectional, **B:** Dogs in Copenhagen, **C:** Dogs referred to the Hospital, **D:** The sample is the 150 dogs, **E:** The dog.

Answer 3: A: Cohort (prospective) study, **B:** Cross-sectional study, **C:** Case–control study.

Answer 4: Study A: A: True, B: True, C: False. **Study B:** A: False, B: False, C: True. **Study C:** A: False, B: False, C: False.

Answer 5: Repeated cross-sectional study.

Answer 6: Cross-sectional design with follow-up.

Chapter 5

Answer 1: Observational: A, C and D. **Experimental:** B, E and F.

Answer 2: With intervention.

Answer 3: A: False, **B:** False, **C:** True.

Answer 4: Parallel group design.

Answer 5: Factorial.

Answer 6: Cross-over.

Chapter 6

Answer 1: True: A, C, D, E, F, G and I. **False:** B and H.

Answer 2: It is only possible to calculate the prevalence at the two days. Prevalence at 4 April $= 100$ pigs with diarrhoea$/5000$ pigs $= 0.02 = 2\%$. Prevalence at 25 April $= 109/4982 = 0.022 = 2.2\%$.

Answer 3: It is possible to calculate the prevalence at 1 May 2003 as well as the incidence risk and incidence rate for the next 30 days. The prevalence of feather pecking on 1 May is $p = 20$ pecked turkeys$/100$ turkeys $= 0.20 = 20\%$. $I_{risk} = 10$ new cases$/(80$ turkeys at risk at the beginning of the period$) = 0.125 = 12.5\%$. $I_{rate} = 10$ new cases$/((80 - 10/2) \times 30$ days at risk$) = 0.0044$ cases per turkey day.

Answer 4: The incidence risk gives the answer: $I_{risk} = 1 - \exp(-I_{rate}) = 1 - \exp(-0.2) = 1 - 0.82 = 0.18 = 18\%$.

Answer 5: Incidence rates can be added over time. Therefore $I_{rate}(3$ months$) = (0.2$ cases$/$animal month$) \times 3 = 0.6$ cases$/3$ animal months $= 0.2$ cases$/$animal month. The incidence rate is constant!

Answer 6: Incidence risk is aggregated over time by multiplication as follows: $I_{risk}(3$ months$) = 1 - (1 - 0.2)^3 = 1 - 0.512 = 0.488$.

Answer 7: We need $1 - I_{risk}$ (May, June, July). Since I_{risk} (May, June, July) $= 1 - \exp(-(0.06 + 0.11 + 0.08)) = 1 - \exp(-0.25) = 0.22$, the answer is $1 - 0.22 = 0.78$.

Answer 8: Prevalence $= 0.2 \times 10/(0.2 \times 10 + 1) = 0.67 = 67\%$ at any given point in time in that herd when assuming the incidence rate and duration of disease are constants.

Answer 9: Incidence risk: $I_{risk} = (6200 + 770)/10\,000 = 0.697 = 69.7\%$. Mortality risk: $M_{risk} = 770/10\,000 = 0.077 = 7.7\%$. Lethality (or case fatality): $CF = 770/(6200 + 770) = 0.110 = 11\%$.

Chapter 7

Answer 1: True: A, B, G, H and J. **False:** C, D, E, F and I.

Answer 2: A: OR, **B:** RR (but OR can be calculated), **C:** RR (but OR can be calculated).

Answer 3: True: B and C. **False:** A.

Answer 4: A: RR $= 3$, $RR_{pop} = 2.14$; use RR rather than OR. **B:** AR $= 0.4$, AF $= 67\%$. **C:** PAR $= 0.23$, PAF $= 53\%$.

Answer 5: A: False, in a case–control study the inference must follow the columns. The OR $= 1.29$ means that odds are 1.29 times higher for having a positive antibody reaction among dogs with a skin reaction than among dogs without skin reaction. **B:** True. **C:** False, this implies that the current study cannot establish a significant association between the presence (or absence) of antibodies against *Borrelia burgdorferi* and skin reactions. **D:** False, it is meaningless to calculate PAF in a case–control study. An estimated PAF may be calculated, but only when the controls are sampled so the ratio between exposed and unexposed is representative for the target population.

Answer 6: A: Relative risk: RR $= 50\%/20\% = 2.5$. **B:** Attributable risk: AR $= 0.50 - 0.20 = 0.30$. This means that the risk of pneumonia among farm B calves that may be attributed to them being from farm B is 0.3 out of 0.5. **C:** Attributable fraction AF $= (0.50 - 0.20)/0.50 = 60\%$. This means that 60% of the risk among farm B calves is due to coming from farm B.

Chapter 8

Answer 1: True: A, C, D and E. **False:** B and F.

Answer 2: $n = \frac{1.96^2 \times 0.15(1 - 0.15)}{0.05^2} = 195.9 \approx 196$ animals.

Answer 3: The sample size adjusted for the population size is: $n_a = \frac{196}{1 + \frac{196}{100}} = 66.2 \approx 67$ animals.

Answer 4: A: Convenience sampling, **B:** Simple random sampling, **C:** Stratified random sampling, **D:** Multistage sampling, **E:** Cluster sampling, **F:** Purposive sampling, **G:** Systematic random sampling.

Answer 5: $n = (1 - (1 - 0.95)^{1/50})(250 - (49/2)) = 13.1 \approx 14$.

Answer 6: A: The required sample size increases from 14 to $n = (1 - (1 - 0.95)^{1/25})(250 - (24/2)) = 26.9 \approx 27$. **B:** The required sample size increases from 14 to $n = (1 - (1 - 0.99)^{1/50})(250 - (49/2)) = 19.9 \approx 20$.

Answer 7: The maximum possible number of detectable cases in the population of mice is $D = (1 - (1 - 0.95)^{1/40})(250 - (39/2)) = 16$, which gives a maximum prevalence of $p = 16/250 = 0.06$.

Answer 8: $n = \frac{2(0.84 + 1.96)^2 100^2}{200^2} = 3.9 \approx 4$ in each group.

Chapter 9

Answer 1: True: B and D. **False:** A, C and E.

Answer 2: Tests are characterised by A, C, D, E, G, H, I and J.

Answer 3: Sensitivity: Se $= 60/70 = 0.86 = 86\%$. Specificity Sp $= 97/100 = 0.97 = 97\%$. Predictive value of a positive test: PPV $= 60/63 = 0.95 = 95\%$. Predictive value of a negative test: NPV $= 97/107 = 0.91 = 91\%$. Likelihood ratio of a positive test: LR+ $= (60/70)/(3/100) = 29$. Likelihood ratio of a negative test: LR$-$ $= (10/70)/(97/100) = 0.15$.

Answer 4: True: A. **False:** B and C.

Answer 5: True: B and C. **False:** A.

Answer 6: A: Positive predictive value: PPV $= \frac{0.3 \times 0.81}{0.3 \times 0.81 + (1 - 0.3) \times (1 - 0.98)} = 0.95$. **B:** Negative predictive value: NPV $= \frac{(1 - 0.3) \times 0.98}{(1 - 0.3) \times 0.98 + 0.3 \times (1 - 0.81)} = 0.92$. **C:** Likelihood ratio of a negative test: LR$-$ $= \frac{1 - 0.81}{0.98} = 0.19$. **D:** Likelihood ratio of a positive test: LR+ $= \frac{0.81}{1 - 0.98} = 40.5$.

Answer 7: The 95% CI is $0.7 \pm 1.96 \times \sqrt{\frac{0.7 \times (1 - 0.7)}{100}} = 0.7 \pm 0.09$, i.e. [0.61; 0.79].

Answer 8: True: B. **False:** A.

Answer 9: True: A. **False:** B.

Answer 10: A: A combination to increase sensitivity is called parallel testing. In this situation the combined sensitivity will be: $Se_{par} = 1 - (1 - 0.70) \times (1 - 0.95) = 0.985$; $Sp_{par} = 0.95 \times 0.95 = 0.90$. **B:** A combination to increase specificity is called serial testing. In this situation the combined sensitivity will be: $Se_{ser} = 0.70 \times 0.95 = 0.67$; $Sp_{ser} = 1 - (1 - 0.95)(1 - 0.95) = 0.998$. **C:** The tests should be independent.

Answer 11: Herd sensitivity: $HSe = 1 - (1 - 0.10)^{10} = 0.65$. Herd specificity: $Hsp = 0.95^{10} = 0.60$.

Chapter 10

Answer 1: True: A, B and D. **False:** C and E.

Answer 2: The correct chronological order is: E, C, B, F, A, D.

Answer 3: The key will be: farm id + bitch id + date + type of event.

Answer 4: Make two tables, one with production records (live and dead born mink) and one with diseases.

Answer 5: A, B, C and D are all important when evaluating the quality of data.

Answer 6: B, C, D, F and H should all be part of a data control. The reentering (A) should not be carried out using the database, but the original data forms. Milk yield is a quantitative (continuous) variable, and frequency tables should not be used to summarize milk yield (E). Comparing milk yield across parity (or any other qualitative trait) (G) is part of the data analysis, not data control. It is OK for some diseases, e.g. mastitis, to occur more than once for a cow (I).

Chapter 11

Answer 1: True: A, B, C, D. **False:** E.

Answer 2: A: Selection bias, **B:** Information bias (misclassification), **C:** Information bias (recall bias), **D:** Confounder bias, **E:** None, **F:** Interaction.

Answer 3: True: A, B, C and D. **False:** None.

Answer 4:

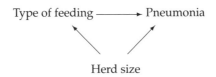

Answer 5: A. Interaction between type of feeding and breed.

Answer 6:

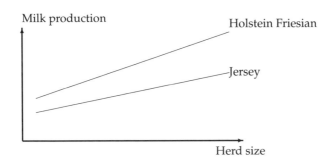

Chapter 12

Answer 1: True: A, C and E. **False:** B and D.

Answer 2: True: A, C and D. **False:** B.

Answer 3: G, F, I, A, H, E, C, B, D, J, K.

Answer 4: A: Closed, **B:** Open ended, **C:** Closed, **D:** Semi-open, **E:** Closed.

Answer 5: A: Dichotomous, **B:** Discrete, **C:** Dichotomous, **D:** Nominal, **E:** Ordinal.

Answer 6: Ordinal scale.

Answer 7: A: Little, **B:** Moderate, **C:** Little, **D:** Very time consuming.

Answer 8: A: False, **B:** False, **C:** True, **D:** True.

Answer 9: A: True, **B:** True, **C:** False, **D:** False.

Chapter 13

Answer 1: True: A, B, D, F and G. **False:** C and E.

Answer 2: A: Type I error, **B:** Correct decision, **C:** Correct decision, **D:** Type II error.

Answer 3: True: A, B, C, D and E. **False:** None.

Answer 4: True: A and C. **False:** B, D, E and F.

Answer 5: True: A and F. **False:** B, C, D and E.

Answer 6: True: A and B. **False:** C and D.

Answer 7: Model A is correct.

Answer 8: True: A, D and G. **False:** B, C, E, F (the expected frequency of positive skin reaction and *Borrelia* antigens is 2.7 (less than 5) under the null hypothesis), H.

Answer 9: B. Logistic analysis should be used.

Answer 10: A: True (as RR_{young} and RR_{old} are very different), **B:** False (as $RR_{crude} = 4.0$ and $RR_{adj} = 3.56$ are not very different), **C:** True, **D:** False, **E:** True.

Answer 11: True: A, B and D. **False:** C and E.

APPENDIX B: BIOSTATISTICS

Annette Kjær Ersbøll and Nils Toft

B.1 Introduction

This appendix is intended to give an overview of the fundamental distributions in biostatistics. As such it contains the essential prerequisites in order to read the rest of the text book.

B.2 The normal distribution

Let us assume a random variable X with a normal distribution with the two population parameters, mean $E(X) = \mu$ and variance $V(X) = \sigma^2$, where σ is the standard deviation

$$X \sim N(\mu, \sigma^2)$$

Based on a random sample of size n drawn from the population, we can estimate the mean and variance, $\bar{x}$ and s^2, as

$$\bar{x} = \frac{1}{n} \sum_{i=1}^{n} x_i$$

$$s^2 = s_x^2 = \frac{1}{n-1} \sum_{i=1}^{n} (x_i - \bar{x})^2$$

that is, the standard deviation $s = \sqrt{s^2}$. The standard error of the mean is calculated as

$$\text{se} = s_{\bar{x}} = \frac{s}{\sqrt{n}}$$

The $(1 - \alpha)100\%$ confidence interval for the mean is

$$\bar{x} \pm t(n-1)_{1-\alpha/2}\text{se}$$

EXAMPLE B.1. The milk yield of 111 dairy cows has been measured. The mean and standard deviation were estimated at $\bar{x} = 21.3\,\text{kg}$ and $s = 6.14\,\text{kg}$. It is assumed that the milk yield is well approximated by a normal distribution

$$x \sim N(21.3;\, 6.14^2)$$

The distribution of the milk yield is shown in Figure B.1 as a histogram. The assumed normal distribution is also shown, as the smooth curve. It is seen that the histogram based on the measured milk yield is similar to the normal distribution.

Let us assume two independent random variables X_1 and X_2 with normal distributions

$$X_1 \sim N\left(\mu_1, \sigma_1^2\right) \quad \text{and} \quad X_2 \sim N\left(\mu_2, \sigma_2^2\right)$$

Based on samples of n_1 and n_2 animals, the $(1 - \alpha)100\%$ confidence interval for the difference between the two means is

$$(\bar{x}_1 - \bar{x}_2) \pm t(n_1 + n_2 - 2)_{1-\alpha/2} s_{\bar{x}_1 - \bar{x}_2}$$

where $\bar{x}_1$ and $\bar{x}_2$ are the estimated means

n_1 and n_2 are number of animals in the two samples

$t(n_1 + n_2 - 2)_{1-\alpha/2}$ is a value from the t-distribution with $(n_1 + n_2 - 2)$ degrees of freedom

$s_{\bar{x}_1 - \bar{x}_2} = \sqrt{s_p^2 \left(\frac{1}{n_1} + \frac{1}{n_2}\right)}$ is the standard error of the mean difference

$s_p^2 = \frac{(n_1-1)s_1^2 + (n_2-1)s_2^2}{n_1 + n_2 - 2}$ is the pooled variance for the difference between the two means

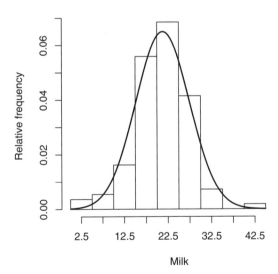

Figure B.1. *The normal distribution of milk yield for dairy cows with mean and standard deviation* $\bar{x} = 21.3$ *and* $s = 6.14$.

Calculation of the pooled estimate of the variance s_p^2 is based on an assumption of approximately equal variances σ_1^2 and σ_2^2 for the two variables x_1 and x_2.

For a paired sample, the $(1 - \alpha)100\%$ confidence interval of the mean difference between the two variables is

$$\bar{d} \pm t(n-1)_{1-\alpha/2} \frac{s_d}{\sqrt{n}}$$

where x_1 and x_2 are two dependent (paired) variables
$d_i = x_{1i} - x_{2i}$
$\bar{d} = \sum_{i=1}^{n} d_i$
n is number of animals in the two samples
$t(n-1)_{1-\alpha/2}$ is a value from the t-distribution with $(n-1)$
     degrees of freedom
s_d is the standard deviation of the difference d

B.3   The binomial distribution

A variable has a Bernoulli distribution if it can take one of only two possible values, e.g. 0 and 1. The two possible outcome levels can be, e.g. infection yes/no. The probability $(\Pr\{\})$ for infection is π and the probability for no infection is $1 - \pi$

$$\Pr\{X = 1\} = \pi \quad \text{and} \quad \Pr\{X = 0\} = 1 - \pi$$

Let us assume n Bernoulli trials, with probability for success (e.g. infection) π in each trial. The number of successes is a random variable X with a binomial distribution with the two parameters n and π

$$X \sim \text{Bin}(n, \pi)$$

The mean and variance of X are

$$E(X) = n\pi$$

$$V(X) = n\pi(1 - \pi)$$

Based on a random sample of size n drawn from the population, we can estimate the probability for success, p, as

$$p = \frac{x}{n}$$

where p is the estimated probability for success in each trial, x is the number of observed successes, n is sample size.

The $(1 - \alpha)100\%$ confidence interval for the probability π has the lower limit

$$\frac{x}{x + (n - x + 1)F(2n - 2x + 2, 2x)_{1-\alpha/2}}$$

and upper limit

$$\frac{(x + 1)F(2x + 2, 2n - 2x)_{1-\alpha/2}}{n - x + (x + 1)F(2x + 2, 2n - 2x)_{1-\alpha/2}}$$

where x is the number of successes, n is sample size, $F(\text{num}, \text{den})_{1-\alpha/2}$ is an F-distribution with parameters, 'num' and 'den', α is the significance level, often set to 0.05.

The approximate $(1 - \alpha)100\%$ confidence interval for the probability π is

$$p \pm z_{1-\alpha/2}\sqrt{\frac{p(1 - p)}{n}}$$

assuming that the number of successes X has a normal distribution. The approximation can be used, if n is large and π is not close to 0 and 1. As a rule of thumb, the approximation can be used when $n\pi > 5$ and $n(1 - \pi) > 5$.

The approximate $(1 - \alpha)100\%$ confidence interval for the difference between probabilities π_1 and π_2 is

$$(p_1 - p_2) \pm z_{1-\alpha/2}\sqrt{\frac{p_1(1 - p_1)}{n_1} + \frac{p_2(1 - p_2)}{n_2}}$$

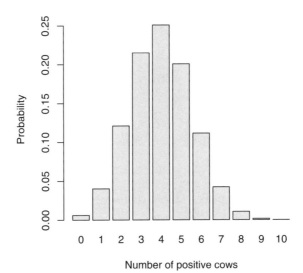

Figure B.2. *The binomial distribution of cows tested positive for* Salmonella Dublin *in a random sample of 10 cows, where four cows were tested positive.*

EXAMPLE B.2. In a study of *Salmonella* Dublin in dairy cows, a random sample of 10 cows were selected in a herd. Four of the cows were tested positive using an ELISA test. The probability for a cow to be tested positive is estimated at $p = 4/10 = 0.40$. The distribution of number of cows tested positive is

$$X \sim \text{Bin}(10; 0.4)$$

The binomial distribution of cows tested positive is shown in Figure B.2. It can be seen (Figure B.2) that the probability for drawing a random sample of 10 cows where none of the cows are tested positive is

$$\Pr\{X = 0\} = (1 - p)^1 0 = 0.006$$

APPENDIX C:
STATISTICAL TABLES

C.1   The normal distribution

In Table C.1, the areas under the standard normal distribution below z are given. This is the probability that a value from the $N(0,1)$ distribution takes on a value less than or equal to z. In Figure C.1, the grey area illustrates the tabled value for a given z. As an example of how to read Table C.1, the probability to

Table C.1. *Probabilities of the $N(0,1)$*

z	$N(0,1)$ *probabilities*									
	0	0.01	0.02	0.03	0.04	0.05	0.06	0.07	0.08	0.09
−3.0	0.0013	0.0013	0.0013	0.0012	0.0012	0.0011	0.0011	0.0011	0.0010	0.0010
−2.9	0.0019	0.0018	0.0018	0.0017	0.0016	0.0016	0.0015	0.0015	0.0014	0.0014
−2.8	0.0026	0.0025	0.0024	0.0023	0.0023	0.0022	0.0021	0.0021	0.0020	0.0019
−2.7	0.0035	0.0034	0.0033	0.0032	0.0031	0.0030	0.0029	0.0028	0.0027	0.0026
−2.6	0.0047	0.0045	0.0044	0.0043	0.0041	0.0040	0.0039	0.0038	0.0037	0.0036
−2.5	0.0062	0.0060	0.0059	0.0057	0.0055	0.0054	0.0052	0.0051	0.0049	0.0048
−2.4	0.0082	0.0080	0.0078	0.0075	0.0073	0.0071	0.0069	0.0068	0.0066	0.0064
−2.3	0.0107	0.0104	0.0102	0.0099	0.0096	0.0094	0.0091	0.0089	0.0087	0.0084
−2.2	0.0139	0.0136	0.0132	0.0129	0.0125	0.0122	0.0119	0.0116	0.0113	0.0110
−2.1	0.0179	0.0174	0.0170	0.0166	0.0162	0.0158	0.0154	0.0150	0.0146	0.0143
−2.0	0.0228	0.0222	0.0217	0.0212	0.0207	0.0202	0.0197	0.0192	0.0188	0.0183
−1.9	0.0287	0.0281	0.0274	0.0268	0.0262	0.0256	0.0250	0.0244	0.0239	0.0233
−1.8	0.0359	0.0351	0.0344	0.0336	0.0329	0.0322	0.0314	0.0307	0.0301	0.0294
−1.7	0.0446	0.0436	0.0427	0.0418	0.0409	0.0401	0.0392	0.0384	0.0375	0.0367
−1.6	0.0548	0.0537	0.0526	0.0516	0.0505	0.0495	0.0485	0.0475	0.0465	0.0455
−1.5	0.0668	0.0655	0.0643	0.0630	0.0618	0.0606	0.0594	0.0582	0.0571	0.0559
−1.4	0.0808	0.0793	0.0778	0.0764	0.0749	0.0735	0.0721	0.0708	0.0694	0.0681
−1.3	0.0968	0.0951	0.0934	0.0918	0.0901	0.0885	0.0869	0.0853	0.0838	0.0823
−1.2	0.1151	0.1131	0.1112	0.1093	0.1075	0.1056	0.1038	0.1020	0.1003	0.0985
−1.1	0.1357	0.1335	0.1314	0.1292	0.1271	0.1251	0.1230	0.1210	0.1190	0.1170
−1.0	0.1587	0.1562	0.1539	0.1515	0.1492	0.1469	0.1446	0.1423	0.1401	0.1379
−0.9	0.1841	0.1814	0.1788	0.1762	0.1736	0.1711	0.1685	0.1660	0.1635	0.1611
−0.8	0.2119	0.2090	0.2061	0.2033	0.2005	0.1977	0.1949	0.1922	0.1894	0.1867
−0.7	0.2420	0.2389	0.2358	0.2327	0.2296	0.2266	0.2236	0.2206	0.2177	0.2148

(continued)

Table C.1. (continued)

z	$N(0,1)$ probabilities									
	0	0.01	0.02	0.03	0.04	0.05	0.06	0.07	0.08	0.09
−0.6	0.2743	0.2709	0.2676	0.2643	0.2611	0.2578	0.2546	0.2514	0.2483	0.2451
−0.5	0.3085	0.3050	0.3015	0.2981	0.2946	0.2912	0.2877	0.2843	0.2810	0.2776
−0.4	0.3446	0.3409	0.3372	0.3336	0.3300	0.3264	0.3228	0.3192	0.3156	0.3121
−0.3	0.3821	0.3783	0.3745	0.3707	0.3669	0.3632	0.3594	0.3557	0.3520	0.3483
−0.2	0.4207	0.4168	0.4129	0.4090	0.4052	0.4013	0.3974	0.3936	0.3897	0.3859
−0.1	0.4602	0.4562	0.4522	0.4483	0.4443	0.4404	0.4364	0.4325	0.4286	0.4247
0.0	0.5000	0.4960	0.4920	0.4880	0.4840	0.4801	0.4761	0.4721	0.4681	0.4641
0.1	0.5398	0.5438	0.5478	0.5517	0.5557	0.5596	0.5636	0.5675	0.5714	0.5753
0.2	0.5793	0.5832	0.5871	0.5910	0.5948	0.5987	0.6026	0.6064	0.6103	0.6141
0.3	0.6179	0.6217	0.6255	0.6293	0.6331	0.6368	0.6406	0.6443	0.6480	0.6517
0.4	0.6554	0.6591	0.6628	0.6664	0.6700	0.6736	0.6772	0.6808	0.6844	0.6879
0.5	0.6915	0.6950	0.6985	0.7019	0.7054	0.7088	0.7123	0.7157	0.7190	0.7224
0.6	0.7257	0.7291	0.7324	0.7357	0.7389	0.7422	0.7454	0.7486	0.7517	0.7549
0.7	0.7580	0.7611	0.7642	0.7673	0.7704	0.7734	0.7764	0.7794	0.7823	0.7852
0.8	0.7881	0.7910	0.7939	0.7967	0.7995	0.8023	0.8051	0.8078	0.8106	0.8133
0.9	0.8159	0.8186	0.8212	0.8238	0.8264	0.8289	0.8315	0.8340	0.8365	0.8389
1.0	0.8413	0.8438	0.8461	0.8485	0.8508	0.8531	0.8554	0.8577	0.8599	0.8621
1.1	0.8643	0.8665	0.8686	0.8708	0.8729	0.8749	0.8770	0.8790	0.8810	0.8830
1.2	0.8849	0.8869	0.8888	0.8907	0.8925	0.8944	0.8962	0.8980	0.8997	0.9015
1.3	0.9032	0.9049	0.9066	0.9082	0.9099	0.9115	0.9131	0.9147	0.9162	0.9177
1.4	0.9192	0.9207	0.9222	0.9236	0.9251	0.9265	0.9279	0.9292	0.9306	0.9319
1.5	0.9332	0.9345	0.9357	0.9370	0.9382	0.9394	0.9406	0.9418	0.9429	0.9441
1.6	0.9452	0.9463	0.9474	0.9484	0.9495	0.9505	0.9515	0.9525	0.9535	0.9545
1.7	0.9554	0.9564	0.9573	0.9582	0.9591	0.9599	0.9608	0.9616	0.9625	0.9633
1.8	0.9641	0.9649	0.9656	0.9664	0.9671	0.9678	0.9686	0.9693	0.9699	0.9706
1.9	0.9713	0.9719	0.9726	0.9732	0.9738	0.9744	0.9750	0.9756	0.9761	0.9767
2.0	0.9772	0.9778	0.9783	0.9788	0.9793	0.9798	0.9803	0.9808	0.9812	0.9817
2.1	0.9821	0.9826	0.9830	0.9834	0.9838	0.9842	0.9846	0.9850	0.9854	0.9857
2.2	0.9861	0.9864	0.9868	0.9871	0.9875	0.9878	0.9881	0.9884	0.9887	0.9890
2.3	0.9893	0.9896	0.9898	0.9901	0.9904	0.9906	0.9909	0.9911	0.9913	0.9916
2.4	0.9918	0.9920	0.9922	0.9925	0.9927	0.9929	0.9931	0.9932	0.9934	0.9936
2.5	0.9938	0.9940	0.9941	0.9943	0.9945	0.9946	0.9948	0.9949	0.9951	0.9952
2.6	0.9953	0.9955	0.9956	0.9957	0.9959	0.9960	0.9961	0.9962	0.9963	0.9964
2.7	0.9965	0.9966	0.9967	0.9968	0.9969	0.9970	0.9971	0.9972	0.9973	0.9974
2.8	0.9974	0.9975	0.9976	0.9977	0.9977	0.9978	0.9979	0.9979	0.9980	0.9981
2.9	0.9981	0.9982	0.9982	0.9983	0.9984	0.9984	0.9985	0.9985	0.9986	0.9986
3.0	0.9987	0.9987	0.9987	0.9988	0.9988	0.9989	0.9989	0.9989	0.9990	0.9990

observe a value of less than or equal to 1.96 from an $N(0.1)$ is 0.975, i.e. 97.5% of all observations from an $N(0,1)$ lies to the left of 1.96. By reading Table C.1 backwards, the value z_p where the proportion p of an $N(0,1)$ lies to left can be found. For example, to find $z_{0.8}$ look in the body of Table C.1 to find the value closest to 0.8, i.e. $p = 0.7995$ corresponding to $z_{0.8} = 0.84$.

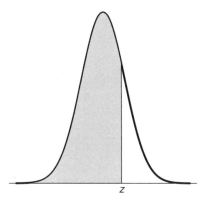

Figure C.1. *The standard normal distribution with mean and standard deviation $\mu = 0$ and $\sigma = 1$, the value of the grey area is given in Table C.1.*

C.2 The *t*-distribution

The critical value $t(k)_q$ is the value below which an area of q lies under the density curve for the $t(k)$-distribution, i.e. the quantile q of the t-distribution with k degrees of freedom. In Table C.2, the critical values $t(k)_q$ are given for selected degrees of freedom k and quantiles q. In Figure C.2, the grey area is q. Note that a t-distribution with ∞ degrees of freedom is an $N(0, 1)$ distribution.

Table C.2. *Critical values of the t-distribution for selected quantiles*

Degrees of freedom, k	Critical values of the t-distribution						
	$t(k)_{0.90}$	$t(k)_{0.95}$	$t(k)_{0.975}$	$t(k)_{0.99}$	$t(k)_{0.995}$	$t(k)_{0.999}$	$t(k)_{0.9995}$
1	3.0777	6.3138	12.7062	31.8205	63.6567	318.3088	636.6192
2	1.8856	2.9200	4.3027	6.9646	9.9248	22.3271	31.5991
3	1.6377	2.3534	3.1824	4.5407	5.8409	10.2145	12.9240
4	1.5332	2.1318	2.7764	3.7470	4.6041	7.1732	8.6103
5	1.4759	2.0150	2.5706	3.3649	4.0322	5.8934	6.8688
6	1.4398	1.9432	2.4469	3.1427	3.7074	5.2076	5.9588
7	1.4149	1.8946	2.3646	2.9980	3.4995	4.7853	5.4079
8	1.3968	1.8595	2.3060	2.8965	3.3554	4.5008	5.0413
9	1.3830	1.8331	2.2622	2.8214	3.2498	4.2968	4.7809
10	1.3722	1.8125	2.2281	2.7638	3.1693	4.1437	4.5869
11	1.3634	1.7959	2.2010	2.7181	3.1058	4.0247	4.4370
12	1.3562	1.7823	2.1788	2.6810	3.0545	3.9296	4.3178
13	1.3502	1.7709	2.1604	2.6503	3.0123	3.8520	4.2208
14	1.3450	1.7613	2.1448	2.6245	2.9768	3.7874	4.1405
15	1.3406	1.7531	2.1314	2.6025	2.9467	3.7328	4.0728
16	1.3368	1.7459	2.1199	2.5835	2.9208	3.6862	4.0150
17	1.3334	1.7396	2.1098	2.5669	2.8982	3.6458	3.9651
18	1.3304	1.7341	2.1009	2.5524	2.8784	3.6105	3.9216

(continued)

Table C.2. (continued)

Degrees of freedom, k	Critical values of the t-distribution						
	$t(k)_{0.90}$	$t(k)_{0.95}$	$t(k)_{0.975}$	$t(k)_{0.99}$	$t(k)_{0.995}$	$t(k)_{0.999}$	$t(k)_{0.9995}$
19	1.3277	1.7291	2.0930	2.5395	2.8609	3.5794	3.8834
20	1.3253	1.7247	2.0860	2.5280	2.8453	3.5518	3.8495
21	1.3232	1.7207	2.0796	2.5176	2.8314	3.5272	3.8193
22	1.3212	1.7171	2.0739	2.5083	2.8188	3.5050	3.7921
23	1.3195	1.7139	2.0687	2.4999	2.8073	3.4850	3.7676
24	1.3178	1.7109	2.0639	2.4922	2.7969	3.4668	3.7454
25	1.3163	1.7081	2.0595	2.4851	2.7874	3.4502	3.7251
26	1.3150	1.7056	2.0555	2.4786	2.7787	3.4350	3.7066
27	1.3137	1.7033	2.0518	2.4727	2.7707	3.4210	3.6896
28	1.3125	1.7011	2.0484	2.4671	2.7633	3.4082	3.6739
29	1.3114	1.6991	2.0452	2.4620	2.7564	3.3962	3.6594
30	1.3104	1.6973	2.0423	2.4573	2.7500	3.3852	3.6460
35	1.3062	1.6896	2.0301	2.4377	2.7238	3.3400	3.5911
40	1.3031	1.6839	2.0211	2.4233	2.7045	3.3069	3.5510
50	1.2987	1.6759	2.0086	2.4033	2.6778	3.2614	3.4960
60	1.2958	1.6706	2.0003	2.3901	2.6603	3.2317	3.4602
70	1.2938	1.6669	1.9944	2.3808	2.6479	3.2108	3.4350
80	1.2922	1.6641	1.9901	2.3739	2.6387	3.1953	3.4163
90	1.2910	1.6620	1.9867	2.3685	2.6316	3.1833	3.4019
100	1.2901	1.6602	1.9840	2.3642	2.6259	3.1737	3.3905
∞	1.2816	1.6449	1.9600	2.3263	2.5758	3.0902	3.2905

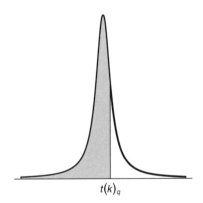

$t(k)_q$

Figure C.2. *The $t(k)$-distribution, the grey area is q, values of $t(k)_q$ are given in Table C.2.*

C.3 The χ^2-distribution

The critical value $\chi^2(k)_q$ is the value below which an area of q lies under the density curve for the $\chi^2(k)$-distribution, i.e. the quantile q of the χ^2-distribution with k degrees of freedom. In Table C.3, the critical values $t(k)_q$ are given for selected degrees of freedom k and quantiles q. In Figure C.3, the grey area is q.

Table C.3. *Critical values of the χ^2-distribution for selected quantiles*

Degrees of freedom, k	Critical values of the χ^2-distribution					
	$\chi^2(k)_{0.025}$	$\chi^2(k)_{0.050}$	$\chi^2(k)_{0.100}$	$\chi^2(k)_{0.900}$	$\chi^2(k)_{0.950}$	$\chi^2(k)_{0.975}$
1	0.0010	0.0039	0.0158	2.7055	3.8415	5.0239
2	0.0506	0.1026	0.2107	4.6052	5.9915	7.3778
3	0.2158	0.3518	0.5844	6.2514	7.8147	9.3484
4	0.4844	0.7107	1.0636	7.7794	9.4877	11.1433
5	0.8312	1.1455	1.6103	9.2364	11.0705	12.8325
6	1.2373	1.6354	2.2041	10.6446	12.5916	14.4494
7	1.6899	2.1673	2.8331	12.0170	14.0671	16.0128
8	2.1797	2.7326	3.4895	13.3616	15.5073	17.5345
9	2.7004	3.3251	4.1682	14.6837	16.9190	19.0228
10	3.2470	3.9403	4.8652	15.9872	18.3070	20.4832
11	3.8157	4.5748	5.5778	17.2750	19.6751	21.9200
12	4.4038	5.2260	6.3038	18.5493	21.0261	23.3367
13	5.0088	5.8919	7.0415	19.8119	22.3620	24.7356
14	5.6287	6.5706	7.7895	21.0641	23.6848	26.1189
15	6.2621	7.2609	8.5468	22.3071	24.9958	27.4884
16	6.9077	7.9616	9.3122	23.5418	26.2962	28.8454
17	7.5642	8.6718	10.0852	24.7690	27.5871	30.1910
18	8.2307	9.3905	10.8649	25.9894	28.8693	31.5264
19	8.9065	10.1170	11.6509	27.2036	30.1435	32.8523
20	9.5908	10.8508	12.4426	28.4120	31.4104	34.1696
21	10.2829	11.5913	13.2396	29.6151	32.6706	35.4789
22	10.9823	12.3380	14.0415	30.8133	33.9244	36.7807
23	11.6886	13.0905	14.8480	32.0069	35.1725	38.0756
24	12.4012	13.8484	15.6587	33.1962	36.4150	39.3641
25	13.1197	14.6114	16.4734	34.3816	37.6525	40.6465
26	13.8439	15.3792	17.2919	35.5632	38.8851	41.9232
27	14.5734	16.1514	18.1139	36.7412	40.1133	43.1945
28	15.3079	16.9279	18.9392	37.9159	41.3371	44.4608
29	16.0471	17.7084	19.7677	39.0875	42.5570	45.7223
30	16.7908	18.4927	20.5992	40.2560	43.7730	46.9792
35	20.5694	22.4650	24.7967	46.0588	49.8018	53.2033
40	24.4330	26.5093	29.0505	51.8051	55.7585	59.3417
50	32.3574	34.7643	37.6886	63.1671	67.5048	71.4202
60	40.4817	43.1880	46.4589	74.3970	79.0819	83.2977
70	48.7576	51.7393	55.3289	85.5270	90.5312	95.0232
80	57.1532	60.3915	64.2778	96.5782	101.8795	106.6286
90	65.6466	69.1260	73.2911	107.5650	113.1453	118.1359
100	74.2219	77.9295	82.3581	118.4980	124.3421	129.5612

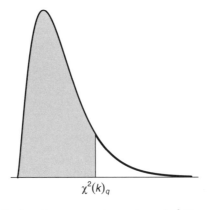

$$\chi^2(k)_q$$

Figure C.3. *The $\chi^2(k)$-distribution, the grey area is q, values of $\chi^2(k)_q$ are given in Table C.2.*

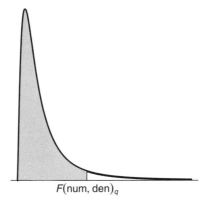

$$F(num, den)_q$$

Figure C.4. *The F(num, den)-distribution, the grey area is q, values of F(num, den)$_q$ are given in Table C.4 for q = 0.95 and Table C.5 for q = 0.99.*

C.4 The *F*-distribution

The critical value $F(num, den)_q$ is the value below which an area of q lies under the density curve for the $F(num, den)$-distribution, i.e. the quantile q of the F-distribution with 'den' degrees of freedom in the denominator and 'num' degrees of freedom in the numerator. In Table C.4, the critical values $F(num, den)_q$ are given for selected degrees of freedom 'den' for the denominator and 'num' for the numerator for $q = 0.95$. For $q = 0.99$ the values are given Table C.5. In Figure C.4, the grey area is q.

Table C.4. *Critical values of the F-distribution for the 95% quantiles*

Critical values of the F-distribution: $F(num, den)_{0.95}$

Denominator degrees of freedom, den	Numerator degrees of freedom, num																	
	1	2	3	4	5	6	7	8	9	10	15	20	25	30	40	50	100	1000
1	161.4	199.5	215.7	224.6	230.2	234.0	236.8	238.9	240.5	241.9	245.9	248.0	249.3	250.1	251.1	251.8	253.0	254.2
2	18.51	19.00	19.16	19.25	19.30	19.33	19.35	19.37	19.38	19.40	19.43	19.45	19.46	19.46	19.47	19.48	19.49	19.49
3	10.13	9.552	9.277	9.117	9.013	8.941	8.887	8.845	8.812	8.786	8.703	8.660	8.634	8.617	8.594	8.581	8.554	8.529
4	7.709	6.944	6.591	6.388	6.256	6.163	6.094	6.041	5.999	5.964	5.858	5.803	5.769	5.746	5.717	5.699	5.664	5.632
5	6.608	5.786	5.409	5.192	5.050	4.950	4.876	4.818	4.772	4.735	4.619	4.558	4.521	4.496	4.464	4.444	4.405	4.369
6	5.987	5.143	4.757	4.534	4.387	4.284	4.207	4.147	4.099	4.060	3.938	3.874	3.835	3.808	3.774	3.754	3.712	3.673
7	5.591	4.737	4.347	4.120	3.972	3.866	3.787	3.726	3.677	3.637	3.511	3.445	3.404	3.376	3.340	3.319	3.275	3.234
8	5.318	4.459	4.066	3.838	3.687	3.581	3.500	3.438	3.388	3.347	3.218	3.150	3.108	3.079	3.043	3.020	2.975	2.932
9	5.117	4.256	3.863	3.633	3.482	3.374	3.293	3.230	3.179	3.137	3.006	2.936	2.893	2.864	2.826	2.803	2.756	2.712
10	4.965	4.103	3.708	3.478	3.326	3.217	3.135	3.072	3.020	2.978	2.845	2.774	2.730	2.700	2.661	2.637	2.588	2.543
11	4.844	3.982	3.587	3.357	3.204	3.095	3.012	2.948	2.896	2.854	2.719	2.646	2.601	2.570	2.531	2.507	2.457	2.410
12	4.747	3.885	3.490	3.259	3.106	2.996	2.913	2.849	2.796	2.753	2.617	2.544	2.498	2.466	2.426	2.401	2.350	2.302
13	4.667	3.806	3.411	3.179	3.025	2.915	2.832	2.767	2.714	2.671	2.533	2.459	2.412	2.380	2.339	2.314	2.261	2.212
14	4.600	3.739	3.344	3.112	2.958	2.848	2.764	2.699	2.646	2.602	2.463	2.388	2.341	2.308	2.266	2.241	2.187	2.136
15	4.543	3.682	3.287	3.056	2.901	2.790	2.707	2.641	2.588	2.544	2.403	2.328	2.280	2.247	2.204	2.178	2.123	2.072
16	4.494	3.634	3.239	3.007	2.852	2.741	2.657	2.591	2.538	2.494	2.352	2.276	2.227	2.194	2.151	2.124	2.068	2.016
17	4.451	3.592	3.197	2.965	2.810	2.699	2.614	2.548	2.494	2.450	2.308	2.230	2.181	2.148	2.104	2.077	2.020	1.967
18	4.414	3.555	3.160	2.928	2.773	2.661	2.577	2.510	2.456	2.412	2.269	2.191	2.141	2.107	2.063	2.035	1.978	1.923
19	4.381	3.522	3.127	2.895	2.740	2.628	2.544	2.477	2.423	2.378	2.234	2.155	2.106	2.071	2.026	1.999	1.940	1.884
20	4.351	3.493	3.098	2.866	2.711	2.599	2.514	2.447	2.393	2.348	2.203	2.124	2.074	2.039	1.994	1.966	1.907	1.850
21	4.325	3.467	3.072	2.840	2.685	2.573	2.488	2.420	2.366	2.321	2.176	2.096	2.045	2.010	1.965	1.936	1.876	1.818
22	4.301	3.443	3.049	2.817	2.661	2.549	2.464	2.397	2.342	2.297	2.151	2.071	2.020	1.984	1.938	1.909	1.849	1.790
23	4.279	3.422	3.028	2.796	2.640	2.528	2.442	2.375	2.320	2.275	2.128	2.048	1.996	1.961	1.914	1.885	1.823	1.764
24	4.260	3.403	3.009	2.776	2.621	2.508	2.423	2.355	2.300	2.255	2.108	2.027	1.975	1.939	1.892	1.863	1.800	1.740
25	4.242	3.385	2.991	2.759	2.603	2.490	2.405	2.337	2.282	2.236	2.089	2.007	1.955	1.919	1.872	1.842	1.779	1.718
26	4.225	3.369	2.975	2.743	2.587	2.474	2.388	2.321	2.265	2.220	2.072	1.990	1.938	1.901	1.853	1.823	1.760	1.698
27	4.210	3.354	2.960	2.728	2.572	2.459	2.373	2.305	2.250	2.204	2.056	1.974	1.921	1.884	1.836	1.806	1.742	1.679
28	4.196	3.340	2.947	2.714	2.558	2.445	2.359	2.291	2.236	2.190	2.041	1.959	1.906	1.869	1.820	1.790	1.725	1.662
29	4.183	3.328	2.934	2.701	2.545	2.432	2.346	2.278	2.223	2.177	2.027	1.945	1.891	1.854	1.806	1.775	1.710	1.645
30	4.171	3.316	2.922	2.690	2.534	2.421	2.334	2.266	2.211	2.165	2.015	1.932	1.878	1.841	1.792	1.761	1.695	1.630
40	4.085	3.232	2.839	2.606	2.449	2.336	2.249	2.180	2.124	2.077	1.924	1.839	1.783	1.744	1.693	1.660	1.589	1.517
50	4.034	3.183	2.790	2.557	2.400	2.286	2.199	2.130	2.073	2.026	1.871	1.784	1.727	1.687	1.634	1.599	1.525	1.448
100	3.936	3.087	2.696	2.463	2.305	2.191	2.103	2.032	1.975	1.927	1.768	1.676	1.616	1.573	1.515	1.477	1.392	1.296
1000	3.851	3.005	2.614	2.381	2.223	2.108	2.019	1.948	1.889	1.840	1.676	1.581	1.517	1.471	1.406	1.363	1.260	1.110

Table C.5. Critical values of the F-distribution for the 99% quantiles

Critical values of the F-distribution: $F(num, den)_{0.99}$

Denominator degrees of freedom, den	Numerator degrees of freedom, num																	
	1	2	3	4	5	6	7	8	9	10	15	20	25	30	40	50	100	1000
1	4052	4999	5403	5625	5764	5859	5928	5981	6022	6056	6157	6209	6240	6261	6287	6303	6334	6363
2	98.50	99.00	99.17	99.25	99.30	99.33	99.36	99.37	99.39	99.40	99.43	99.45	99.46	99.47	99.47	99.48	99.49	99.50
3	34.12	30.82	29.46	28.71	28.24	27.91	27.67	27.49	27.35	27.23	26.87	26.69	26.58	26.50	26.41	26.35	26.24	26.14
4	21.20	18.00	16.69	15.98	15.52	15.21	14.98	14.80	14.66	14.55	14.20	14.02	13.91	13.84	13.75	13.69	13.58	13.47
5	16.26	13.27	12.06	11.39	10.97	10.67	10.46	10.29	10.16	10.05	9.722	9.553	9.449	9.379	9.291	9.238	9.130	9.031
6	13.75	10.92	9.780	9.148	8.746	8.466	8.260	8.102	7.976	7.874	7.559	7.396	7.296	7.229	7.143	7.091	6.987	6.891
7	12.25	9.547	8.451	7.847	7.460	7.191	6.993	6.840	6.719	6.620	6.314	6.155	6.058	5.992	5.908	5.858	5.755	5.660
8	11.26	8.649	7.591	7.006	6.632	6.371	6.178	6.029	5.911	5.814	5.515	5.359	5.263	5.198	5.116	5.065	4.963	4.869
9	10.56	8.022	6.992	6.422	6.057	5.802	5.613	5.467	5.351	5.257	4.962	4.808	4.713	4.649	4.567	4.517	4.415	4.321
10	10.04	7.559	6.552	5.994	5.636	5.386	5.200	5.057	4.942	4.849	4.558	4.405	4.311	4.247	4.165	4.115	4.014	3.920
11	9.646	7.206	6.217	5.668	5.316	5.069	4.886	4.744	4.632	4.539	4.251	4.099	4.005	3.941	3.860	3.810	3.708	3.613
12	9.330	6.927	5.953	5.412	5.064	4.821	4.640	4.499	4.388	4.296	4.010	3.858	3.765	3.701	3.619	3.569	3.467	3.372
13	9.074	6.701	5.739	5.205	4.862	4.620	4.441	4.302	4.191	4.100	3.815	3.665	3.571	3.507	3.425	3.375	3.272	3.176
14	8.862	6.515	5.564	5.035	4.695	4.456	4.278	4.140	4.030	3.939	3.656	3.505	3.412	3.348	3.266	3.215	3.112	3.015
15	8.683	6.359	5.417	4.893	4.556	4.318	4.142	4.004	3.895	3.805	3.522	3.372	3.278	3.214	3.132	3.081	2.977	2.880
16	8.531	6.226	5.292	4.773	4.437	4.202	4.026	3.890	3.780	3.691	3.409	3.259	3.165	3.101	3.018	2.967	2.863	2.764
17	8.400	6.112	5.185	4.669	4.336	4.102	3.927	3.791	3.682	3.593	3.312	3.162	3.068	3.003	2.920	2.869	2.764	2.664
18	8.285	6.013	5.092	4.579	4.248	4.015	3.841	3.705	3.597	3.508	3.227	3.077	2.983	2.919	2.835	2.784	2.678	2.577
19	8.185	5.926	5.010	4.500	4.171	3.939	3.765	3.631	3.523	3.434	3.153	3.003	2.909	2.844	2.761	2.709	2.602	2.501
20	8.096	5.849	4.938	4.431	4.103	3.871	3.699	3.564	3.457	3.368	3.088	2.938	2.843	2.778	2.695	2.643	2.535	2.433
21	8.017	5.780	4.874	4.369	4.042	3.812	3.640	3.506	3.398	3.310	3.030	2.880	2.785	2.720	2.636	2.584	2.475	2.372
22	7.945	5.719	4.817	4.313	3.988	3.758	3.587	3.453	3.346	3.258	2.978	2.827	2.733	2.667	2.583	2.531	2.422	2.317
23	7.881	5.664	4.765	4.264	3.939	3.710	3.539	3.406	3.299	3.211	2.931	2.781	2.686	2.620	2.535	2.483	2.373	2.268
24	7.823	5.614	4.718	4.218	3.895	3.667	3.496	3.363	3.256	3.168	2.889	2.738	2.643	2.577	2.492	2.440	2.329	2.223
25	7.770	5.568	4.675	4.177	3.855	3.627	3.457	3.324	3.217	3.129	2.850	2.699	2.604	2.538	2.453	2.400	2.289	2.182
26	7.721	5.526	4.637	4.140	3.818	3.591	3.421	3.288	3.182	3.094	2.815	2.664	2.569	2.503	2.417	2.364	2.252	2.144
27	7.677	5.488	4.601	4.106	3.785	3.558	3.388	3.256	3.149	3.062	2.783	2.632	2.536	2.470	2.384	2.330	2.218	2.109
28	7.636	5.453	4.568	4.074	3.754	3.528	3.358	3.226	3.120	3.032	2.753	2.602	2.506	2.440	2.354	2.300	2.187	2.077
29	7.598	5.420	4.538	4.045	3.725	3.499	3.330	3.198	3.092	3.005	2.726	2.574	2.478	2.412	2.325	2.271	2.158	2.047
30	7.562	5.390	4.510	4.018	3.699	3.473	3.304	3.173	3.067	2.979	2.700	2.549	2.453	2.386	2.299	2.245	2.131	2.019
40	7.314	5.179	4.313	3.828	3.514	3.291	3.124	2.993	2.888	2.801	2.522	2.369	2.271	2.203	2.114	2.058	1.938	1.819
50	7.171	5.057	4.199	3.720	3.408	3.186	3.020	2.890	2.785	2.698	2.419	2.265	2.167	2.098	2.007	1.949	1.825	1.698
100	6.895	4.824	3.984	3.513	3.206	2.988	2.823	2.694	2.590	2.503	2.223	2.067	1.965	1.893	1.797	1.735	1.598	1.447
1000	6.660	4.626	3.801	3.338	3.036	2.820	2.657	2.529	2.425	2.339	2.056	1.897	1.791	1.716	1.613	1.544	1.383	1.159

APPENDIX D:
DATA SETS FOR
THE EXAMPLES IN
CHAPTER 13

In this appendix we give a brief description of the data sets used for some of the examples in Chapter 13. The data sets can be found at www.itve.dk as SAS data sets and comma separated text files.

SOWS **Production Results of Sows**

Source

Data from a Danish pig herd.

Used in

Examples 13.2 and 13.16.

Description

These data are a part of the production records from a sow herd. They contain information about the litters of individual sows regarding the litter size at birth and weaning as well as information regarding the sows themselves. The data set contains 379 records with six variables.

Table of variables

Variable	Description	Scale	Unit
sowid	Sow identification		
parity	The parity of the sow	Discrete	
liveborn	No. of piglets born alive	Discrete	Piglets
stillborn	No. of stillborn piglets	Discrete	Piglets
weanno	No. of piglets weaned	Discrete	Piglets
weanwgt	Total weight of the weaned piglets	Continuous	kg
farrowmonth	Month of farrowing	Ordinal	Jan, Feb, Mar, Apr, May, Jun

milk1   Milk Yield in a Danish Dairy Herd

Source

Data from a Danish dairy herd.

Used in

Examples 13.3–13.5 and 13.13.

Description

These data are modified production records from a Danish dairy herd. Data consist of information regarding breed and parity of the individual cows as well as the milk yield of the cows at two subsequent milk recordings. The data set contains 111 records with five variables.

Table of variables

Variable	Description	Scale	Unit
cowid	Cow identification		
parity	The parity of the cow	Discrete	
breed	The breed of the cow	Nominal	2 = Danish Holstein Friesians 8 = Cross-breed
kgmilk1	Milk yield at control in Jan	Continuous	kg
kgmilk2	Milk yield at control in Feb	Continuous	kg

`milk2` **Somatic Cell Count and Milk Yield in Danish Dairy Herds**

Source

Data from Danish dairy herds.

Used in

Examples 13.11, 13.12 and 13.14.

Description

These data are modified production records from Danish dairy herds. Data consist of information regarding breed and parity, milk yield of the individual cows as well as the somatic cell count. The data set contains 1140 records with five variables.

Table of variables

Variable	Description	Scale	Unit
cowid	Cow identification		
parity	The parity of the cow	Discrete	
breed	The breed of the cow	Nominal	1 = Red Danish Milk race 2 = Danish Holstein Friesians 3 = Jersey 8 = Cross-breed
kgmilk	Milk yield at control	Continuous	kg
cellcount	The somatic cell count at control	Discrete	1000 cells/ml

`colic` **Colic in Horses**

Source

Thøfner, M. B., Ersbøll, A. K., and Hesselholt, M. (2000). Prognostic indicators in a Danish hospital-based population of colic horses. *Equine Colic II, Equine Veterinary Journal*, 32(Suppl.):11–18.

Used in

Examples 13.6 and 13.7.

Description

Data are from a study of colic horses referred to the hospital at The Royal Veterinary and Agricultural University, Copenhagen, Denmark. During the study several clinical findings thought to be influenced by colic were recorded. These data are a subset of these recordings. The data set contains 472 records with six variables.

Table of variables

Variable	Description	Scale	Unit
horseid	Horse identification		
temp	Temperature	Continuous	°C
pulse	Pulse	Discrete	Heart beats per minute
crt	Capillary refill time	Discrete	Seconds
sbe	Standard base excess	Continuous	mmol/l
pcv	Packed cell volume	Continuous	Hematocrit percentage

bpcats   Blood Pressure in Cats

Source

Pedersen, K.-M. (2002). *Hypertension in Polycystic Kidney Disease in Persian Cats – Prevalence, Diagnosis, Pathophysiology and Pathology*. PhD thesis, The Royal Veterinary and Agricultural University, Copenhagen, Denmark.

Used in

Example 13.19.

Description

These data were collected to compare a direct and an indirect method for measuring blood pressure in cats. To compare the methods, the systolic arterial blood pressure was measured during hypotension, normotension and hypertension. The data set contains 18 records with four variables.

Table of variables

Variable	Description	Scale	Unit
catid	Cat identification		
level	Phase where blood pressure is measured	Nominal	Hypotension Normotension Hypertension
saps	Direct measure of blood pressure	Continuous	mlHg
sapc	Indirect measure of blood pressure	Continuous	mlHg

APPENDIX E: SAS CODE AND OUTPUT FOR THE EXAMPLES IN CHAPTER 13

Annette Kjær Ersbøll and Nils Toft

In this appendix, we give the SAS code for the examples used in Chapter 13. The programs have been written for the SAS system for Windows, Version 8.2, but should work on most versions of SAS. The output has been generated using the above version of SAS and differences in appearance might occur between SAS versions. All programs assume that the data sets are located in the SAS library 'c'. This library can be constructed by the SAS code:

```
libname c 'c:\some\directory\with\the\data\sets';
```

All examples and data sets can be found at www.itve.dk. For the different plots produced by the SAS code, we refer to the examples in Chapter 13.

Example 13.2

Program

```
data sowdata;
  set c.sowdata;
  meanweanweight=weanwgt/weanno;

proc ttest data=sowdata h0=7.0;
  var meanweanweight;
run;
```

Output

The TTEST Procedure

Statistics

Variable	N	Lower CL Mean	Mean	Upper CL Mean	Lower CL Std Dev	Std Dev
meanweanweight	379	7.1268	7.2666	7.4065	1.2929	1.3849

Statistics

Variable	Upper CL Std Dev	Std Err	Minimum	Maximum
meanweanweight	1.4912	0.0711	4	17.727

T-Tests

Variable	DF	t Value	Pr > |t|
meanweanweight	378	3.75	0.0002

Example 13.3

Program

```
* Descriptive statistics;
proc univariate data=c.milk1 noprint;
  var kgmilk1;
  output out=stat1 mean=mean n=n std=std stderr=se
               median=median q1=q1 q3=q3;
proc print data=stat1;
run;

proc sort data=c.milk1;
  by breed;
proc univariate data=c.milk1 noprint;
  var kgmilk1;
  by breed;
  output out=stat2 mean=mean n=n std=std stderr=se
               median=median q1=q1 q3=q3;
proc print data=stat2;
run;

proc sort data=c.milk1;
  by parity;
proc univariate data=c.milk1 noprint;
  var kgmilk1;
  by parity;
  output out=stat3 mean=mean n=n std=std stderr=se
               median=median q1=q1 q3=q3;
proc print data=stat3;
run;
```

```
proc ttest data=c.milk1;
  var kgmilk1;
  class breed;
run;
```

Output

Obs	n	mean	std	se	q3	median	q1
1	111	21.3036	6.13692	0.58249	25.4	21.9	17.7

Obs	breed	n	mean	std	se	q3	median	q1
1	2	31	22.0194	7.77206	1.39590	26.4	21.9	18.00
2	8	80	21.0263	5.40583	0.60439	24.9	22.0	17.45

Obs	parity	n	mean	std	se	q3	median	q1
1	1	33	18.5606	4.95000	0.86168	22.2	18.00	15.60
2	2	36	21.9778	5.56207	0.92701	26.4	22.60	18.90
3	3	20	21.8800	6.18058	1.38202	25.8	24.35	21.05
4	4	22	23.7909	7.37673	1.57272	29.3	23.10	18.90

The TTEST Procedure

Statistics

Variable	breed		N	Lower CL Mean	Mean	Upper CL Mean	Lower CL Std Dev
kgmilk1		2	31	19.169	22.019	24.87	6.2107
kgmilk1		8	80	19.823	21.026	22.229	4.6785
kgmilk1	Diff (1-2)			-1.585	0.9931	3.5713	5.4295

Statistics

Variable	breed		Std Dev	Upper CL Std Dev	Std Err	Minimum	Maximum
kgmilk1		2	7.7721	10.389	1.3959	4.1	43.1
kgmilk1		8	5.4058	6.4031	0.6044	4.8	31.3
kgmilk1	Diff (1-2)		6.1486	7.089	1.3008		

T-Tests

Variable	Method	Variances	DF	t Value	Pr > |t|
kgmilk1	Pooled	Equal	109	0.76	0.4468
kgmilk1	Satterthwaite	Unequal	41.7	0.65	0.5174

                        Equality of Variances

    Variable   Method   Num DF   Den DF   F Value   Pr > F

     kgmilk1   Folded F   30   79   2.07   0.0111

Example 13.4

Program

```
proc ttest data=c.milk1;
  paired kgmilk1*kgmilk2;
run;
```

Output

                        The TTEST Procedure

                            Statistics

                                Lower CL   Upper CL   Lower CL
    Difference   N   Mean   Mean   Mean   Std Dev

    kgmilk1 - kgmilk2   104   -0.487   1.5212   3.5289   9.0863

                            Statistics

                                Upper CL
    Difference   Std Dev   Std Dev   Std Err   Minimum   Maximum

    kgmilk1 - kgmilk2 10.324   11.955   1.0124   -10.1   32.6

                              T-Tests

            Difference   DF   t Value   Pr > |t|

            kgmilk1 - kgmilk2   103   1.50   0.1360

Example 13.5

Program

```
proc mixed data=c.milk1;
  class parity breed;
  model kgmilk1=parity breed;
  lsmeans parity breed /pdiff;
run;
```

Output

```
                    The Mixed Procedure

                    Model Information

Data Set                       C.MILK1
Dependent Variable             kgmilk1
Covariance Structure           Diagonal
Estimation Method              REML
Residual Variance Method       Profile
Fixed Effects SE Method        Model-Based
Degrees of Freedom Method      Residual


                 Class Level Information

   Class      Levels    Values

   parity        4      1 2 3 4
   breed         2      2 8


                       Dimensions

        Covariance Parameters          1
        Columns in X                   7
        Columns in Z                   0
        Subjects                       1
        Max Obs Per Subject          111
        Observations Used            111
        Observations Not Used          0
        Total Observations           111


                 Covariance Parameter
                      Estimates

            Cov Parm      Estimate

            Residual       33.9379


                     Fit Statistics

        -2 Res Log Likelihood        689.6
        AIC (smaller is better)      691.6
        AICC (smaller is better)     691.7
        BIC (smaller is better)      694.3
```

```
                    Type 3 Tests of Fixed Effects

                        Num      Den
            Effect       DF       DF      F Value    Pr > F

            parity        3      106       5.14      0.0023
            breed         1      106       4.07      0.0463


                        Least Squares Means

                                    Standard
   Effect  parity  breed  Estimate    Error    DF   t Value   Pr > |t|

   parity  1                16.5719   1.4146   106    11.71    <.0001
   parity  2                19.9783   1.3878   106    14.40    <.0001
   parity  3                21.4566   1.3195   106    16.26    <.0001
   parity  4                25.7155   1.5664   106    16.42    <.0001
   breed           2        18.8135   1.4733   106    12.77    <.0001
   breed           8        23.0476   0.9357   106    24.63    <.0001


                   Differences of Least Squares Means

                                                        Standard
   Effect  parity  breed  _parity  _breed  Estimate      Error     DF

   parity  1                2               -3.4065     1.4040     106
   parity  1                3               -4.8847     1.8243     106
   parity  1                4               -9.1436     2.5175     106
   parity  2                3               -1.4782     1.8029     106
   parity  2                4               -5.7371     2.5045     106
   parity  3                4               -4.2589     2.1437     106
   breed           2                8       -4.2341     2.0999     106

                   Differences of Least Squares Means

   Effect  parity  breed  _parity  _breed  t Value    Pr > |t|

   parity  1                2               -2.43      0.0169
   parity  1                3               -2.68      0.0086
   parity  1                4               -3.63      0.0004
   parity  2                3               -0.82      0.4141
   parity  2                4               -2.29      0.0240
   parity  3                4               -1.99      0.0495
   breed           2                8       -2.02      0.0463
```

Example 13.6

Program

```
proc corr data=c.colic pearson spearman;
  var temp crt pulse sbe pcv;
run;
```

Output

The CORR Procedure

5 Variables: temp   crt   pulse   SBE   PCV

Simple Statistics

Variable	N	Mean	Std Dev	Median
temp	423	37.96856	0.63259	38.00000
crt	440	2.93182	1.37498	3.00000
pulse	458	59.16594	20.36867	52.50000
SBE	419	-2.20310	5.11222	-1.70000
PCV	414	39.34541	8.94963	37.50000

Simple Statistics

Variable	Minimum	Maximum	Label
temp	35.70000	40.20000	
crt	1.00000	10.00000	
pulse	30.00000	122.00000	
SBE	-28.20000	8.30000	Standard Base Excess
PCV	23.00000	75.00000	Hematokrit %

Pearson Correlation Coefficients
Prob > |r| under H0: Rho=0
Number of Observations

	temp	crt	pulse	SBE	PCV
temp	1.00000	0.03661	0.16973	0.02245	0.07159
		0.4653	0.0005	0.6593	0.1631
	423	400	414	388	381
crt	0.03661	1.00000	0.59222	-0.42461	0.53027
	0.4653		<.0001	<.0001	<.0001
	400	440	436	401	396
pulse	0.16973	0.59222	1.00000	-0.40220	0.56081
	0.0005	<.0001		<.0001	<.0001
	414	436	458	412	407
SBE	0.02245	-0.42461	-0.40220	1.00000	-0.26903
Standard Base Excess	0.6593	<.0001	<.0001		<.0001
	388	401	412	419	403
PCV	0.07159	0.53027	0.56081	-0.26903	1.00000
Hematokrit %	0.1631	<.0001	<.0001	<.0001	
	381	396	407	403	414

```
                    Spearman Correlation Coefficients
                       Prob > |r| under H0: Rho=0
                         Number of Observations

                          temp        crt       pulse        SBE        PCV

temp                   1.00000    0.01828    0.16522   -0.02551    0.04185
                                   0.7155     0.0007     0.6164     0.4154
                           423        400        414        388        381

crt                    0.01828    1.00000    0.51553   -0.36587    0.45333
                        0.7155                <.0001     <.0001     <.0001
                           400        440        436        401        396

pulse                  0.16522    0.51553    1.00000   -0.35882    0.46294
                        0.0007     <.0001                <.0001     <.0001
                           414        436        458        412        407

SBE                   -0.02551   -0.36587   -0.35882    1.00000   -0.22343
Standard Base Excess    0.6164     <.0001     <.0001                <.0001
                           388        401        412        419        403

PCV                    0.04185    0.45333    0.46294   -0.22343    1.00000
Hematokrit %            0.4154     <.0001     <.0001     <.0001
                           381        396        407        403        414
```

Example 13.7

Program

```
proc reg data=c.colic;
  model pulse=pcv;
  plot pulse*pcv;
run;
```

Output

```
                       The REG Procedure
                         Model: MODEL1
                   Dependent Variable: pulse

                      Analysis of Variance

                              Sum of        Mean
Source               DF      Squares      Square   F Value   Pr > F

Model                 1        53380       53380    185.82   <.0001
Error               405       116344   287.26998
Corrected Total     406       169724


              Root MSE            16.94904   R-Square     0.3145
              Dependent Mean      59.99509   Adj R-Sq     0.3128
              Coeff Var           28.25071
```

```
                          Parameter Estimates

                               Parameter        Standard
      Variable    Label          DF   Estimate      Error    t Value

      Intercept   Intercept       1    9.78068     3.77830      2.59
      PCV         Hematokrit %    1    1.27542     0.09356     13.63

                          Parameter Estimates

             Variable    Label          DF   Pr > |t|

             Intercept   Intercept       1    0.0100
             PCV         Hematokrit %    1    <.0001
```

Example 13.8

Program

```
data farm;
input endo$ number;
cards;
endo_neg 590
endo_pos 110
;
proc freq data=farm;
table endo /binomialc(p=0.1 level=2) chisq testp=(0.9,0.1);
weight number;
run;
```

Output

```
                      The FREQ Procedure

                                  Test    Cumulative  Cumulative
   endo      Frequency   Percent  Percent   Frequency   Percent
   ----------------------------------------------------------------
   endo_neg       590     84.29    90.00         590     84.29
   endo_pos       110     15.71    10.00         700    100.00

                      Chi-Square Test
                  for Specified Proportions
                  -------------------------
                  Chi-Square        25.3968
                  DF                      1
                  Pr > ChiSq        <.0001
```

```
        Binomial Proportion
          for endo = endo_pos
    -------------------------------
    Proportion                  0.1571
    ASE                         0.0138
    95% Lower Conf Limit        0.1295
    95% Upper Conf Limit        0.1848

    Exact Conf Limits
    95% Lower Conf Limit        0.1310
    95% Upper Conf Limit        0.1863

       Test of H0: Proportion = 0.1

    ASE under H0                0.0113
    Z                          4.9765
    One-sided Pr >   Z          <.0001
    Two-sided Pr > |Z|          <.0001

    The asymptotic confidence limits and test
       include a continuity correction.

          Sample Size = 700
```

Example 13.9

Program

```
data metritis;
  input breed$ metritis$ number;
  cards;
  holstein + 100
  holstein - 400
  jersey   + 10
  jersey   - 190
  ;

proc freq data=metritis;
  tables breed*metritis / relrisk;
  exact fisher;
  weight number;
run;
```

Output

```
                    The FREQ Procedure

              Table of breed by metritis

         breed      metritis

         Frequency|
         Percent  |
         Row Pct  |
         Col Pct  |+        |-        |  Total
         ---------+---------+---------+
         holstein |    100  |    400  |    500
                  |  14.29  |  57.14  |  71.43
                  |  20.00  |  80.00  |
                  |  90.91  |  67.80  |
         ---------+---------+---------+
         jersey   |     10  |    190  |    200
                  |   1.43  |  27.14  |  28.57
                  |   5.00  |  95.00  |
                  |   9.09  |  32.20  |
         ---------+---------+---------+
         Total         110       590       700
                     15.71     84.29    100.00


         Statistics for Table of breed by metritis

Statistic                        DF       Value       Prob
----------------------------------------------------------
Chi-Square                        1     24.2681     <.0001
Likelihood Ratio Chi-Square       1     29.0537     <.0001
Continuity Adj. Chi-Square        1     23.1488     <.0001
Mantel-Haenszel Chi-Square        1     24.2334     <.0001
Phi Coefficient                          0.1862
Contingency Coefficient                  0.1830
Cramer's V                               0.1862


                  Fisher's Exact Test
          ----------------------------------
          Cell (1,1) Frequency (F)        100
          Left-sided Pr <= F           1.0000
          Right-sided Pr >= F       8.496E-08

          Table Probability (P)     6.784E-08
          Two-sided Pr <= P         1.371E-07
```

```
              Estimates of the Relative Risk (Row1/Row2)

  Type of Study                    Value         95% Confidence Limits
  ----------------------------------------------------------------------
  Case-Control (Odds Ratio)       4.7500          2.4243        9.3067
  Cohort (Col1 Risk)              4.0000          2.1324        7.5031
  Cohort (Col2 Risk)              0.8421          0.7977        0.8890

                        Sample Size = 700
```

Example 13.10

Program

```
data turkey;
  input conv$ eiafoss$ number;
  cards;
  + + 32
  + - 21
  - + 4
  - - 4
  ;

proc freq data=turkey;
  tables conv*eiafoss;
  exact mcnemar;
  weight number;
run;
```

Output

```
                        The FREQ Procedure

                      Table of conv by eiafoss

               conv        eiafoss

               Frequency|
               Percent  |
               Row Pct  |
               Col Pct  |+        |-        | Total
               ---------+--------+--------+
               +        |     32 |     21 |    53
                        |  52.46 |  34.43 | 86.89
                        |  60.38 |  39.62 |
                        |  88.89 |  84.00 |
               ---------+--------+--------+
               -        |      4 |      4 |     8
                        |   6.56 |   6.56 | 13.11
                        |  50.00 |  50.00 |
                        |  11.11 |  16.00 |
               ---------+--------+--------+
               Total          36       25      61
                            59.02    40.98   100.00
```

```
             Statistics for Table of conv by eiafoss

                       McNemar's Test
               -------------------------------
               Statistic (S)             11.5600
               DF                              1
               Asymptotic Pr >  S         0.0007
               Exact       Pr >= S     9.105E-04


                   Simple Kappa Coefficient
               -------------------------------
               Kappa                      0.0546
               ASE                        0.1005
               95% Lower Conf Limit      -0.1424
               95% Upper Conf Limit       0.2515

                       Sample Size = 61
```

Example 13.11

Program

```
data a;
  set c.milk2;
  if cellcount>125 then scc='high';
  if cellcount<=125 then scc='low';
run;

proc sort data=a;
  by scc;
proc univariate data=a noprint;
  var kgmilk;
  by scc;
  output out=stat2 mean=mean n=n std=std stderr=stderr
                   median=median q1=q1 q3=q3;
proc print data=stat2;
run;

proc genmod data=a;
  model scc = kgmilk / dist=bin link=logit type3;
  output out=pred p=p;
  estimate 'Milk change: 2 kg' kgmilk 2 / exp;
  estimate 'Milk change: 5 kg' kgmilk 5 / exp;
run;
proc gplot data=pred;
  plot p*kgmilk;
run;
```

Output

Obs	scc	n	mean	std	stderr	q3	median	q1
1	high	600	19.2345	6.97362	0.28470	23.25	18.8	14.4
2	low	540	20.7267	5.84870	0.25169	24.20	20.4	16.6

The GENMOD Procedure

Model Information

Data Set	WORK.A
Distribution	Binomial
Link Function	Logit
Dependent Variable	scc
Observations Used	1140

Response Profile

Ordered Value	scc	Total Frequency
1	high	600
2	low	540

PROC GENMOD is modeling the probability that scc='high'. One way to change this to model the probability that scc='low' is to specify the DESCENDING option in the PROC statement.

Parameter Information

Parameter	Effect
Prm1	Intercept
Prm2	kgmilk

Criteria For Assessing Goodness Of Fit

Criterion	DF	Value	Value/DF
Deviance	1138	1562.1602	1.3727
Scaled Deviance	1138	1562.1602	1.3727
Pearson Chi-Square	1138	1139.3361	1.0012
Scaled Pearson X2	1138	1139.3361	1.0012
Log Likelihood		-781.0801	

Algorithm converged.

Analysis Of Parameter Estimates

Parameter	DF	Estimate	Standard Error	Wald 95% Confidence Limits		Chi-Square
Intercept	1	0.8191	0.1954	0.4362	1.2020	17.58
kgmilk	1	-0.0357	0.0093	-0.0540	-0.0175	14.75
Scale	0	1.0000	0.0000	1.0000	1.0000	

Analysis Of Parameter Estimates

Parameter	Pr > ChiSq
Intercept	<.0001
kgmilk	0.0001
Scale	

NOTE: The scale parameter was held fixed.

LR Statistics For Type 3 Analysis

Source	DF	Chi-Square	Pr > ChiSq
kgmilk	1	15.06	0.0001

Contrast Estimate Results

Label	Estimate	Standard Error	Alpha	Confidence Limits	
Milk change: 2 kg	-0.0715	0.0186	0.05	-0.1080	-0.0350
Exp(Milk change: 2 kg)	0.9310	0.0173	0.05	0.8977	0.9656
Milk change: 5 kg	-0.1787	0.0465	0.05	-0.2699	-0.0875
Exp(Milk change: 5 kg)	0.8364	0.0389	0.05	0.7635	0.9162

Contrast Estimate Results

Label	Chi-Square	Pr > ChiSq
Milk change: 2 kg	14.75	0.0001
Exp(Milk change: 2 kg)		
Milk change: 5 kg	14.75	0.0001
Exp(Milk change: 5 kg)		

Example 13.12

Program

```
data milk;
set c.milk2;
  if cellcount>125 then scc='high';
  if cellcount<=125 then scc='low';
run;

proc freq data=milk;
  tables breed*scc;
run;

proc genmod data=milk ;
  class breed;
  model scc=breed   / dist=bin link=logit type3;
  lsmeans breed / diff;
  estimate 'RDM vs CB' breed 1 0   0 -1 / exp;
  estimate 'SDM vs CB' breed 0 1   0 -1 / exp;
  estimate 'Jersey vs CB' breed 0 0   1 -1 / exp;
run;

proc genmod data=milk;
  class breed;
  model scc= kgmilk breed   / dist=bin link=logit type3;
  lsmeans breed / diff;
  output out=stat_pred p=p;
  estimate 'RDM vs CB' breed 1 0   0 -1 / exp;
  estimate 'SDM vs CB' breed 0 1   0 -1 / exp;
  estimate 'Jersey vs CB' breed 0 0   1 -1 / exp;
  estimate 'Milk change: 5 kg' kgmilk 5 / exp;
run;

proc gplot data=stat_pred;
  plot p*kgmilk=breed;
run;
```

Output

```
                        The FREQ Procedure

                     Table of breed by scc

            breed      scc

            Frequency|
            Percent  |
            Row Pct  |
            Col Pct  |high    |low     |    Total
            ---------+--------+--------+
                1 |     92 |     69 |      161
                  |   8.07 |   6.05 |    14.12
                  |  57.14 |  42.86 |
                  |  15.33 |  12.78 |
            ---------+--------+--------+
                2 |    296 |    222 |      518
                  |  25.96 |  19.47 |    45.44
                  |  57.14 |  42.86 |
                  |  49.33 |  41.11 |
            ---------+--------+--------+
                3 |     85 |    111 |      196
                  |   7.46 |   9.74 |    17.19
                  |  43.37 |  56.63 |
                  |  14.17 |  20.56 |
            ---------+--------+--------+
                8 |    127 |    138 |      265
                  |  11.14 |  12.11 |    23.25
                  |  47.92 |  52.08 |
                  |  21.17 |  25.56 |
            ---------+--------+--------+
            Total          600      540      1140
                         52.63    47.37    100.00


                     The GENMOD Procedure

                      Model Information

            Data Set                  WORK.MILK
            Distribution               Binomial
            Link Function                 Logit
            Dependent Variable              scc
            Observations Used              1140


                  Class Level Information

             Class      Levels     Values

             breed          4      1 2 3 8
```

```
                         Response Profile

                 Ordered                    Total
                 Value        scc         Frequency

                    1         high            600
                    2         low             540
```

PROC GENMOD is modeling the probability that scc='high'. One way to change this to model the probability that scc='low' is to specify the DESCENDING option in the PROC statement.

```
                    Parameter Information

             Parameter        Effect        breed

             Prm1             Intercept
             Prm2             breed          1
             Prm3             breed          2
             Prm4             breed          3
             Prm5             breed          8
```

```
          Criteria For Assessing Goodness Of Fit

     Criterion              DF          Value        Value/DF

     Deviance              1136      1562.5550        1.3755
     Scaled Deviance       1136      1562.5550        1.3755
     Pearson Chi-Square    1136      1140.0000        1.0035
     Scaled Pearson X2     1136      1140.0000        1.0035
     Log Likelihood                  -781.2775
```

Algorithm converged.

```
                    Analysis Of Parameter Estimates

                              Standard      Wald 95%           Chi-
     Parameter     DF  Estimate   Error  Confidence Limits    Square

     Intercept      1  -0.0831  0.1230  -0.3241   0.1579      0.46
     breed      1   1   0.3707  0.2012  -0.0236   0.7651      3.40
     breed      2   1   0.3707  0.1517   0.0735   0.6680      5.98
     breed      3   1  -0.1838  0.1895  -0.5551   0.1875      0.94
     breed      8   0   0.0000  0.0000   0.0000   0.0000       .
     Scale          0   1.0000  0.0000   1.0000   1.0000
```

```
                   Analysis Of Parameter
                         Estimates

               Parameter      Pr > ChiSq

               Intercept         0.4993
               breed      1      0.0654
               breed      2      0.0145
               breed      3      0.3319
               breed      8        .
               Scale

NOTE: The scale parameter was held fixed.


               LR Statistics For Type 3 Analysis

                                   Chi-
          Source          DF      Square     Pr > ChiSq

          breed            3      14.66         0.0021


                    Least Squares Means

                             Standard          Chi-
Effect    breed  Estimate     Error     DF    Square    Pr > ChiSq

breed      1      0.2877      0.1593      1     3.26       0.0709
breed      2      0.2877      0.0888      1    10.50       0.0012
breed      3     -0.2669      0.1441      1     3.43       0.0641
breed      8     -0.0831      0.1230      1     0.46       0.4993


                 Differences of Least Squares Means

                              Standard          Chi-
Effect  breed  _breed  Estimate   Error    DF   Square  Pr > ChiSq

breed    1      2      0.0000    0.1823     1    0.00     1.0000
breed    1      3      0.5546    0.2148     1    6.67     0.0098
breed    1      8      0.3707    0.2012     1    3.40     0.0654
breed    2      3      0.5546    0.1693     1   10.73     0.0011
breed    2      8      0.3707    0.1517     1    5.98     0.0145
breed    3      8     -0.1838    0.1895     1    0.94     0.3319
```

Contrast Estimate Results

Label	Estimate	Standard Error	Alpha	Confidence Limits	
RDM vs CB	0.3707	0.2012	0.05	-0.0236	0.7651
Exp(RDM vs CB)	1.4488	0.2915	0.05	0.9767	2.1492
SDM vs CB	0.3707	0.1517	0.05	0.0735	0.6680
Exp(SDM vs CB)	1.4488	0.2197	0.05	1.0763	1.9504
Jersey vs CB	-0.1838	0.1895	0.05	-0.5551	0.1875
Exp(Jersey vs CB)	0.8321	0.1576	0.05	0.5740	1.2063

Contrast Estimate Results

Label	Chi-Square	Pr > ChiSq
RDM vs CB	3.40	0.0654
Exp(RDM vs CB)		
SDM vs CB	5.98	0.0145
Exp(SDM vs CB)		
Jersey vs CB	0.94	0.3319
Exp(Jersey vs CB)		

The GENMOD Procedure

Model Information

Data Set	WORK.MILK
Distribution	Binomial
Link Function	Logit
Dependent Variable	scc
Observations Used	1140

Class Level Information

Class	Levels	Values
breed	4	1 2 3 8

Response Profile

Ordered Value	scc	Total Frequency
1	high	600
2	low	540

PROC GENMOD is modeling the probability that scc='high'. One way to change this to model the probability that scc='low' is to specify the DESCENDING option in the PROC statement.

```
                    Parameter Information

          Parameter          Effect        breed

          Prm1               Intercept
          Prm2               kgmilk
          Prm3               breed         1
          Prm4               breed         2
          Prm5               breed         3
          Prm6               breed         8


            Criteria For Assessing Goodness Of Fit

    Criterion              DF          Value        Value/DF

    Deviance              1135       1538.6011       1.3556
    Scaled Deviance       1135       1538.6011       1.3556
    Pearson Chi-Square    1135       1138.2508       1.0029
    Scaled Pearson X2     1135       1138.2508       1.0029
    Log Likelihood                   -769.3006

Algorithm converged.


              Analysis Of Parameter Estimates

                              Standard     Wald 95%           Chi-
  Parameter      DF  Estimate    Error  Confidence Limits    Square

  Intercept      1    0.9053    0.2396   0.4358    1.3749    14.28
  kgmilk         1   -0.0478    0.0099  -0.0673   -0.0284    23.17
  breed    1     1    0.2752    0.2041  -0.1247    0.6752     1.82
  breed    2     1    0.4135    0.1536   0.1125    0.7145     7.25
  breed    3     1   -0.3988    0.1959  -0.7828   -0.0148     4.14
  breed    8     0    0.0000    0.0000   0.0000    0.0000     .
  Scale          0    1.0000    0.0000   1.0000    1.0000

              Analysis Of Parameter
                    Estimates

          Parameter      Pr > ChiSq

          Intercept         0.0002
          kgmilk            <.0001
          breed    1        0.1774
          breed    2        0.0071
          breed    3        0.0418
          breed    8          .
          Scale

NOTE: The scale parameter was held fixed.
```

```
          LR Statistics For Type 3 Analysis

                                     Chi-
           Source          DF       Square    Pr > ChiSq

           kgmilk           1       23.95       <.0001
           breed            3       23.56       <.0001


                   Least Squares Means

                              Standard           Chi-
   Effect    breed   Estimate    Error    DF    Square    Pr > ChiSq

   breed      1       0.2265    0.1615     1     1.97       0.1607
   breed      2       0.3647    0.0916     1    15.85       <.0001
   breed      3      -0.4476    0.1498     1     8.92       0.0028
   breed      8      -0.0488    0.1242     1     0.15       0.6945


              Differences of Least Squares Means

                                  Standard      Chi-
   Effect  breed  _breed  Estimate   Error   DF  Square  Pr > ChiSq

   breed    1      2      -0.1383   0.1867    1   0.55     0.4588
   breed    1      3       0.6740   0.2183    1   9.53     0.0020
   breed    1      8       0.2752   0.2041    1   1.82     0.1774
   breed    2      3       0.8123   0.1793    1  20.52     <.0001
   breed    2      8       0.4135   0.1536    1   7.25     0.0071
   breed    3      8      -0.3988   0.1959    1   4.14     0.0418


                 Contrast Estimate Results

                                Standard
   Label                Estimate   Error   Alpha   Confidence Limits

   RDM vs CB             0.2752   0.2041   0.05   -0.1247    0.6752
   Exp(RDM vs CB)        1.3168   0.2687   0.05    0.8827    1.9644
   SDM vs CB             0.4135   0.1536   0.05    0.1125    0.7145
   Exp(SDM vs CB)        1.5121   0.2322   0.05    1.1191    2.0431
   Jersey vs CB         -0.3988   0.1959   0.05   -0.7828   -0.0148
   Exp(Jersey vs CB)     0.6711   0.1315   0.05    0.4571    0.9853
   Milk change: 5 kg    -0.2392   0.0497   0.05   -0.3366   -0.1418
   Exp(Milk change: 5 kg) 0.7872  0.0391   0.05    0.7142    0.8678
```

```
                  Contrast Estimate Results

                                  Chi-
            Label                Square    Pr > ChiSq

            RDM vs CB             1.82       0.1774
            Exp(RDM vs CB)
            SDM vs CB             7.25       0.0071
            Exp(SDM vs CB)
            Jersey vs CB          4.14       0.0418
            Exp(Jersey vs CB)
            Milk change: 5 kg    23.17      <.0001
            Exp(Milk change: 5 kg)
```

Example 13.13

Program

```
proc mixed data=c.milk1;
  class parity breed;
  model kgmilk1=parity breed / s outp=stat;

symbol v=dot c=black;

proc univariate data=stat normal noprint;
  var resid;
  histogram resid / normal;
  qqplot resid / normal(mu=est sigma=est);
  * Jeg har erstattet det med et qqplot;
  *probplot resid / normal (mu=0 sigma=5.72 color=black l=1);
run;
proc gplot data=stat;
  plot resid*pred / vref=0;
run;
```

Output

```
                  The Mixed Procedure

                    Model Information

     Data Set                    C.MILK1
     Dependent Variable          kgmilk1
     Covariance Structure        Diagonal
     Estimation Method           REML
     Residual Variance Method    Profile
     Fixed Effects SE Method     Model-Based
     Degrees of Freedom Method   Residual
```

Class Level Information

Class	Levels	Values
parity	4	1 2 3 4
breed	2	2 8

Dimensions

Covariance Parameters	1
Columns in X	7
Columns in Z	0
Subjects	1
Max Obs Per Subject	111
Observations Used	111
Observations Not Used	0
Total Observations	111

Covariance Parameter Estimates

Cov Parm	Estimate
Residual	33.9379

Fit Statistics

-2 Res Log Likelihood	689.6
AIC (smaller is better)	691.6
AICC (smaller is better)	691.7
BIC (smaller is better)	694.3

Solution for Fixed Effects

Effect	parity	breed	Estimate	Standard Error	DF	t Value	Pr > |t|
Intercept			27.8325	2.3581	106	11.80	<.0001
parity	1		-9.1436	2.5175	106	-3.63	0.0004
parity	2		-5.7371	2.5045	106	-2.29	0.0240
parity	3		-4.2589	2.1437	106	-1.99	0.0495
parity	4		0	.	.	.	.
breed		2	-4.2341	2.0999	106	-2.02	0.0463
breed		8	0	.	.	.	.

Type 3 Tests of Fixed Effects

Effect	Num DF	Den DF	F Value	Pr > F
parity	3	106	5.14	0.0023

```
    breed              1      106       4.07      0.0463
                    The UNIVARIATE Procedure
                  Fitted Distribution for Resid

           Parameters for Normal Distribution

           Parameter    Symbol    Estimate

           Mean         Mu               0
           Std Dev      Sigma      5.71872


        Goodness-of-Fit Tests for Normal Distribution

   Test                   ---Statistic----    -----p Value-----

   Kolmogorov-Smirnov    D     0.06971676    Pr > D      >0.150
   Cramer-von Mises      W-Sq  0.09516580    Pr > W-Sq    0.132
   Anderson-Darling      A-Sq  0.81822726    Pr > A-Sq    0.035


           Quantiles for Normal Distribution

                      -------Quantile-------
           Percent    Observed     Estimated

              1.0    -15.23955    -13.303732
              5.0    -11.18891     -9.406457
             10.0     -6.66131     -7.328834
             25.0     -3.33955     -3.857218
             50.0      0.60461     -0.000000
             75.0      3.80461      3.857218
             90.0      6.10461      7.328834
             95.0      7.50155      9.406457
             99.0      9.51109     13.303732
```

Example 13.15

Program

```
data a;
  input bordetella$ pmtox$ rhinitis$ number;
  cards;
  + + + 22
  + + - 0
  + - + 5
  + - - 11
  - + + 12
  - + - 3
  - - + 5
  - - - 10
  ;
```

```
proc sort data=a;
  by pmtox;

proc freq data=a;
  weight number;
  tables bordetella*rhinitis / relrisk;
run;

proc freq data=a;
  weight number;
  tables bordetella*rhinitis / relrisk;
  by pmtox;
run;

proc freq data=a;
  weight number;
  tables pmtox*bordetella*rhinitis / cmh;
run;

proc genmod data=a;
  weight number;
  class bordetella pmtox;
  model rhinitis=bordetella pmtox / dist=bin link=logit type3;
run;
```

Output

```
                    The FREQ Procedure

                Table of bordetella by rhinitis

            bordetella      rhinitis

            Frequency|
            Percent  |
            Row Pct  |
            Col Pct  |+        |-       |    Total
            ---------+--------+--------+
            +        |     27 |     11 |      38
                     |  39.71 |  16.18 |   55.88
                     |  71.05 |  28.95 |
                     |  61.36 |  45.83 |
            ---------+--------+--------+
            -        |     17 |     13 |      30
                     |  25.00 |  19.12 |   44.12
                     |  56.67 |  43.33 |
                     |  38.64 |  54.17 |
            ---------+--------+--------+
            Total          44       24        68
                        64.71    35.29    100.00
```

```
              Statistics for Table of bordetella by rhinitis

              Estimates of the Relative Risk (Row1/Row2)

Type of Study                     Value      95% Confidence Limits
-------------------------------------------------------------------
Case-Control (Odds Ratio)         1.8770        0.6861        5.1353
Cohort (Col1 Risk)                1.2539        0.8635        1.8207
Cohort (Col2 Risk)                0.6680        0.3506        1.2728

                      Sample Size = 68


---------------------------- pmtox=+ ------------------------------

                      The FREQ Procedure

              Table of bordetella by rhinitis

              bordetella      rhinitis

              Frequency|
              Percent  |
              Row Pct  |
              Col Pct  |+        |-         |  Total
              ---------+--------+--------+
              +        |     22 |      0 |     22
                       |  59.46 |   0.00 |  59.46
                       | 100.00 |   0.00 |
                       |  64.71 |   0.00 |
              ---------+--------+--------+
              -        |     12 |      3 |     15
                       |  32.43 |   8.11 |  40.54
                       |  80.00 |  20.00 |
                       |  35.29 | 100.00 |
              ---------+--------+--------+
              Total          34        3       37
                          91.89     8.11   100.00


              Statistics for Table of bordetella by rhinitis

              Estimates of the Relative Risk (Row1/Row2)

Type of Study                     Value      95% Confidence Limits
-------------------------------------------------------------------
Cohort (Col1 Risk)                1.2500        0.9706        1.6099

      One or more risk estimates not computed --- zero cell.

                      Sample Size = 37
```

```
----------------------------- pmtox=- -------------------------------

                      The FREQ Procedure

                  Table of bordetella by rhinitis

              bordetella      rhinitis

              Frequency|
              Percent  |
              Row Pct  |
              Col Pct  |+         |-        |  Total
              ---------+--------+--------+
              +        |      5 |     11 |     16
                       |  16.13 |  35.48 |  51.61
                       |  31.25 |  68.75 |
                       |  50.00 |  52.38 |
              ---------+--------+--------+
              -        |      5 |     10 |     15
                       |  16.13 |  32.26 |  48.39
                       |  33.33 |  66.67 |
                       |  50.00 |  47.62 |
              ---------+--------+--------+
              Total           10       21       31
                           32.26    67.74   100.00


        Statistics for Table of bordetella by rhinitis

           Estimates of the Relative Risk (Row1/Row2)

Type of Study                    Value        95% Confidence Limits
-----------------------------------------------------------------
Case-Control (Odds Ratio)       0.9091       0.2015       4.1014
Cohort (Col1 Risk)              0.9375       0.3381       2.5999
Cohort (Col2 Risk)              1.0313       0.6337       1.6783

                      Sample Size = 31
```

The FREQ Procedure

Table 1 of bordetella by rhinitis
Controlling for pmtox=+

bordetella   rhinitis

```
Frequency|
Percent  |
Row Pct  |
Col Pct  |+        |-        |  Total
---------+--------+--------+
+        |     22 |      0 |      22
         |  59.46 |   0.00 |   59.46
         | 100.00 |   0.00 |
         |  64.71 |   0.00 |
---------+--------+--------+
-        |     12 |      3 |      15
         |  32.43 |   8.11 |   40.54
         |  80.00 |  20.00 |
         |  35.29 | 100.00 |
---------+--------+--------+
Total           34        3        37
             91.89     8.11   100.00
```

Table 2 of bordetella by rhinitis
Controlling for pmtox=-

bordetella   rhinitis

```
Frequency|
Percent  |
Row Pct  |
Col Pct  |+        |-        |  Total
---------+--------+--------+
+        |      5 |     11 |      16
         |  16.13 |  35.48 |   51.61
         |  31.25 |  68.75 |
         |  50.00 |  52.38 |
---------+--------+--------+
-        |      5 |     10 |      15
         |  16.13 |  32.26 |   48.39
         |  33.33 |  66.67 |
         |  50.00 |  47.62 |
---------+--------+--------+
Total           10       21        31
             32.26    67.74   100.00
```

The FREQ Procedure

Summary Statistics for bordetella by rhinitis
Controlling for pmtox

```
Cochran-Mantel-Haenszel Statistics (Based on Table Scores)

Statistic    Alternative Hypothesis    DF      Value      Prob
-------------------------------------------------------------
    1        Nonzero Correlation        1      1.0828    0.2981
    2        Row Mean Scores Differ     1      1.0828    0.2981
    3        General Association        1      1.0828    0.2981


        Estimates of the Common Relative Risk (Row1/Row2)

        Type of Study     Method                    Value
        ------------------------------------------------------
        Case-Control      Mantel-Haenszel          1.9145
           (Odds Ratio)   Logit **                 1.5255

        Cohort            Mantel-Haenszel          1.1670
           (Col1 Risk)    Logit                    1.2293

        Cohort            Mantel-Haenszel          0.7664
           (Col2 Risk)    Logit **                 0.9669

    Type of Study     Method               95% Confidence Limits
    -----------------------------------------------------------
    Case-Control      Mantel-Haenszel      0.5377        6.8166
       (Odds Ratio)   Logit **             0.3954        5.8857

    Cohort            Mantel-Haenszel      0.8561        1.5907
       (Col1 Risk)    Logit                0.9616        1.5715

    Cohort            Mantel-Haenszel      0.4642        1.2653
       (Col2 Risk)    Logit **             0.5981        1.5630

** These logit estimators use a correction of 0.5 in every cell
   of those tables that contain a zero.


                    Breslow-Day Test for
                 Homogeneity of the Odds Ratios
                 ------------------------------
                 Chi-Square             3.6025
                 DF                          1
                 Pr > ChiSq             0.0577


              Total Sample Size = 68
```

The GENMOD Procedure

Model Information

Data Set   WORK.A
Distribution   Binomial
Link Function   Logit
Dependent Variable   rhinitis
Scale Weight Variable   number
Observations Used   7
Missing Values   1

Class Level Information

Class	Levels	Values
bordetella	2	+ -
pmtox	2	+ -

Response Profile

Ordered Value	rhinitis	Total Frequency
1	+	44
2	-	24

PROC GENMOD is modeling the probability that rhinitis='+'. One way to change this to model the probability that rhinitis='-' is to specify the DESCENDING option in the PROC statement.

Criteria For Assessing Goodness Of Fit

Criterion	DF	Value	Value/DF
Deviance	4	58.6913	14.6728
Scaled Deviance	4	58.6913	14.6728
Pearson Chi-Square	4	60.0183	15.0046
Scaled Pearson X2	4	60.0183	15.0046
Log Likelihood		-29.3457	

Algorithm converged.

Analysis Of Parameter Estimates

Parameter		DF	Estimate	Standard Error	Wald 95% Confidence Limits		Chi- Square
Intercept		1	-1.1209	0.5459	-2.1908	-0.0510	4.22
bordetella	+	1	0.6925	0.6613	-0.6037	1.9887	1.10
bordetella	-	0	0.0000	0.0000	0.0000	0.0000	.
pmtox	+	1	3.1862	0.7243	1.7666	4.6057	19.35
pmtox	-	0	0.0000	0.0000	0.0000	0.0000	.
Scale		0	1.0000	0.0000	1.0000	1.0000	

Analysis Of Parameter
Estimates

Parameter		Pr > ChiSq
Intercept		0.0400
bordetella	+	0.2950
bordetella	-	.
pmtox	+	<.0001
pmtox	-	.
Scale		

NOTE: The scale parameter was held fixed.

LR Statistics For Type 3 Analysis

Source	DF	Chi- Square	Pr > ChiSq
bordetella	1	1.12	0.2904
pmtox	1	28.09	<.0001

Example 13.16

Program

```
data sows;
  set c.sows;
  still_born='-stillborn';
  if stillborn>0 then still_born='+stillborn';
  if parity>1 then paritygrp='More than one';
  if parity=1 then paritygrp='One';

proc freq data=sows;
 tables paritygrp*still_born / relrisk chisq;

proc freq data=sows;
 tables farrowmonth*paritygrp*still_born / relrisk cmh chisq;
run;
```

Output

```
                    The FREQ Procedure

            Table of paritygrp by still_born

        paritygrp        still_born

        Frequency      |
        Percent        |
        Row Pct        |
        Col Pct        |+stillbo|-stillbo|  Total
                       |rn      |rn      |
        ---------------+--------+--------+
        More than one  |    103 |     78 |    181
                       |  27.18 |  20.58 |  47.76
                       |  56.91 |  43.09 |
                       |  55.98 |  40.00 |
        ---------------+--------+--------+
        One            |     81 |    117 |    198
                       |  21.37 |  30.87 |  52.24
                       |  40.91 |  59.09 |
                       |  44.02 |  60.00 |
        ---------------+--------+--------+
        Total               184      195      379
                          48.55    51.45   100.00


        Statistics for Table of paritygrp by still_born

Statistic                         DF       Value      Prob
-----------------------------------------------------------
Chi-Square                         1      9.6874     0.0019
Likelihood Ratio Chi-Square        1      9.7268     0.0018
Continuity Adj. Chi-Square         1      9.0576     0.0026
Mantel-Haenszel Chi-Square         1      9.6618     0.0019
Phi Coefficient                           0.1599
Contingency Coefficient                   0.1579
Cramer's V                                0.1599


                  Fisher's Exact Test
          -----------------------------------
          Cell (1,1) Frequency (F)        103
          Left-sided Pr <= F           0.9994
          Right-sided Pr >= F          0.0013

          Table Probability (P)     6.491E-04
          Two-sided Pr <= P            0.0020
```

```
                Estimates of the Relative Risk (Row1/Row2)

Type of Study                     Value         95% Confidence Limits
-------------------------------------------------------------------
Case-Control (Odds Ratio)        1.9074          1.2679      2.8696
Cohort (Col1 Risk)               1.3910          1.1276      1.7161
Cohort (Col2 Risk)               0.7293          0.5949      0.8940

                         Sample Size = 379
                         The FREQ Procedure

                   Table 1 of paritygrp by still_born
                      Controlling for farrowmonth=1

              paritygrp        still_born

              Frequency    |
              Percent      |
              Row Pct      |
              Col Pct      |+stillbo|-stillbo|  Total
                           |rn      |rn      |
              -------------+--------+--------+
              More than one|    11 |      9 |     20
                           |  45.83 |  37.50 |  83.33
                           |  55.00 |  45.00 |
                           |  91.67 |  75.00 |
              -------------+--------+--------+
              One          |     1 |      3 |      4
                           |   4.17 |  12.50 |  16.67
                           |  25.00 |  75.00 |
                           |   8.33 |  25.00 |
              -------------+--------+--------+
              Total             12       12       24
                              50.00    50.00   100.00


          Statistics for Table 1 of paritygrp by still_born
                      Controlling for farrowmonth=1

     Statistic                          DF      Value        Prob
     ---------------------------------------------------------------
     Chi-Square                          1      1.2000      0.2733
     Likelihood Ratio Chi-Square         1      1.2468      0.2642
     Continuity Adj. Chi-Square          1      0.3000      0.5839
     Mantel-Haenszel Chi-Square          1      1.1500      0.2835
     Phi Coefficient                            0.2236
     Contingency Coefficient                    0.2182
     Cramer's V                                 0.2236

     WARNING: 50% of the cells have expected counts less
              than 5. Chi-Square may not be a valid test.
```

```
                     Fisher's Exact Test
          ----------------------------------
          Cell (1,1) Frequency (F)          11
          Left-sided Pr <= F           0.9534
          Right-sided Pr >= F          0.2950

          Table Probability (P)        0.2484
          Two-sided Pr <= P            0.5901


         Estimates of the Relative Risk (Row1/Row2)

Type of Study                  Value        95% Confidence Limits
------------------------------------------------------------------
Case-Control (Odds Ratio)     3.6667        0.3233        41.5901
Cohort (Col1 Risk)            2.2000        0.3850        12.5725
Cohort (Col2 Risk)            0.6000        0.2849         1.2637

                    Sample Size = 24


               Table 2 of paritygrp by still_born
                 Controlling for farrowmonth=2

          paritygrp         still_born

          Frequency      |
          Percent        |
          Row Pct        |
          Col Pct        |+stillbo|-stillbo|  Total
                         |rn      |rn      |
          --------------+--------+--------+
          More than one |    12  |     8  |    20
                        |  40.00 |  26.67 | 66.67
                        |  60.00 |  40.00 |
                        |  66.67 |  66.67 |
          --------------+--------+--------+
          One           |     6  |     4  |    10
                        |  20.00 |  13.33 | 33.33
                        |  60.00 |  40.00 |
                        |  33.33 |  33.33 |
          --------------+--------+--------+
          Total               18       12       30
                           60.00    40.00   100.00
```

```
          Statistics for Table 2 of paritygrp by still_born
                    Controlling for farrowmonth=2

     Statistic                        DF        Value        Prob
     ------------------------------------------------------------
     Chi-Square                       1        0.0000       1.0000
     Likelihood Ratio Chi-Square      1        0.0000       1.0000
     Continuity Adj. Chi-Square       1        0.0000       1.0000
     Mantel-Haenszel Chi-Square       1        0.0000       1.0000
     Phi Coefficient                           0.0000
     Contingency Coefficient                   0.0000
     Cramer's V                                0.0000

        WARNING: 25% of the cells have expected counts less
                 than 5. Chi-Square may not be a valid test.


                    Fisher's Exact Test
              -------------------------------
              Cell (1,1) Frequency (F)          12
              Left-sided Pr <= F              0.6559
              Right-sided Pr >= F             0.6500

              Table Probability (P)           0.3058
              Two-sided Pr <= P               1.0000


          Estimates of the Relative Risk (Row1/Row2)

     Type of Study                 Value      95% Confidence Limits
     ------------------------------------------------------------
     Case-Control (Odds Ratio)    1.0000      0.2124      4.7091
     Cohort (Col1 Risk)           1.0000      0.5381      1.8585
     Cohort (Col2 Risk)           1.0000      0.3947      2.5337

                    Sample Size = 30
```

```
        Table 3 of paritygrp by still_born
          Controlling for farrowmonth=3

    paritygrp         still_born

    Frequency    |
    Percent      |
    Row Pct      |
    Col Pct      |+stillbo|-stillbo|  Total
                 |rn      |rn      |
    -------------+--------+--------+
    More than one|     26 |     27 |     53
                 |  26.80 |  27.84 |  54.64
                 |  49.06 |  50.94 |
                 |  65.00 |  47.37 |
    -------------+--------+--------+
    One          |     14 |     30 |     44
                 |  14.43 |  30.93 |  45.36
                 |  31.82 |  68.18 |
                 |  35.00 |  52.63 |
    -------------+--------+--------+
    Total              40       57       97
                    41.24    58.76   100.00


    Statistics for Table 3 of paritygrp by still_born
            Controlling for farrowmonth=3
```

Statistic	DF	Value	Prob
Chi-Square	1	2.9482	0.0860
Likelihood Ratio Chi-Square	1	2.9778	0.0844
Continuity Adj. Chi-Square	1	2.2797	0.1311
Mantel-Haenszel Chi-Square	1	2.9178	0.0876
Phi Coefficient		0.1743	
Contingency Coefficient		0.1717	
Cramer's V		0.1743	

```
                Fisher's Exact Test
        -----------------------------------
        Cell (1,1) Frequency (F)        26
        Left-sided Pr <= F          0.9734
        Right-sided Pr >= F         0.0651

        Table Probability (P)       0.0385
        Two-sided Pr <= P           0.1006
```

Estimates of the Relative Risk (Row1/Row2)

Type of Study	Value	95% Confidence Limits	
Case-Control (Odds Ratio)	2.0635	0.8979	4.7424
Cohort (Col1 Risk)	1.5418	0.9238	2.5732
Cohort (Col2 Risk)	0.7472	0.5358	1.0419

Sample Size = 97

Table 4 of paritygrp by still_born
Controlling for farrowmonth=4

paritygrp   still_born

Frequency Percent Row Pct Col Pct	+stillbo rn	-stillbo rn	Total
More than one	15 21.13 45.45 50.00	18 25.35 54.55 43.90	33 46.48
One	15 21.13 39.47 50.00	23 32.39 60.53 56.10	38 53.52
Total	30 42.25	41 57.75	71 100.00

Statistics for Table 4 of paritygrp by still_born
Controlling for farrowmonth=4

Statistic	DF	Value	Prob
Chi-Square	1	0.2589	0.6109
Likelihood Ratio Chi-Square	1	0.2589	0.6109
Continuity Adj. Chi-Square	1	0.0718	0.7887
Mantel-Haenszel Chi-Square	1	0.2553	0.6134
Phi Coefficient		0.0604	
Contingency Coefficient		0.0603	
Cramer's V		0.0604	

```
                 Fisher's Exact Test
          ---------------------------------
          Cell (1,1) Frequency (F)           15
          Left-sided Pr <= F             0.7732
          Right-sided Pr >= F            0.3942

          Table Probability (P)          0.1674
          Two-sided Pr <= P              0.6379


          Estimates of the Relative Risk (Row1/Row2)

Type of Study                   Value      95% Confidence Limits
-----------------------------------------------------------------
Case-Control (Odds Ratio)       1.2778       0.4968       3.2868
Cohort (Col1 Risk)              1.1515       0.6691       1.9817
Cohort (Col2 Risk)              0.9012       0.6019       1.3493

                     Sample Size = 71


               Table 5 of paritygrp by still_born
                 Controlling for farrowmonth=5

          paritygrp        still_born

          Frequency     |
          Percent       |
          Row Pct       |
          Col Pct       |+stillbo|-stillbo|  Total
                        |rn      |rn      |
          --------------+--------+--------+
          More than one |     24 |     12 |     36
                        |  33.33 |  16.67 |  50.00
                        |  66.67 |  33.33 |
                        |  60.00 |  37.50 |
          --------------+--------+--------+
          One           |     16 |     20 |     36
                        |  22.22 |  27.78 |  50.00
                        |  44.44 |  55.56 |
                        |  40.00 |  62.50 |
          --------------+--------+--------+
          Total               40       32       72
                            55.56    44.44   100.00
```

```
         Statistics for Table 5 of paritygrp by still_born
                  Controlling for farrowmonth=5

Statistic                            DF      Value      Prob
------------------------------------------------------------
Chi-Square                           1      3.6000     0.0578
Likelihood Ratio Chi-Square          1      3.6322     0.0567
Continuity Adj. Chi-Square           1      2.7563     0.0969
Mantel-Haenszel Chi-Square           1      3.5500     0.0595
Phi Coefficient                             0.2236
Contingency Coefficient                     0.2182
Cramer's V                                  0.2236

                    Fisher's Exact Test
              ---------------------------------
              Cell (1,1) Frequency (F)        24
              Left-sided Pr <= F          0.9840
              Right-sided Pr >= F         0.0481

              Table Probability (P)       0.0321
              Two-sided Pr <= P           0.0962

         Estimates of the Relative Risk (Row1/Row2)
Type of Study                     Value      95% Confidence Limits
-----------------------------------------------------------------
Case-Control (Odds Ratio)        2.5000      0.9619        6.4978
Cohort (Col1 Risk)               1.5000      0.9737        2.3108
Cohort (Col2 Risk)               0.6000      0.3473        1.0364

                    Sample Size = 72

          Table 6 of paritygrp by still_born
             Controlling for farrowmonth=6

         paritygrp        still_born

         Frequency   |
         Percent     |
         Row Pct     |
         Col Pct     |+stillbo|-stillbo|  Total
                     |rn      |rn      |
         ------------+--------+--------+
         More than one|     15 |      4 |     19
                     |  17.65 |   4.71 |  22.35
                     |  78.95 |  21.05 |
                     |  34.09 |   9.76 |
         ------------+--------+--------+
         One         |     29 |     37 |     66
                     |  34.12 |  43.53 |  77.65
                     |  43.94 |  56.06 |
                     |  65.91 |  90.24 |
         ------------+--------+--------+
         Total            44       41        85
                       51.76    48.24    100.00
```

```
       Statistics for Table 6 of paritygrp by still_born
                Controlling for farrowmonth=6

       Statistic                      DF       Value       Prob
       ------------------------------------------------------------
       Chi-Square                      1       7.2413      0.0071
       Likelihood Ratio Chi-Square     1       7.6490      0.0057
       Continuity Adj. Chi-Square      1       5.9071      0.0151
       Mantel-Haenszel Chi-Square      1       7.1561      0.0075
       Phi Coefficient                         0.2919
       Contingency Coefficient                 0.2802
       Cramer's V                              0.2919


                      Fisher's Exact Test
              ------------------------------------
              Cell (1,1) Frequency (F)          15
              Left-sided Pr <= F            0.9988
              Right-sided Pr >= F           0.0067

              Table Probability (P)        0.0055
              Two-sided Pr <= P            0.0090


          Estimates of the Relative Risk (Row1/Row2)

Type of Study                   Value       95% Confidence Limits
------------------------------------------------------------------
Case-Control (Odds Ratio)      4.7845        1.4334        15.9695
Cohort (Col1 Risk)             1.7967        1.2560         2.5702
Cohort (Col2 Risk)             0.3755        0.1532         0.9205

                      Sample Size = 85
                      The FREQ Procedure

          Summary Statistics for paritygrp by still_born
                 Controlling for farrowmonth

      Cochran-Mantel-Haenszel Statistics (Based on Table Scores)

   Statistic    Alternative Hypothesis    DF      Value       Prob
   ---------------------------------------------------------------
       1        Nonzero Correlation        1      11.2337     0.0008
       2        Row Mean Scores Differ     1      11.2337     0.0008
       3        General Association        1      11.2337     0.0008
```

```
            Estimates of the Common Relative Risk (Row1/Row2)

         Type of Study      Method                      Value
         ---------------------------------------------------------
         Case-Control       Mantel-Haenszel            2.1211
            (Odds Ratio)    Logit                      2.0837

         Cohort             Mantel-Haenszel            1.4528
            (Col1 Risk)     Logit                      1.4799

         Cohort             Mantel-Haenszel            0.6959
            (Col2 Risk)     Logit                      0.7310

     Type of Study      Method              95% Confidence Limits
     ---------------------------------------------------------------
     Case-Control       Mantel-Haenszel        1.3642        3.2978
        (Odds Ratio)    Logit                  1.3284        3.2684

     Cohort             Mantel-Haenszel        1.1697        1.8043
        (Col1 Risk)     Logit                  1.2030        1.8207

     Cohort             Mantel-Haenszel        0.5586        0.8669
        (Col2 Risk)     Logit                  0.5927        0.9016


                    Breslow-Day Test for
                 Homogeneity of the Odds Ratios
                 ------------------------------
                 Chi-Square               4.1558
                 DF                            5
                 Pr > ChiSq               0.5272


                 Total Sample Size = 379
```

Example 13.17

Program

```
data a;
  input conv$ eiafoss$ number;
  cards;
  + + 32
  + - 21
  - + 4
  - - 4
  ;

proc freq data=a;
  tables conv*eiafoss;
  exact agree;
  weight number;
run;
```

Output

```
                    The FREQ Procedure
               Table of conv by eiafoss

          conv        eiafoss

          Frequency|
          Percent  |
          Row Pct  |
          Col Pct  |+        |-        |     Total
          ---------+--------+--------+
          +        |      32 |      21 |        53
                   |   52.46 |   34.43 |     86.89
                   |   60.38 |   39.62 |
                   |   88.89 |   84.00 |
          ---------+--------+--------+
          -        |       4 |       4 |         8
                   |    6.56 |    6.56 |     13.11
                   |   50.00 |   50.00 |
                   |   11.11 |   16.00 |
          ---------+--------+--------+
          Total           36       25        61
                       59.02    40.98    100.00


        Statistics for Table of conv by eiafoss

                   McNemar's Test
          ------------------------------------
          Statistic (S)              11.5600
          DF                               1
          Asymptotic Pr >  S          0.0007
          Exact      Pr >= S      9.105E-04

              Simple Kappa Coefficient
          ------------------------------------
          Kappa (K)                   0.0546
          ASE                         0.1005
          95% Lower Conf Limit       -0.1424
          95% Upper Conf Limit        0.2515

              Test of H0: Kappa = 0

          ASE under H0                0.0981
          Z                           0.5563
          One-sided Pr >   Z          0.2890
          Two-sided Pr > |Z|          0.5780

          Exact Test
          One-sided Pr >=  K          0.4260
          Two-sided Pr >= |K|         0.7056

                Sample Size = 61
```

Example 13.18

Program

```
data udder;
   do clinician1=0 to 4 by 1;
      do clinician2=0 to 4 by 1;
         input number @@;
         output;
      end;
   end;
   cards;
   7 3 2 0 0
   0 1 0 0 0
   1 0 0 1 0
   0 0 1 0 0
   1 0 0 0 3
   ;

proc freq data=udder;
   tables clinician1*clinician2;
   exact agree;
   weight number;
run;
```

Output

```
                         The FREQ Procedure

                  Table of clinician1 by clinician2

        clinician1      clinician2

        Frequency|
        Percent  |
        Row Pct  |
        Col Pct  |       0|       1|       2|       3|       4|  Total
        ---------+--------+--------+--------+--------+--------+
              0  |     7  |     3  |     2  |     0  |     0  |    12
                 |  35.00 |  15.00 |  10.00 |   0.00 |   0.00 |  60.00
                 |  58.33 |  25.00 |  16.67 |   0.00 |   0.00 |
                 |  77.78 |  75.00 |  66.67 |   0.00 |   0.00 |
        ---------+--------+--------+--------+--------+--------+
              1  |     0  |     1  |     0  |     0  |     0  |     1
                 |   0.00 |   5.00 |   0.00 |   0.00 |   0.00 |   5.00
                 |   0.00 | 100.00 |   0.00 |   0.00 |   0.00 |
                 |   0.00 |  25.00 |   0.00 |   0.00 |   0.00 |
        ---------+--------+--------+--------+--------+--------+
              2  |     1  |     0  |     0  |     1  |     0  |     2
                 |   5.00 |   0.00 |   0.00 |   5.00 |   0.00 |  10.00
                 |  50.00 |   0.00 |   0.00 |  50.00 |   0.00 |
                 |  11.11 |   0.00 |   0.00 | 100.00 |   0.00 |
        ---------+--------+--------+--------+--------+--------+
              3  |     0  |     0  |     1  |     0  |     0  |     1
                 |   0.00 |   0.00 |   5.00 |   0.00 |   0.00 |   5.00
                 |   0.00 |   0.00 | 100.00 |   0.00 |   0.00 |
                 |   0.00 |   0.00 |  33.33 |   0.00 |   0.00 |
        ---------+--------+--------+--------+--------+--------+
              4  |     1  |     0  |     0  |     0  |     3  |     4
                 |   5.00 |   0.00 |   0.00 |   0.00 |  15.00 |  20.00
                 |  25.00 |   0.00 |   0.00 |   0.00 |  75.00 |
                 |  11.11 |   0.00 |   0.00 |   0.00 | 100.00 |
        ---------+--------+--------+--------+--------+--------+
        Total          9        4        3        1        3       20
                   45.00    20.00    15.00     5.00    15.00   100.00


              Statistics for Table of clinician1 by clinician2

                          Test of Symmetry
                      ----------------------
                      Statistic (S)     4.3333
                      DF                    10
                      Pr > S            0.9311
```

```
            Simple Kappa Coefficient
       ---------------------------------
       Kappa (K)                  0.3309
       ASE                        0.1480
       95% Lower Conf Limit       0.0408
       95% Upper Conf Limit       0.6209

           Test of H0: Kappa = 0

       ASE under H0               0.1218
       Z                          2.7157
       One-sided Pr >  Z          0.0033
       Two-sided Pr > |Z|         0.0066

       Exact Test
       One-sided Pr >=  K         0.0130
       Two-sided Pr >= |K|        0.0154


           Weighted Kappa Coefficient
       ---------------------------------
       Weighted Kappa (K)         0.5327
       ASE                        0.1611
       95% Lower Conf Limit       0.2169
       95% Upper Conf Limit       0.8485

       Test of H0: Weighted Kappa = 0

       ASE under H0               0.1705
       Z                          3.1241
       One-sided Pr >  Z          0.0009
       Two-sided Pr > |Z|         0.0018

       Exact Test
       One-sided Pr >=  K         0.0026
       Two-sided Pr >= |K|        0.0026

            Sample Size = 20
```

Example 13.19

Program

```
data bp;
  set c.bpcats;
  diffsap = sapc - saps;
  meansap = (saps + sapc)/2;

proc univariate data=bp noprint;
  var diffsap;
  output out=stat n=n mean=meandiff std=stddiff;
data stat;
  set stat;
  lower=meandiff-1.96*stddiff;
  upper=meandiff+1.96*stddiff;
proc print;
run;

goptions reset=all ftext=swiss;

axis1 label=(h=1.5 'Mean blood pressure')
      value=(h=1.3)
  ;
axis2 label=(h=1.5 angle=90
      'Difference between direct and indirect blood pressure')
      value=(h=1.3)
      order=(-40 to 40 by 10)
  ;
axis3 label=none
      value=none
    order=(-40 to 40 by 10)
    minor=none
    major=none
  ;
legend1 label=none
        value=(h=1.3)
  ;
symbol1 h=2 v=dot c=black;
symbol2 h=2 v=circle c=black;
symbol3 h=2 v=star c=black;
symbol4 h=2 v=dot c=black;
symbol5 h=2 v=circle c=black;
symbol6 h=2 v=star c=black;

proc gplot data=bp;
  plot diffsap*meansap=level
      / haxis=axis1 vaxis=axis2 legend=legend1 vref=-11.94 lvref=1;
  plot2 diffsap*meansap=level
      / vref=-27.7 3.81 lvref=3 vaxis=axis3 nolegend;

run;
```

Output

Obs	n	meandiff	stddiff	lower	upper
1	18	-11.9444	8.04014	-27.7031	3.81422

APPENDIX F: R-CODE AND OUTPUT FOR THE EXAMPLES IN CHAPTER 13

Nils Toft

In this appendix we give the R-code for the examples in Chapter 13. R (R Development Core Team, 2004) is a statistical computer program, which can be downloaded and used for free under the General Public Licence (GPL). In the examples R-code is preceded by a '>', while output is not. If a command uses more than one line it is continued on the next line where a '+' indicates that it is a continuation from the previous line. The R-code and data sets used in the examples can be found at www.itve.dk. For the different plots produced by the R code, we refer to the examples in Chapter 13.

Example 13.2

```
> sowdata <- read.csv('sows.csv',header=T)
> attach(sowdata)
> avg.weight <- weanwgt/weanno
> t.test(avg.weight,mu=7.0)

One-sample t-test

data:  avg.weight
t = 3.7481, df = 378, p-value = 0.0002060
alternative hypothesis: true mean is not equal to 7
95 percent confidence interval:
7.126757 7.406512
sample estimates:
mean of x
7.266635
```

Example 13.3

```
> milk <- read.csv('milk1.csv',header=T)
> milk$parity <- factor(milk$parity)
> milk$breed <- factor(milk$breed)
> sem <- function(x) { return(sd(x)/sqrt(length(x)));}
> attach(milk)
> summary(kgmilk1)
   Min. 1st Qu.  Median    Mean 3rd Qu.    Max.
   4.10   17.75   21.90   21.30   25.20   43.10
> sd(kgmilk1)
[1] 6.136921
> length(kgmilk1)
[1] 111
> sem(kgmilk1)
[1] 0.5824908
>
> tapply(kgmilk1,breed,summary)
$"2"
   Min. 1st Qu.  Median    Mean 3rd Qu.    Max.
   4.10   18.35   21.90   22.02   26.10   43.10

$"8"
   Min. 1st Qu.  Median    Mean 3rd Qu.    Max.
   4.80   17.48   22.00   21.03   24.85   31.30


> tapply(kgmilk1,breed,sd)
       2        8
7.772062 5.405828
> tapply(kgmilk1,breed,sem)
        2         8
1.3959035 0.6043899
> tapply(kgmilk1,breed,length)
  2   8
 31  80
>
>
> tapply(kgmilk1,parity,summary)
$"1"
   Min. 1st Qu.  Median    Mean 3rd Qu.    Max.
   7.50   15.60   18.00   18.56   22.20   28.20

$"2"
   Min. 1st Qu.  Median    Mean 3rd Qu.    Max.
   4.80   18.95   22.60   21.98   26.30   31.30

$"3"
   Min. 1st Qu.  Median    Mean 3rd Qu.    Max.
   4.10   21.18   24.35   21.88   25.80   28.60

$"4"
   Min. 1st Qu.  Median    Mean 3rd Qu.    Max.
   9.10   19.05   23.10   23.79   28.83   43.10
```

```
> tapply(kgmilk1,parity,sd)
       1        2        3        4
4.949996 5.562071 6.180581 7.376727
> tapply(kgmilk1,parity,sem)
        1         2         3         4
0.8616837 0.9270118 1.3820199 1.5727235
> tapply(kgmilk1,parity,length)
 1  2  3  4
33 36 20 22
>
> t.test(kgmilk1~breed)

Welch two-sample t-test

data:  kgmilk1 by breed
t = 0.6529, df = 41.745, p-value = 0.5174
alternative hypothesis: true difference in means is not equal to 0
95 percent confidence interval:
 -2.077213  4.063423
sample estimates:
mean in group 2 mean in group 8
      22.01935        21.02625


> t.test(kgmilk1~breed,var.equal=T)

Two-sample t-test

data:  kgmilk1 by breed
t = 0.7635, df = 109, p-value = 0.4468
alternative hypothesis: true difference in means is not equal to 0
95 percent confidence interval:
 -1.585043  3.571252
sample estimates:
mean in group 2 mean in group 8
      22.01935        21.02625


> var.test(kgmilk1~breed)

F test to compare two variances

data:  kgmilk1 by breed
F = 2.067, num df = 30, denom df = 79, p-value = 0.01111
alternative hypothesis: true ratio of variances is not equal to 1
95 percent confidence interval:
 1.177995 3.938268
sample estimates:
ratio of variances
          2.067036
```

Example 13.4

```
> milk <- read.csv('milk1.csv',header=T)
> attach(milk)
> t.test(kgmilk1,kgmilk2,paired=T)

Paired t-test

data:  kgmilk1 and kgmilk2
t = 1.5026, df = 103, p-value = 0.136
alternative hypothesis: true difference in means is not equal to 0
95 percent confidence interval:
 -0.4866195  3.5289271
sample estimates:
mean of the differences
              1.521154
```

Example 13.5

```
> milk <- read.csv('milk1.csv',header=T)
> milk$parity <- factor(milk$parity)
> milk$breed <- factor(milk$breed)
> model <- lm(kgmilk1~parity+breed,data=milk)
> anova(model)

Analysis of variance table

Response: kgmilk1
           Df Sum Sq Mean Sq  F value   Pr(>F)
parity      3  407.4   135.8   4.0015 0.009636 **
breed       1  138.0   138.0   4.0656 0.046294 *
Residuals 106 3597.4    33.9
---
Signif. codes:  0 '***' 0.001 '**' 0.01 '*' 0.05 '.' 0.1 ' ' 1
> #load extra function
> library(gregmisc)
> #Least squares means of parity
> estimable(model,c(1,0,0,0,0.5))
              Estimate Std. Error  t value  DF Pr(>|t|)
(1 0 0 0 0.5) 16.57187   1.414649 11.71448 106        0
> estimable(model,c(1,1,0,0,0.5))
              Estimate Std. Error  t value  DF Pr(>|t|)
(1 1 0 0 0.5) 19.97835   1.387811 14.39559 106        0
> estimable(model,c(1,0,1,0,0.5))
              Estimate Std. Error  t value  DF Pr(>|t|)
(1 0 1 0 0.5) 21.45659   1.319465 16.26158 106        0
> estimable(model,c(1,0,0,1,0.5))
              Estimate Std. Error  t value  DF Pr(>|t|)
(1 0 0 1 0.5) 25.71549   1.566426 16.41666 106        0
> #Least squares means of breed
> estimable(model,c(1,0.25,0.25,0.25,0))
                    Estimate Std. Error  t value  DF Pr(>|t|)
(1 0.25 0.25 0.25 0) 18.81353   1.473311 12.76956 106        0
```

```
> estimable(model,c(1,0.25,0.25,0.25,1))
                       Estimate Std. Error  t value  DF Pr(>|t|)
(1 0.25 0.25 0.25 1) 23.04762  0.9357468 24.63019 106        0
>
> # Pairwise comparison
> summary(model)

Call:
lm(formula = kgmilk1 ~ parity + breed, data = milk)

Residuals:
     Min       1Q   Median       3Q      Max
-17.2954  -3.3175   0.6046   3.8031  19.5015

Coefficients:
            Estimate Std. Error t value Pr(>|t|)
(Intercept)   14.455      2.275   6.354 5.36e-09 ***
parity2        3.406      1.404   2.426 0.016942 *
parity3        4.885      1.824   2.678 0.008595 **
parity4        9.144      2.517   3.632 0.000435 ***
breed8         4.234      2.100   2.016 0.046294 *
---
Signif. codes:  0 '***' 0.001 '**' 0.01 '*' 0.05 '.' 0.1 ' ' 1

Residual standard error: 5.826 on 106 degrees of freedom
Multiple R-Squared: 0.1316,     Adjusted R-squared: 0.09888
F-statistic: 4.018 on 4 and 106 DF,  p-value: 0.004495

> # parity = 2 vs parity = 3
> fit.contrast(model,"parity",c(0,-1,1,0))
                       Estimate Std. Error    t value   Pr(>|t|)
parity c=( 0 -1 1 0 ) 1.478242   1.802928 0.8199119 0.4141062
> # parity = 2 vs parity >3
> fit.contrast(model,"parity",c(0,-1,0,1))
                       Estimate Std. Error  t value    Pr(>|t|)
parity c=( 0 -1 0 1 ) 5.737143   2.504535 2.290702 0.02395942
> # parity = 3 vs parity >3
> fit.contrast(model,"parity",c(0,0,-1,1))
                       Estimate Std. Error  t value Pr(>|t|)
parity c=( 0 0 -1 1 ) 4.258901   2.143723 1.986685 0.049538
```

Example 13.6

```
> colic <- read.csv('colic.csv',header=T)
> round(cor(colic,use="pairwise.complete",method="pearson"),3)
           SBE    PCV horseid   temp  pulse    crt
SBE      1.000 -0.269   0.130  0.022 -0.402 -0.425
PCV     -0.269  1.000  -0.020  0.072  0.561  0.530
horseid  0.130 -0.020   1.000 -0.009  0.006 -0.054
temp     0.022  0.072  -0.009  1.000  0.170  0.037
pulse   -0.402  0.561   0.006  0.170  1.000  0.592
crt     -0.425  0.530  -0.054  0.037  0.592  1.000
```

```
> round(cor(colic,use="pairwise.complete",method="spearman"),3)
            SBE     PCV horseid    temp   pulse     crt
SBE       1.000   0.081   0.007   0.056  -0.316  -0.246
PCV       0.081   1.000  -0.124   0.069   0.295   0.323
horseid   0.007  -0.124   1.000  -0.088  -0.002  -0.037
temp      0.056   0.069  -0.088   1.000   0.137   0.062
pulse    -0.316   0.295  -0.002   0.137   1.000   0.488
crt      -0.246   0.323  -0.037   0.062   0.488   1.000
> # Make plot of pairwise variables
> pairs(colic)
```

Example 13.7

```
> colic <- read.csv('colic.csv',header=T)
> attach(colic)
> reg <- lm(pulse~PCV)
> summary(reg)

Call:
lm(formula = pulse ~ PCV)

Residuals:
    Min      1Q  Median      3Q     Max
-36.276 -11.783  -3.696  10.275  56.101

Coefficients:
            Estimate Std. Error t value Pr(>|t|)
(Intercept)  9.78068    3.77830   2.589  0.00998 **
PCV          1.27542    0.09356  13.631  < 2e-16 ***
---
Signif. codes:  0 '***' 0.001 '**' 0.01 '*' 0.05 '.' 0.1 ' ' 1

Residual standard error: 16.95 on 405 degrees of freedom
Multiple R-Squared: 0.3145,     Adjusted R-squared: 0.3128
F-statistic: 185.8 on 1 and 405 DF,   p-value: < 2.2e-16

> #Make plot
> plot(PCV,pulse)
> abline(reg)
```

Example 13.8

```
> prop.test(110,700,0.1)

One-sample proportions test with continuity correction

data:  110 out of 700, null probability 0.1
X-squared = 24.7659, df = 1, p-value = 6.473e-07
alternative hypothesis: true p is not equal to 0.1
95 percent confidence interval:
 0.1314016 0.1867253
sample estimates:
       p
0.1571429
> binom.test(110,700,0.1)
```

```
Exact binomial test

data:  110 and 700
number of successes = 110, number of trials = 700, p-value = 2.698e-06
alternative hypothesis: true probability of success is not equal to 0.1
95 percent confidence interval:
 0.1309594 0.1862536
sample estimates:
probability of success
             0.1571429
```

Example 13.9

```
> metritis <- matrix(c(100,400,10,190),byrow=T,nrow=2)
> rownames(metritis) <- c("Holstein","Jersey")
> colnames(metritis) <- c("Positive","Negative")
> chisq.test(metritis)

Pearson's chi-squared test with Yates' continuity correction

data:  metritis
X-squared = 23.1488, df = 1, p-value = 1.499e-06

> chisq.test(metritis)$expected
         Positive Negative
Holstein 78.57143 421.4286
Jersey   31.42857 168.5714
> fisher.test(metritis)

Fisher's exact test for count data

data:  metritis
p-value = 1.371e-07
alternative hypothesis: true odds ratio is not equal to 1
95 percent confidence interval:
  2.402586 10.429514
sample estimates:
odds ratio
  4.742021
```

Example 13.10

```
> turkey <- matrix(c(32,21,4,4),byrow=T,nrow=2)
> rownames(turkey) <- c("Conv.pos","Conv.neg")
> colnames(turkey) <- c("Eiafoss.pos","Eiafoss.neg")
> mcnemar.test(turkey)

McNemar's chi-squared test with continuity correction

data:  turkey
McNemar's chi-squared = 10.24, df = 1, p-value = 0.001374
```

Example 13.11

```
> milk <- read.csv('milk2.csv',header=T)
> milk$breed <- factor(milk$breed)
> milk$scc <-milk$cellcount
> milk$scc[milk$cellcount > 125] <- 1;
> milk$scc[milk$cellcount <= 125] <- 0;
> attach(milk)
> tapply(kgmilk,scc,summary)
$"0"
   Min. 1st Qu.  Median    Mean 3rd Qu.     Max.
   6.80   16.60   20.40   20.73   24.20    43.10

$"1"
   Min. 1st Qu.  Median    Mean 3rd Qu.     Max.
   3.20   14.40   18.80   19.23   23.23    40.20

> tapply(kgmilk,scc,sd)
        0        1
5.848698 6.973620
> tapply(kgmilk,scc,length)
  0   1
540 600
>
> model <- glm(scc~kgmilk,data=milk,family=binomial(link=logit))
> summary(model)

Call:
glm(formula = scc ~ kgmilk, family = binomial(link = logit),
    data = milk)

Deviance Residuals:
    Min      1Q  Median      3Q     Max
-1.4298 -1.2101  0.9637  1.1193  1.4484

Coefficients:
            Estimate Std. Error z value Pr(>|z|)
(Intercept)  0.819109   0.195370   4.193 2.76e-05 ***
kgmilk      -0.035740   0.009306  -3.841 0.000123 ***
---
Signif. codes:  0 '***' 0.001 '**' 0.01 '*' 0.05 '.' 0.1 ' ' 1

(Dispersion parameter for binomial family taken to be 1)

    Null deviance: 1577.2  on 1139  degrees of freedom
Residual deviance: 1562.2  on 1138  degrees of freedom
AIC: 1566.2

Number of Fisher Scoring iterations: 4

> # Make OR for change in 1 kg milk
> exp(ci(model)[2,1:3])
 Estimate  CI lower  CI upper
0.9648915 0.9474340 0.9826706
> # Make OR for change in 5 kg milk
```

```
> exp(ci(model)[2,1:3]*5)
 Estimate  CI lower  CI upper
0.8363582 0.7633871 0.9163044
>
> plot(kgmilk,fitted(model),type="l")
```

Example 13.12

```
> milk <- read.csv('milk2.csv',header=T)
> milk$breed <- factor(milk$breed)
> milk$scc <-milk$cellcount
> milk$scc[milk$cellcount > 125] <- 1;
> milk$scc[milk$cellcount <= 125] <- 0;
> milk$scc <- factor(milk$scc)
> milk$breed <- relevel(milk$breed,ref=4)
> attach(milk)
>
> table(breed,scc)
     scc
breed 0    1
    8 138 127
    1  69  92
    2 222 296
    3 111  85
> prop.table(table(breed,scc),1)
     scc
breed 0         1
    8 0.5207547 0.4792453
    1 0.4285714 0.5714286
    2 0.4285714 0.5714286
    3 0.5663265 0.4336735
>
> model <- glm(scc~breed,data=milk,family=binomial(link=logit))
> summary(model)

Call:
glm(formula = scc ~ breed,
    family = binomial(link = logit), data = milk)

Deviance Residuals:
   Min     1Q Median     3Q    Max
-1.302 -1.302  1.058  1.058  1.293

Coefficients:
            Estimate Std. Error z value Pr(>|z|)
(Intercept) -0.08307    0.12297  -0.676   0.4993
breed1       0.37075    0.20120   1.843   0.0654 .
breed2       0.37075    0.15167   2.444   0.0145 *
breed3      -0.18381    0.18946  -0.970   0.3319
---
Signif. codes:  0 '***' 0.001 '**' 0.01 '*' 0.05 '.' 0.1 ' ' 1

(Dispersion parameter for binomial family taken to be 1)
```

```
    Null deviance: 1577.2  on 1139  degrees of freedom
Residual deviance: 1562.6  on 1136  degrees of freedom
AIC: 1570.6

Number of Fisher Scoring iterations: 4

> library(gregmisc)
> fit.contrast(model,"breed",c(0,-1,1,0))
                          Estimate Std. Error        z value Pr(>|z|)
breed c=( 0 -1 1 0 ) -2.587764e-16  0.1823327 -1.419254e-15        1

> fit.contrast(model,"breed",c(0,-1,0,1))
                        Estimate Std. Error   z value      Pr(>|z|)
breed c=( 0 -1 0 1 ) -0.554561   0.214793 -2.581839 0.009827533
> fit.contrast(model,"breed",c(0,0,-1,1))
                        Estimate Std. Error   z value      Pr(>|z|)
breed c=( 0 0 -1 1 ) -0.554561   0.1692826 -3.275948 0.001053079
> exp(ci(model)[2:4,1:3])
       Estimate  CI lower CI upper
breed1 1.448819 0.9762634 2.150113
breed2 1.448819 1.0759104 1.950977
breed3 0.832092 0.5737634 1.206729
>
> model <- glm(scc~breed + kgmilk,
+data=milk,family=binomial(link=logit))
> summary(model)

Call:
glm(formula = scc ~ breed + kgmilk, family = binomial(link = logit),
    data = milk)

Deviance Residuals:
    Min      1Q   Median      3Q      Max
-1.5940  -1.1732   0.8436   1.1138   1.5986

Coefficients:
            Estimate Std. Error z value Pr(>|z|)
(Intercept)  0.905308   0.239574   3.779 0.000158 ***
breed1       0.275224   0.204062   1.349 0.177426
breed2       0.413513   0.153559   2.693 0.007084 **
breed3      -0.398810   0.195936  -2.035 0.041810 *
kgmilk      -0.047844   0.009939  -4.814 1.48e-06 ***
---
Signif. codes:  0 '***' 0.001 '**' 0.01 '*' 0.05 '.' 0.1 ' ' 1

(Dispersion parameter for binomial family taken to be 1)

    Null deviance: 1577.2  on 1139  degrees of freedom
Residual deviance: 1538.6  on 1135  degrees of freedom
AIC: 1548.6

Number of Fisher Scoring iterations: 4

> fit.contrast(model,"breed",c(0,-1,1,0))
                        Estimate Std. Error   z value  Pr(>|z|)
breed c=( 0 -1 1 0 ) 0.1382896   0.1866907 0.740742 0.4588499
```

```
> fit.contrast(model,"breed",c(0,-1,0,1))
                        Estimate Std. Error    z value      Pr(>|z|)
breed c=( 0 -1 0 1 ) -0.6740334  0.2182884 -3.087811 0.002016367
> fit.contrast(model,"breed",c(0,0,-1,1))
                        Estimate Std. Error    z value      Pr(>|z|)
breed c=( 0 0 -1 1 ) -0.812323   0.1793369 -4.529592 5.909763e-06
> exp(ci(model)[2:4,1:3])
        Estimate  CI lower  CI upper
breed1 1.3168254 0.8823575 1.9652230
breed2 1.5121213 1.1187623 2.0437861
breed3 0.6711185 0.4569198 0.9857312
> exp(ci(model)[5,1:3]*5)
 Estimate  CI lower  CI upper
0.7872401 0.7141074 0.8678624
>
> plot(kgmilk,fitted(model),pch=as.numeric(breed),type="p")
```

Example 13.13

```
> milk <- read.csv('milk1.csv',header=T)
> milk$parity <- factor(milk$parity)
> milk$breed <- factor(milk$breed)
> attach(milk)
> model <- lm(kgmilk1~parity+breed,data=milk)
> anova(model)

Analysis of variance table

Response: kgmilk1
           Df Sum Sq Mean Sq F value   Pr(>F)
parity      3  407.4   135.8  4.0015 0.009636 **
breed       1  138.0   138.0  4.0656 0.046294 *
Residuals 106 3597.4    33.9
---
Signif. codes:  0 '***' 0.001 '**' 0.01 '*' 0.05 '.' 0.1 ' ' 1
>
> qqnorm(model$res)
> qqline(model$res)
>
> hist(model$res,xlab="Residual",main="Histogram",col="yellow")
>
> plot(predict(model),resid(model),
+xlab="Predicted milk yield (kg)",ylab="Residuals")
> abline(h=0)
>
> shapiro.test(model$res)

Shapiro-Wilk normality test

data:  model$res
W = 0.9692, p-value = 0.01132

> ks.test(model$res,"pnorm",mean=mean(model$res),sd=sd(model$res))
```

```
One-sample Kolmogorov-Smirnov test

data:  model$res
D = 0.0697, p-value = 0.6533
alternative hypothesis: two.sided

Warning message:
cannot compute correct p-values with ties in:
ks.test(model$res, "pnorm", mean = mean(model$res), sd = sd(model$res))
>
```

Example 13.15

```
> mhn <- array(c(22,12,0,3,5,5,11,10),
+ dim=c(2,2,2),
+ dimnames=list(
+ bordetella=c("Pos","Neg"),
+ rhinitis=c("Pos","Neg"),
+ pmtox=c("Pos","Neg")))
>
>
> rr.2x2(mhn[,,1])
$RR
[1] 1.25

$U.RR
[1] 1.609903

$L.RR
[1] 0.9705555

> rr.2x2(mhn[,,2])
$RR
[1] 0.9375

$U.RR
[1] 2.599864

$L.RR
[1] 0.3380586

> rr.2x2(mhn[,,1]+mhn[,,2])
$RR
[1] 1.25387

$U.RR
[1] 1.820666

$L.RR
[1] 0.8635247
```

```
>
> rr.mh(mhn)
$RR
[1] 1.166996

$U.RR
[1] 1.450629

$L.RR
[1] 0.9388195

> mantelhaen.test(mhn)

        Mantel-Haenszel chi-squared test with continuity correction

data:  mhn
Mantel-Haenszel X-squared = 0.5183, df = 1, p-value = 0.4716
alternative hypothesis: true common odds ratio is not equal to 1
95 percent confidence interval:
 0.5377024 6.8165885
sample estimates:
common odds ratio
        1.914496


>
> pos.neg <- c('Pos','Neg')
> bordetella <- gl(2,1,4,pos.neg)
> pmtox <- gl(2,2,4,pos.neg)
> n.tot <- c(22,15,16,15)
> n.hyp <- c(22,12,5,5)
> hyp.rhinitis <- cbind(n.hyp,n.tot-n.hyp)
> model <- glm(hyp.rhinitis~bordetella+pmtox,family=binomial(link=logit))
> summary(model)

Call:
glm(formula = hyp.rhinitis ~ bordetella + pmtox,
    family = binomial(link = logit))

Deviance Residuals:
[1]   1.6450  -0.9801  -0.6813   0.7604

Coefficients:
              Estimate Std. Error z value Pr(>|z|)
(Intercept)     2.7578     0.7054   3.910 9.24e-05 ***
bordetellaNeg  -0.6925     0.6613  -1.047    0.295
pmtoxNeg       -3.1862     0.7243  -4.399 1.09e-05 ***
---
Signif. codes:  0 '***' 0.001 '**' 0.01 '*' 0.05 '.' 0.1 ' ' 1

(Dispersion parameter for binomial family taken to be 1)

    Null deviance: 34.3155  on 3  degrees of freedom
Residual deviance:  4.7091  on 1  degrees of freedom
AIC: 19.672

Number of Fisher Scoring iterations: 5
```

Example 13.16

```
> sowdata <- read.csv('sows.csv',header=T)
> attach(sowdata)
>
> still.born <- stillborn
> still.born[stillborn > 0] <- 'Stillborn +'
> still.born[stillborn == 0] <- 'Stillborn -'
> still.born <- relevel(factor(still.born),ref=2)
> paritygrp <- parity
> paritygrp[parity == 1] <- 'One'
> paritygrp[parity > 1] <- 'More than one'
>
> crude <-table(paritygrp,still.born)
> rr.2x2(crude)
$RR
[1] 1.391037

$U.RR
[1] 1.716077

$L.RR
[1] 1.127563

> or.2x2(crude)
$OR
[1] 1.907407

$U.OR
[1] 2.869566

$L.OR
[1] 1.267858

> chisq.test(crude)

Pearson's chi-squared test with Yates' continuity correction

data:  crude
X-squared = 9.0576, df = 1, p-value = 0.002616

> fisher.test(crude)

Fisher's exact test for count data

data:  crude
p-value = 0.002049
alternative hypothesis: true odds ratio is not equal to 1
95 percent confidence interval:
 1.242216 2.930113
sample estimates:
odds ratio
  1.904119
```

```
>
> farrow <- table(paritygrp,still.born,farrowmonth)
> or <- matrix(0,nrow=6,ncol=3)
> for (i in 1:6) {
+ or.tmp <- or.2x2(farrow[,,i])
+ or[i,1] <- or.tmp$L.OR
+ or[i,2] <- or.tmp$OR
+ or[i,3] <- or.tmp$U.OR
+ }
> or
          [,1]      [,2]       [,3]
[1,] 0.3232607 3.666667 41.590105
[2,] 0.2123568 1.000000  4.709057
[3,] 0.8978574 2.063492  4.742401
[4,] 0.4967502 1.277778  3.286795
[5,] 0.9618685 2.500000  6.497770
[6,] 1.4334404 4.784483 15.969464
> rr <- matrix(0,nrow=6,ncol=3)
> for (i in 1:6) {
+ rr.tmp <- rr.2x2(farrow[,,i])
+ rr[i,1] <- rr.tmp$L.RR
+ rr[i,2] <- rr.tmp$RR
+ rr[i,3] <- rr.tmp$U.RR
+ }
> rr
          [,1]      [,2]       [,3]
[1,] 0.3849666 2.200000 12.572520
[2,] 0.5380547 1.000000  1.858547
[3,] 0.9237939 1.541779  2.573174
[4,] 0.6691278 1.151515  1.981665
[5,] 0.9736861 1.500000  2.310806
[6,] 1.2560278 1.796733  2.570206
> rr.mh(farrow)
$RR
[1] 1.452762

$U.RR
[1] 1.806013

$L.RR
[1] 1.168605


> mantelhaen.test(farrow)

Mantel-Haenszel chi-squared test with continuity correction

data:  farrow
Mantel-Haenszel X-squared = 10.5144, df = 1, p-value = 0.001184
alternative hypothesis: true common odds ratio is not equal to 1
95 percent confidence interval:
 1.364217 3.297790
sample estimates:
common odds ratio
        2.121061
```

Example 13.17

```
> turkey <- matrix(c(32,21,4,4),byrow=T,nrow=2)
> rownames(turkey) <- c("Conv.pos","Conv.neg")
> colnames(turkey) <- c("Eiafoss.pos","Eiafoss.neg")
> cohens.kappa(turkey)
$po
[1] 0.5901639

$pe
[1] 0.5665144

$cohens.kappa
[1] 0.05455673

$ase
[1] 0.06260377
```

Example 13.18

```
> clin <- matrix(
c(7,3,2,0,0,0,1,0,0,0,1,0,0,1,0,0,0,1,0,0,1,0,0,0,3),
+ byrow=T,nrow=5)
> cohens.kappa(clin)
$po
[1] 0.55

$pe
[1] 0.3275

$cohens.kappa
[1] 0.330855

$ase
[1] 0.09177522

> weighted.kappa(clin)
$po
[1] 0.8125

$pe
[1] 0.59875

$weighted.kappa
[1] 0.5327103

$ase
[1] 0.1942474
```

Example 13.19

```
> bp.cats <- read.csv('bpcats.csv',header=T)
> attach(bp.cats)
> diffsap <- sapc - saps
> meansap = (sapc+saps)/2
> upper.diffsap <- mean(diffsap) + 1.96*sd(diffsap)
> lower.diffsap <- mean(diffsap) - 1.96*sd(diffsap)
> plot(meansap,diffsap,pch=as.numeric(level)+5,
+ ylim=c(-40,10),xlim=c(70,210),xlab="Mean blood pressure",
+ ylab="Difference between direct and indirect blood pressure",cex=1.5)
> abline(h=lower.diffsap,lty=2)
> abline(h=upper.diffsap,lty=2)
> abline(h=mean(diffsap))
> legend(80,-30,c("Hyperten","Hypotens","Normoten"),pch=c(6,7,8),cex=1.5)
>
```

REFERENCES

Alban, L. and Agger, J. F. (1996). Welfare in Danish dairy herds 1. Disease management routines in 1983 and 1994. *Acta Veterinaria Scandinavica*, 37:49–63.

Altman, D. G. (1995). *Practical Statistics for Medical Research*. Chapman & Hall, London.

Armitage, P., Berry, G., and Matthews, J. N. S. (2002). *Statistical Methods in Medical Research*, 4th ed. Blackwell Science, Oxford.

Asch, D. A., Jedrziewski, M. K., and Christakis, N. A. (1997). Response rates to mail surveys published in medical journals. *Journal of Clinical Epidemiology*, 50(10): 1129–1136.

Bland, J. M. and Altman, D. G. (1986). Statistical methods for assessing agreement between two methods of clinical measurements. *Lancet*, I:307–310.

Borck, B., Stryhn, H., Ersbøll, A. K., and Pedersen, K. (2002). Thermophilic *Campylobacter* spp in turkey samples: evaluation of two automated enzyme immunoassays and conventional microbiological techniques. *Journal of Applied Microbiology*, 92:574–582.

Bruun, J., Ersbøll, A. K., and Alban, L. (2002). Risk factors for metritis in Danish dairy cows. *Preventive Veterinary Medicine*, 54(2):179–190.

Christensen, J. and Gardner, I. (2000). Herd-level interpretation of test results for epidemiological studies of animal diseases. *Preventive Veterinary Medicine*, 45:83–106.

Cleveland-Nielsen, A., Nielsen, E. O., and Ersbøll, A. K. (2002). Chronic pleuritis in Danish slaughter pig herds. *Preventive Veterinary Medicine*, 55:121–135.

Cochran, W. G. and Cox, G. M. (1992). *Experimental Designs*, 2nd ed. John Wiley & Sons, New York.

Coste, J. and Pouchot, J. (2003). A grey zone for quantitative diagnostic and screening tests. *International Journal of Epidemiology*, 32(2):304–313.

Cox, D. R. (1992). *Planning of Experiments*. John Wiley & Sons, New York.

Creswell, J. W. (1998). *Qualitative Inquiry and Research Design – Choosing among Five Traditions*. Sage Publications, London.

Daniel, W. W. (1995). *Biostatistics: A Foundation for Analysis in the Health Sciences*. John Wiley & Sons, New York.

Dohoo, I., Martin, W., and Stryhn, H. (2003). *Veterinary Epidemiologic Research*. AVC, Charlottetown, Prince Edwards Island, Canada.

Ely, J. W. (1992). Confounding bias and effect modification in epidemiologic research. *Family Medicine*, 24:222–225.

Enøe, C., Georgiadis, M. P., and Johnson, W. O. (2000). Estimation of sensitivity and specificity of diagnostic tests and disease prevalence when the true state of disease is unknown. *Preventive Veterinary Medicine*, 45:61–81.

Ettinger, S. J. and Feldman, E. C. (1995). *Textbook of Veterinary Internal Medicine: Diseases of the Dog and Cat*. W.B. Saunders Co, Philadelphia, PA, USA.

Fleiss, J. L. (1981). *Statistical Methods for Rates and Proportions*. John Wiley & Sons, New York.

Fleiss, J. L. (1986). *The Design and Analysis of Clinical Experiments*. Wiley & Sons, New York.

Gardner, I., Stryhn, H., Lind, P., and Collins, M. (2000). Conditional dependence between tests affects the diagnosis and surveillance of animal diseases. *Preventive Veterinary Medicine*, 45:107–122.

Gardner, I. A. and Greiner, M., eds. (2000). *Validation and Application of Diagnostic Tests Used in Veterinary Epidemiologic Studies. Preventive Veterinary Medicine*, 45(Special issue):1–262.

Greiner, M., Pfeiffer, D., and Smith, R. (2000). Principles and practical application of the receiver-operating characteristic analysis for diagnostic test. *Preventive Veterinary Medicine*, 45:23–41.

Hansen, S. S. (2002). Investigation of ionised calcium in dairy cattle – with special emphasis on subclinical hypocalcaemia. Ph.D. thesis at The Royal Veterinary and Agricultural University, Department of Clinical Studies, Frederiksberg, Denmark. Printed by: Samfundslitteratur Grafik, Frederiksberg, Denmark. ISBN: 87-989531-0-9.

Hardman, P. M., Wathes, C. M., and Wray, C. (1991). Transmission of salmonellae among calves penned individually. *Veterinary Record*, 129:327–329.

Hicks, C. R. (1982). *Fundamental Concepts in the Design of Experiments*, Holt-saunders international edition. CBS College Publishing, New York.

Hosmer, D. W. J. and Lemeshow, S. (2000). *Applied Logistic Regression*. Wiley Series in Probability and Statistics, 2nd ed. Wiley Interscience, New York.

Houe, H. (1994). Bovine virus diarrhoea virus: detection of Danish dairy herds with persistently infected animals by means of a screening test of ten young stock. *Preventive Veterinary Medicine*, 19:241–248.

Houe, H. (1996). *Bovine Virus Diarrhoea Virus (BVDV). Epidemiological Studies of the Infection among Cattle in Denmark and USA*. Thesis for the dr.med.vet degree, The Royal Veterinary and Agricultural University, Copenhagen, Denmark.

Houe, H. and Meyling, A. (1991). Prevalence of bovine virus diarrhoea (BVD) in 19 Danish dairy herds and estimation of incidence of infection in early pregnancy. *Preventive Veterinary Medicine*, 11:9–16.

Houe, H., Vaarst, M., and Enevoldsen, C. (2002). Clinical parameters for assessment of udder health in Danish dairy herds. *Acta Veterinaria Scandinavica*, 43:173–184.

Hui, S. L. and Walter, S. D. (1980). Estimating the error rates of diagnostic tests. *Biometrics*, 36:167–171.

Jensen, A. L. (1994). *Methods for the Evaluation of Laboratory Tests and Test Results with Special Emphasis on the Relative Operating Characteristic (ROC) Curve, Differential Positive Rate, Logistic Regression Model and Critical Difference.* DSR Tryk, Frederiksberg, Denmark.

Jensen, A. L. and Poulsen, J. S. D. (1992). Evaluation of diagnostic tests using relative operating characteristic (ROC) curves and the differential positive rate. An example using the total serum bile acid concentration and the alanine aminotransferase activity in the diagnosis of canine hepatobiliary diseases. *Journal of Veterinary Medicine A*, 39:656–668.

Katz, D., Baptista, J., Azen, S., and Pike, M. (1978). Obtaining confidence intervals for the risk ratio in cohort studies. *Biometrics*, 34:469–474.

Kleinbaum, D. G., Kupper, L. L., and Morgenstern, H. (1982). *Epidemiological Research.* Van Nostrand Reinhold, New York.

Korth, H. F. and Silberschatz, A. (1991). *Database System Concepts,* international edition. Computer Sciences Series. McGraw-Hill, New York.

Kraemer, H. C. (1992). *Evaluating Medical Tests. Objective and Quantitative Guidelines.* Sage Publications, Newbury Park, CA, USA.

Landis, J. R. and Koch, G. G. (1977). The measurement of observer agreement for categorical data. *Biometrics*, 33:159–174.

Miettinen, O. (1974). Confounding and effect-modification. *American Journal of Epidemiology*, 141(12):350–353.

Nielsen, S. S., Grønbæk, C., Agger, J. F., and Houe, H. (2002). Maximum-likelihood estimation of sensitivity and specificity of ELISAs and faecal culture for diagnosis of paratuberculosis. *Preventive Veterinary Medicine*, 53:191–204.

Nielsen, S. S., Thamsborg, S. M., Houe, H., and Bitsch, V. (2000). Bulk-tank milk ELISA antibodies for estimating the prevalence of paratuberculosis in Danish diary herds. *Preventive Veterinary Medicine*, 44:1–7 (with corrigendum in Preventive Veterinary Medicine 46 (2000) 297).

Oppenheim, A. N. (1992). *Questionnaire Design, Interviewing and Attitude Measurement.* Cassell, New York.

Pedersen, K.-M. (2002). *Hypertension in Polycystic Kidney Disease in Persian Cats – Prevalence, Diagnosis, Pathophysiology and Pathology.* PhD thesis, The Royal Veterinary and Agricultural University, Copenhagen, Denmark.

Petrie, A. and Watson, P. (1999). *Statistics for Veterinary and Animal Science.* Blackwell Science, London.

Pocock, S. J. (1983). *Clinical Trials – A Practical Approach.* Wiley & Sons, New York.

R Development Core Team (2004). *R: A Language and Environment for Statistical Computing.* R Foundation for Statistical Computing, Vienna, Austria.

Robertsson, J. A. (1984). Humoral antibody responses to experimental and spontaneous Salmonella infections in cattle measured by ELISA. *Zentralblatt für Veterinär Medizine B*, 31:367–380.

Rothman, K. J. and Greenland, S. (1998). *Modern Epidemiology*, 2nd edn. Lippincott-Raven, Philadelphia.

Rothman, K. J., Greenland, S., and Walker, A. M. (1980). Concepts of interaction. *American Journal of Epidemiology*, 112(4):467–470.

Sallander, M. H., Hedhammar, A., Rundgren, M., and Lindberg, J. E. (2001). Repeatability and validity of a combined mail and telephone questionnaire on demographics, diet, exercise and health status in an insured-dog population. *Preventive Veterinary Medicine*, 50:35–51.

Samuels, M. L. and Witmer, J. A. (1999). *Statistics for the Life Sciences*, 2nd ed. Prentice-Hall, Englewood Cliffs, NJ, USA.

Schukken, Y. H., Geer, D. V. D., Grommers, F. J., and Brand, A. (1989). Assessing the repeatability of questionnaire data from dairy farms. *Acta Veterinaria Scandinavica*, 228–230. Proceedings of the 5th ISVEE Conference.

Senn, S. (1993). *Cross-over Trials in Clinical Research*. Statistics in Practice. John Wiley & Sons, New York.

Smith, R. D. (1991). *Veterinary Clinical Epidemiology. A Problem-Oriented Approach*. Butterworth-Heineman, Boston, MA, USA.

Smith, R. D. and Slenning, B. D. (2000). Decision analysis: dealing with uncertainty in diagnostic testing. *Preventive Veterinary Medicine*, 45:139–162.

Snedecor, G. W. and Cochran, W. G. (1967). *Statistical Methods*, 6th ed. Iowa State University Press, Ames, IA, USA.

Sokal, R. R. and Rohlf, F. J. (1981). *Biometry*. W H Freeman and Company, New York.

Spiegelhalter, D. J., Myles, J. P., Jones, D. R., and Abrams, K. R. (2000). Bayesian methods in health technology assessment: a review. *Health Technology Assessment*, 4(38):1–130.

Thamsborg, S. M., Mejer, H., Roepstorff, A., Ersbøll, A. K., and Eriksen, L. (2001). Effects of nematodes on health and productivity of outdoor sows and suckling piglets. In *Proceedings from the 18th International Conference of WAAVP, Stresa, Italy*, p. 53.

Thøfner, M. B., Ersbøll, A. K., and Hesselholt, M. (2000). Prognostic indicators in a Danish hospital-based population of colic horses. *Equine Colic II, Equine Veterinary Journal*, 32(Suppl.):11–18.

Thrusfield, M. (1995). *Veterinary Epidemiology*, 2nd ed. Butterworth & Co., London.

Toma, B., Vaillancourt, J.-P., Dufour, B., Eloit, M., Moutou, F., Marsh, W., Bénet, J.-J., Sanaa, M., and Michel, P. (1999). *Dictionary of Veterinary Epidemiology*. Iowa State University Press, Ames, IA, USA.

Vaarst, M., Paarup-Laursen, B., Houe, H., Fossing, C., and Andersen, H. J. (2002). Farmers' choice of medical treatment of mastitis in Danish dairy herds based on qualitative research interviews. *Journal of Dairy Science*, 85:992–1001.

Vaillancourt, J.-P., Martineau, G., Morrow, M., Marsh, W., and Robinson, A. (1991). Construction of questionnaires and their use in veterinary medicine. In *Proceedings of Society for Veterinary Epidemiology and Preventive Medicine, London, England*, pp. 94–106.

Waltner-Toews, D. (1983). Questionnaire design and administration. In *Proceedings of the 3rd International Symposium on Veterinary Epidemiology and Economics, Arlington, VA, USA*, pp. 31–37.

Weisberg, S. W. (1985). *Applied Linear Regression*. Wiley & Sons, New York.

West, M. and Harrison, J. (1997). *Bayesian Forecasting and Dynamic Models*, 2nd ed. Springer, New York.

Woodward, M. (1999). *Epidemiology: Study Design and Data Analysis*. Texts in Statistical Science. Chapman & Hall, London.

Woolf, B. (1955). On estimating the relationship between blood group and disease. *Human Genetics*, 19:251–253.

INDEX

Bland–Altman plot, 259
block randomisation, 130
bovine virus diarrhoea (BVD) virus, 7, 18
box plot, 42
box-and-whisker plot, 43
breed, 25
BVDV register, 171

carrier
    active, 30
    latent, 30
    passive, 30
carriers, 33
carry-over effect, 72
case fatality, 91
case–control study, 96
casuality, 58
categorical variable, 38
causal association, 23
causal diagram, 178
causal relationship, 22, 56
causality, 22, 221
causation, 22
    disease, 22
cause
    necessary, 23
    sufficient, 24
cell mediated immune response, 28
Central Farm Animal Register, 170
Centrale Husdyrbrugs Register, 170
CHR-register, 170
chronic infections, 30
climate, 31
clinical data, 160
clinical epidemiology, 5
clinical trial, 73
closed, 192
closed population, 89
cluster sampling, 127
coefficient of determination, 224
Cohen's kappa, *see* kappa
cohort study, 54, 96
communication forms, 190
conformation, 26
confounder, 181
confounding, 181
    control of, 183
confounding bias, 181
confounding variable, 181
content analysis, 189
continuous outcomes, 208

continuous scale, 38
control
    model, 236
control of confounding, 183
control of dates, 164
convenience sampling, 128
correlation, 218
correlation coefficient, 218
    Pearson, 218
    Spearman, 219
critical value, 206
cross-over design, 71
cross-over effect, 72
cross-sectional study, 96
cross-sectional study with follow-up, 58
crude estimate of the association, 241
crude mortality rate, 91
crude odds ratio, 242
crude relative risk, 242
cut-off value, 142, 143

Danish Cattle Database, 171
Danish SPF Company Database, 172
DANMAP, 170
data
    control, 163
    demographic, 154
    location of, 43
    recording of, 154
    sources of, 155
    spread of, 43
data analysis, 205
data control, 163
    control of dates, 164
    dates, 163
    extreme values, 163
    frequency distribution, 163
    graphical illustrations, 163, 164
    logical, 164
    logical checks, 163
    missing values, 163
    proofreading, 163
data editing, 165
data levels, 43
data quality, 160
data recording, 154
database, 157
    examples of, 168
    key, 157
    record, 157
    structure, 157